5TH EDITION

Nolte's
THE
HUMAN BRAIN
IN PHOTOGRAPHS AND DIAGRAMS

Todd W. Vanderah, PhD

Professor and Chair of Pharmacology
Department of Pharmacology, Anesthesiology,
 and Neurology
University of Arizona, College of Medicine
Tucson, Arizona

ELSEVIER

ELSEVIER

1600 John F. Kennedy Blvd.
Ste 1800
Philadelphia, PA 19103-2899

Content Strategist: Marybeth Thiel
Publishing Services Manager: Catherine Jackson
Senior Project Manager: Amanda Mincher
Design Direction: Amy Buxton

Printed in the United States of America

Last digit is the print number: 9 8 7 6 5 4 3

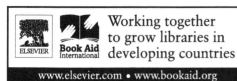

Working together
to grow libraries in
developing countries

www.elsevier.com • www.bookaid.org

To Our Students

Whose enthusiasm excites me to be a better teacher

Whose inquisitiveness drives me to dig deeper for answers

Whose joy to learn thrusts my dedication towards
the educational mission

Whose rich personalities demonstrate how the human
brain has incredible capability and compassion

-John Nolte, PhD, Todd W. Vanderah, PhD, and Jay B. Angevine Jr., PhD

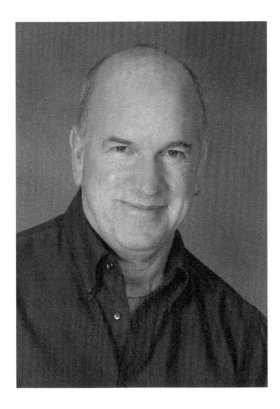

When it comes to learning the anatomy and basic functions of the human nervous system, John "Jack" Nolte has played a role as an author and/or a professor for hundreds of thousands of students, residents, and physicians. Jack viewed the human brain as an endlessly fascinating playground that is forever changing. His lifetime goal was not only to educate students but to educate future teachers as well. He continually scoured the primary literature and behaved with childhood excitement when discovering new explanations for human brain function. His own love and excitement for the nervous system would naturally bleed over to his students and colleagues, encouraging them to explore and question the human nervous system.

In working with Jack for over 15 years, my career and take on life changed from teaching as a "job" to teaching as an enjoyable hobby with benefits. His ability to make teaching fun, telling jokes and giving examples, led to an enriched student environment that resulted in students wanting more. Our meetings most often included discussions of how we could better educate students. Jack was on the cutting edge of designing "case-based" instruction, showing videos of patients for teaching purposes, having patients present in the classroom, and pushing ideas of working and taking exams as groups, using innovative technology, including the virtual brain and interconnected vocabulary terms across multiple fields of science. Jack's desire to create a textbook that was cutting edge yet to the point for learning purposes was his continual love. He shared with me chapters, images, and novel ideas while writing the next edition to continually produce a product that students would enjoy.

Our time together was not all work. Although most know him as a professor of the nervous system, Jack also enjoyed playing handball, woodworking, traveling, cooking, wonderful deep red wines, a martini with blue cheese olives, and the joy of eating oysters (things that often appeared in his textbook as examples of nervous system function). In closing, I dedicate this new edition to my teacher, colleague, and friend. I dearly miss Jack's enthusiasm for teaching, his humor, his friendship, and of course his infamous Birkenstocks.

Learning about the functional anatomy of the human central nervous system (CNS) is usually a daunting task. Structures that interdigitate and overlap in three dimensions contribute to the difficulty, as does a long list of intimidating names, many with origins in descriptive terminology derived from Latin and Greek. Here we have attempted to make the task a little easier by presenting a systematic series of whole-brain sections in three different sets of planes (coronal, sagittal, and axial—similar to what is seen in medical imaging), by relating these sections to three-dimensional reconstructions, and by trying to restrain ourselves when indicating structures.

Unlabeled photographs are presented throughout the book, juxtaposed with faded-out versions of the same photographs with important structures outlined and labeled. This circumvents the common need to mentally superimpose a labeled drawing on a photograph or to inspect a photograph through a thicket of lead lines. Photos of the CNS are comprehensive sets in each plane; sections illustrating major structures or major transitions are shown in greater detail and at a higher magnification. Every labeled structure is discussed briefly in an illustrated glossary at the end of the book. For this edition, minor adjustments were made to sections and photographs throughout the book; the functional pathways in chapter 8 were redone in color; an important new imaging modality (diffusion tensor imaging) was added to Chapter 9; and a number of new illustrations were added to the glossary. Chapter 10 is brand new in this edition as an introduction to neuropathology. Common types of CNS derived tumors and neuro-diseases/disorders are displayed as representative images of what might be detected upon diagnosis.

The methods used in this book inevitably involve compromises. We labeled only structures that we believe are important for the knowledge base of undergraduate and professional students, and we omitted others dear to our hearts but perhaps not critical for these students. Hence the fasciola cinerea so prominent in Figure 7.8 is not labeled, and the indusium griseum is mentioned only briefly in a footnote. In addition, explicitly outlining structures required some simplifications, and complex entities are sometimes indicated more simply as single structures. We think the resulting pedagogical utility for students justifies these anatomical liberties.

Current technological methods allowed us to approach the construction of this atlas differently than we could have when it was first discussed. All the photographs of brains and sections used in the book were retouched digitally. Mounting medium, staining artifacts, and small cracks, folds, and scratches were removed from the digitized versions of the sections. The profiles of many small blood vessels were removed as well. The color balance was changed as appropriate to make the sections as uniform as possible. These procedures improved the illustrations aesthetically while leaving their essential content unchanged. In addition, computer-based surface-reconstruction techniques made possible the beautiful three-dimensional images that appear in Chapter 4 and elsewhere in the book.

John Nolte and Todd W. Vanderah

ACKNOWLEDGMENTS

This book could never have happened without the hard work and endless efforts of Jack Nolte. He loved to teach and mentor colleagues of which I am forever indebted. Many colleagues and friends have helped with previous versions of the book, and that work is presented in this edition, including the photographic expertise of Nathan Nitzky and Jeb Zirato in the UofA Biocommunications. Grant Dahmer and Dr. Norman Koelling of the UofA prepared the prosections shown in Chapter 1. The sections shown in Chapter 2 were cut by Shelley Rowley, and those in Chapter 3 by Pam Eller. John Sundsten produced the three-dimensional images shown in Chapter 4. Paul Yakovlev, as detailed shortly, was the central figure in the production of the sections shown in Chapters 5 through 7. Cody Thorstenson played a major role in retouching the images of these sections. Cheryl Cotman produced the three-dimensional reconstructions of the limbic system shown in Chapter 8. Drs. Ray Carmody, Robert Handy, Elena Plante, and Joe Seeger provided the images shown in Chapters 9 and 10. Drs. Agamanolis and Carmody supplied many of the pathology images in chapter 10 and helped with the description of the neuropathology.

I thank the co-author on the first three editions of this atlas, Jay B. Angevine Jr., who passed away in October 2011. Dr. Angevine was responsible for producing the whole-brain sections in Chapters 5 through 7.

Drs. Nolte and Angevine both had an infectious love for the central nervous system and its incredible capability. Their personalities and enthusiasm made learning about the nervous system fun and exciting. I hope this enjoyment for the nervous system feeds forward to future students of the human nervous system.

Todd W. Vanderah

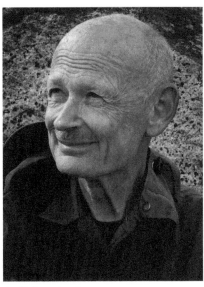

Jay B. Angevine Jr.
June 29, 1928–October 18, 2011.

As crucial as computer technology is to our book, the whole-brain serial sections are its foundation. They were prepared during 1966–1967 in the Warren Anatomical Museum at Harvard Medical School. The work, in which I took part, was performed under the direction of Dr. Paul I. Yakovlev (1894–1983), who was curator of the museum from 1955 to 1961 and then Emeritus Clinical Professor of Neuropathology until 1969. Each brain, embedded whole in celloidin, was sectioned in coronal, horizontal, or sagittal planes on a giant microtome with a standing oblique 36-inch blade and a sliding brain holder. The sections, each 35 μm thick, were rolled and stored in test tubes in a console of 100 numbered receptacles. After processing pilot sections for suitability and quality, we stained every twentieth section with Weigert's hematoxylin (Loyez method) for myelin and mounted it between sheets of window glass. Each preparation is thus about 4 mm thick, yet great depth and detail of cells and fibers are visible.

Such preparations illustrate the white matter and tracts of the brain by staining the myelin sheaths of axons black; gray matter and nuclei appear as more or less pale areas, depending on the number and caliber of myelinated fibers present. These sections, all from essentially normal brains, were added to an already huge collection representing more than 900 cerebra that Dr. Yakovlev had been building since 1930. Now a national resource known and available to neurological scholars worldwide, this priceless compilation known as the Yakovlev-Haleem Collection is graciously housed in the National Museum of Health and Medicine by the Armed Forces Institute of Pathology in Washington, DC. Today it comprises about 1600 specimens, normal and pathological, processed in a rigorously consistent manner from the start.

In mid-1967, with Dr. Yakovlev's blessing, I took with me to The University of Arizona some 1000 of the 8741 sections cut from the three normal brains used in Chapters 5 through 7 of this book. I had left Boston to join the faculty of the University's new College of Medicine in Tucson. Paul, my mentor from the time I came to Harvard in 1956, wanted to support me as I began teaching in a far-off land that he believed (perhaps correctly) to be a frontier: the "Wild West." As with everything else he did, it was thoughtful, kind, and generous. How he would have loved to see students studying the sections illustrated on these pages!

Unlike the fairly simple task of sectioning the brainstem, cutting perfect gapless whole-brain serial sections is difficult. The procedure was never more carefully undertaken or widely employed than by Paul, who used it at or in association with Harvard Medical School for 40 years. A central theme for him was this holistic method ("every part of the brain is there, nothing is left out..."), but no aspect of neuroanatomy or neuropathology failed to intrigue him. Although such sections had been made since the late 19th century (they are found in small numbers at many medical schools and in profusion at a few research institutes), Paul's are unique—in uniformity of preparation at every step from fixation to mounting, and in unity of general neurological interest and comparability. Of this legacy (he called it "over 40 tons of glass"), Derek Denny-Brown, Emeritus Professor of Neurology at Harvard, wrote in 1972: "The perspective given by serial whole brain sections provides at once an arresting view of anatomical relationships in patterns of striking beauty. After working in the collection for years, one still finds every occasion to view it illuminating and rewarding."

In 2000, artist-scientist Cheryl Cotman, computer programmer Kevin Head, and I, an anatomist, traced and digitized structures from the serial sagittal sections shown in this atlas. We made a computer reconstruction and large hologram (three by five feet) of the human limbic system. We are indebted to Cheryl for her help in selecting images from her large collection of color-coded overall and regional views of the system. We are enlightened by her discovery that several limbic structures are quite differently shaped than traditionally believed. Although Paul and I would find this hard to accept, we would accept her fantastic findings with glee and laughter.

-Jay B. Angevine Jr.

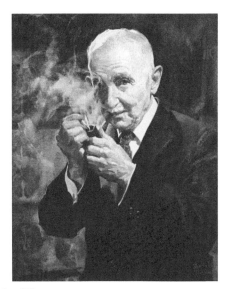

Paul I. Yakovlev, MD
1894–1983.
An autographed copy of an oil portrait of Paul Yakovlev by Bettina Steinke. The original portrait was presented to the Warren Anatomical Museum at Harvard Medical School in 1978. (Courtesy the Warren Museum in the Francis A. Countway Library of Medicine, Boston, Massachusetts.)

CONTENTS

External Anatomy of the Brain

This atlas emphasizes views of the interior of the human **central nervous system (CNS)**, sectioned in various planes. Here in the first chapter we lay some of the groundwork for understanding the arrangements of these interior structures by presenting the surface features with which they are continuous, and by giving a broad overview of the components of the CNS.

The CNS is composed of the **spinal cord** and the **brain**, the major components of which are indicated in Fig. 1.1. The human brain is dominated by two very large **cerebral hemispheres**, separated from each other by a deep **longitudinal fissure**. Each hemisphere is convoluted externally in a fairly consistent pattern into a series of **gyri**, separated from each other by a series of **sulci** (an adaptation that makes more area available for the cortex that covers each cerebral hemisphere). Several prominent sulci are used as major landmarks to divide each hemisphere into five **lobes**[a]—**frontal**, **parietal**, **occipital**, **temporal**, and **limbic**—each of which contains a characteristic set of gyri (Figs. 1.3 to 1.8). The two hemispheres are interconnected by a massive bundle of nerve fibers, the **corpus callosum,** and two smaller bundles of fibers called the **anterior** and **posterior commissures**. Finally, certain areas of gray matter are embedded in the interior of each cerebral hemisphere. These include major components of the **basal ganglia** (or, more properly, basal nuclei) and **limbic system** (primarily the **amygdala**

[a]In addition, the **insula**, an area of cerebral cortex buried deep in the **lateral sulcus** (see Fig. 5.7A), is usually considered as a separate lobe.

and **hippocampus**). They are apparent in the brain sections shown in Chapters 5 through 7.

The cerebral hemispheres of humans are so massive that they overshadow or almost conceal the remaining major subdivisions of the brain—the **diencephalon** (made up of the thalamus, hypothalamus, epithalamus), **brainstem**, and **cerebellum**. Hemisecting a brain in the midsagittal plane, as in Fig. 1.1B, reveals these components.

The diencephalon (literally the "in-between brain") is interposed between each cerebral hemisphere and the brainstem. The diencephalon contains the left and right **thalamus**, major waystations for information seeking access to the cerebral cortex; the **hypothalamus**, a major control center for visceral and drive-related functions; and the epithalamus, which includes the pineal gland and a set of nuclei called the habenula.

The brainstem, continuous caudally with the spinal cord, serves as a conduit for pathways traveling between the cerebellum or spinal cord and more rostral levels of the CNS. It also contains the neurons that receive or give rise to most of the **cranial nerves**.

The cerebellum (literally the "little brain") is even more intricately convoluted than the cerebral hemispheres, to make room for an extensive covering of its own cortex. It plays a major role in the planning and coordination of movement. A deep **transverse fissure** (normally occupied over most of its extent by the **tentorium cerebelli**) separates the cerebellum from the overlying occipital and parietal lobes and then continues deeper into the brain, partially separating the diencephalon from the cerebral hemispheres.

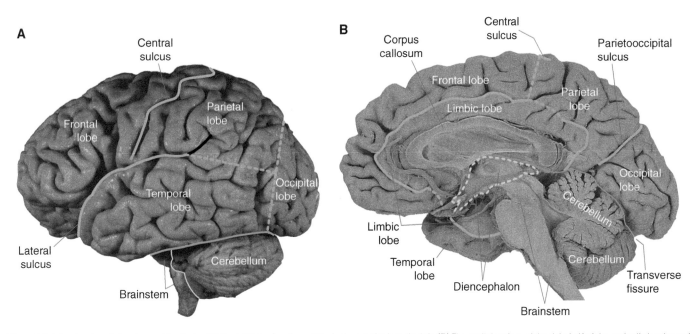

Figure 1.1 Lateral and medial surfaces of the brain. **(A)** The left lateral surface of the brain; anterior is to the left. **(B)** The medial surface of the right half of the sagittally hemisected brain; anterior is to the left. (Dissections by Grant Dahmer, Department of Cell Biology and Anatomy, The University of Arizona College of Medicine.)

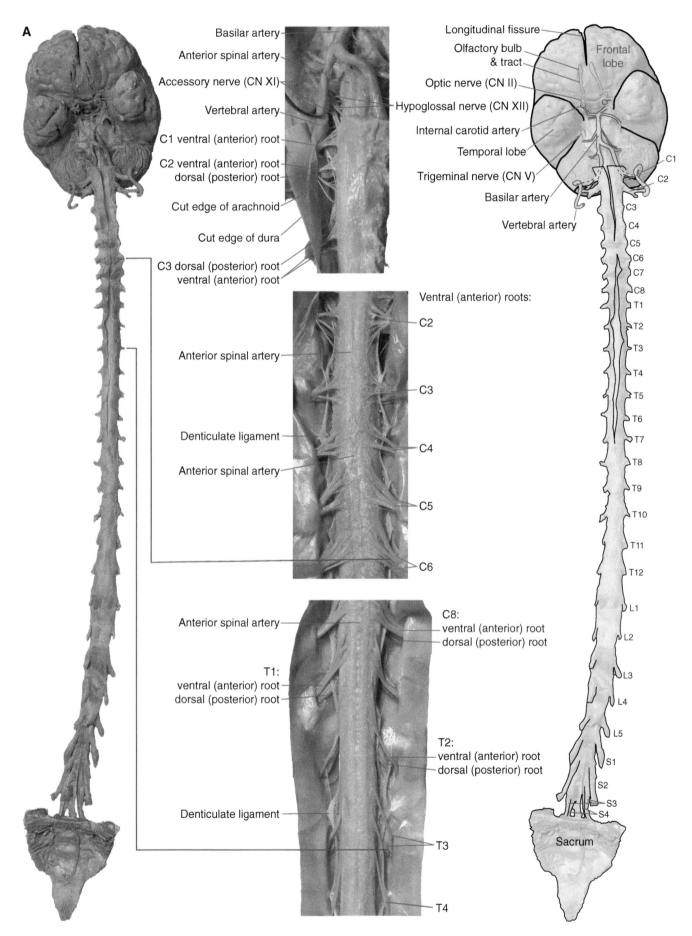

A

Basilar artery
Anterior spinal artery
Accessory nerve (CN XI)
Vertebral artery
C1 ventral (anterior) root
C2 ventral (anterior) root
dorsal (posterior) root
Cut edge of arachnoid
Cut edge of dura
C3 dorsal (posterior) root
ventral (anterior) root

Longitudinal fissure
Olfactory bulb & tract
Optic nerve (CN II)
Hypoglossal nerve (CN XII)
Internal carotid artery
Temporal lobe
Trigeminal nerve (CN V)
Basilar artery
Vertebral artery
Frontal lobe

Ventral (anterior) roots:
Anterior spinal artery
C2
Denticulate ligament
C3
Anterior spinal artery
C4
C5
C6

Anterior spinal artery
C8:
ventral (anterior) root
dorsal (posterior) root
T1:
ventral (anterior) root
dorsal (posterior) root
T2:
ventral (anterior) root
dorsal (posterior) root
Denticulate ligament
T3
T4

C1
C2
C3
C4
C5
C6
C7
C8
T1
T2
T3
T4
T5
T6
T7
T8
T9
T10
T11
T12
L1
L2
L3
L4
L5
S1
S2
S3
S4
Sacrum

Figure 1.2 A masterful dissection of the entire CNS, with the spinal cord still encased in dura mater and arachnoid. **(A)** The anterior/inferior surface. Regions enlarged in the *insets*, after the dura mater and arachnoid were spread apart.

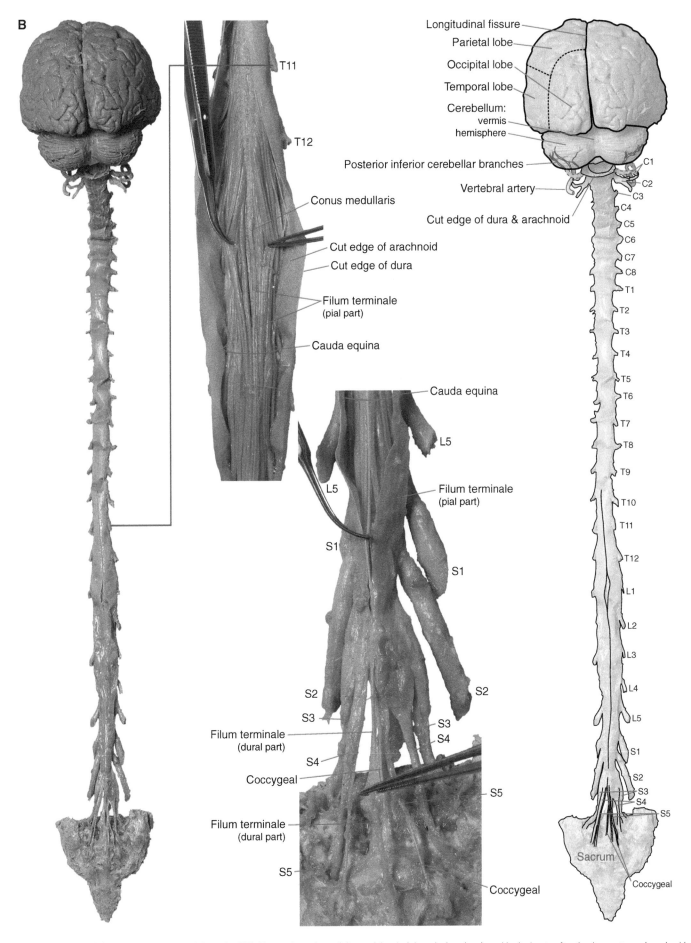

B

Longitudinal fissure

Parietal lobe

Occipital lobe

Temporal lobe

Cerebellum:
vermis
hemisphere

Posterior inferior cerebellar branches

Vertebral artery

Cut edge of dura & arachnoid

C1
C2
C3
C4
C5
C6
C7
C8
T1
T2
T3
T4
T5
T6
T7
T8
T9
T10
T11
T12
L1
L2
L3
L4
L5
S1
S2
S3
S4
S5

Sacrum

Coccygeal

T11

T12

Conus medullaris

Cut edge of arachnoid

Cut edge of dura

Filum terminale
(pial part)

Cauda equina

Cauda equina

L5

L5

Filum terminale
(pial part)

S1

S1

S2

S2

S3

S3

S4

Filum terminale
(dural part)

S4

Coccygeal

S5

Filum terminale
(dural part)

S5

Coccygeal

Figure 1.2 (Continued) **(B)** The posterior surface of the entire CNS. The cauda equina and the caudal end of the spinal cord, enlarged in the insets after the dura mater and arachnoid were spread apart. (Dissection by Dr. Norman Koelling, Department of Cell Biology and Anatomy, The University of Arizona College of Medicine.)

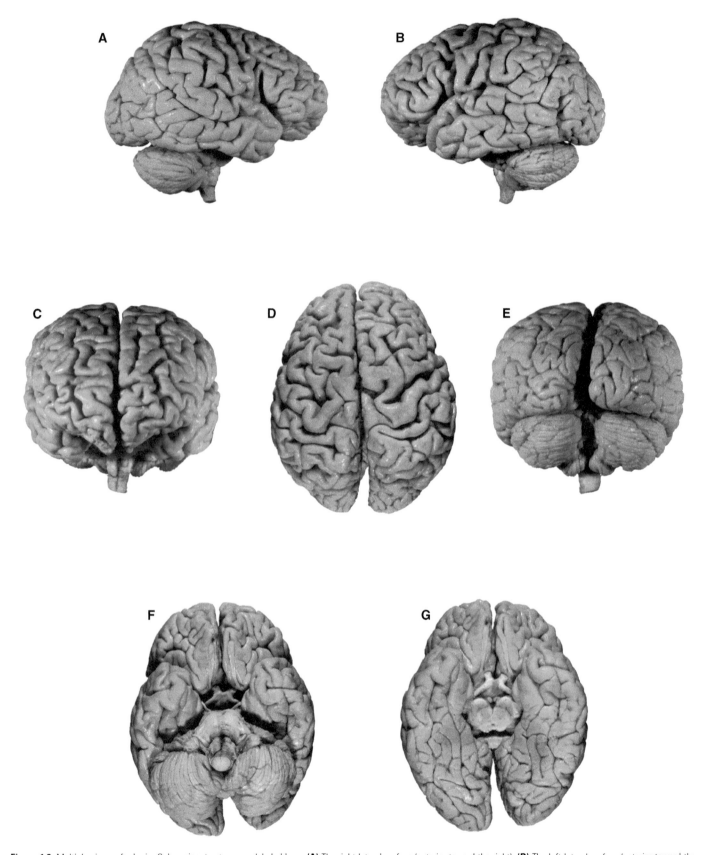

Figure 1.3 Multiple views of a brain. Only major structures are labeled here. **(A)** The right lateral surface (anterior toward the right). **(B)** The left lateral surface (anterior toward the left). **(C)** The anterior surface. **(D)** The superior surface (anterior toward the top of the page). **(E)** The posterior surface. **(F)** The inferior surface (anterior toward the top of the page). **(G)** The same inferior surface after removal of the cerebellum and most of the brainstem; the latter are shown in more detail in Fig. 1.9.

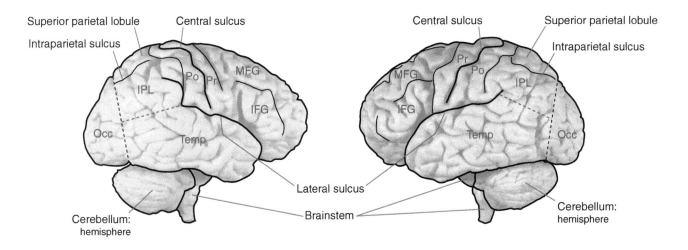

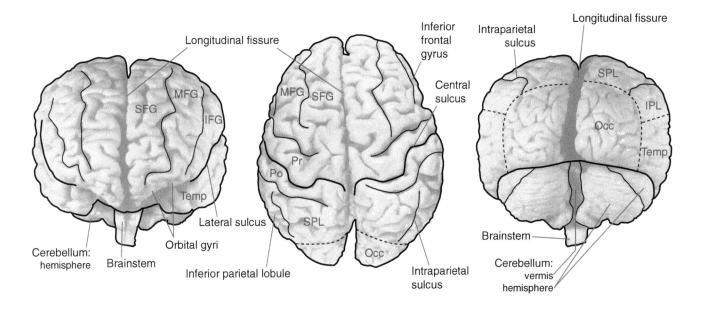

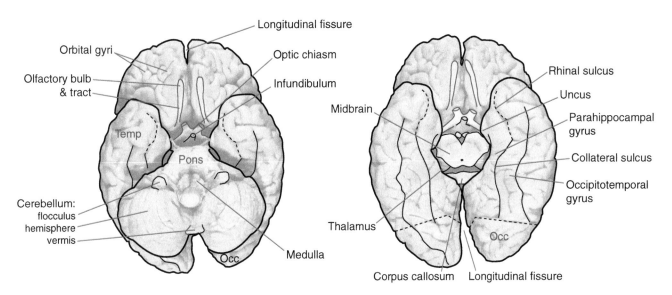

Figure 1.3 (Continued) (The rhinal sulcus is drawn as a *dashed line* to indicate that it is separate from the collateral sulcus, even though in this particular brain the two are continuous.) *IFG*, Inferior frontal gyrus; *IPL*, inferior parietal lobule; *MFG*, middle frontal gyrus; *Occ*, occipital lobe; *Po*, postcentral gyrus; *Pr*, precentral gyrus; *SFG*, superior frontal gyrus; *SPL*, superior parietal lobule; *Temp*, temporal lobe. (Dissection by Grant Dahmer, Department of Cell Biology and Anatomy, The University of Arizona College of Medicine.)

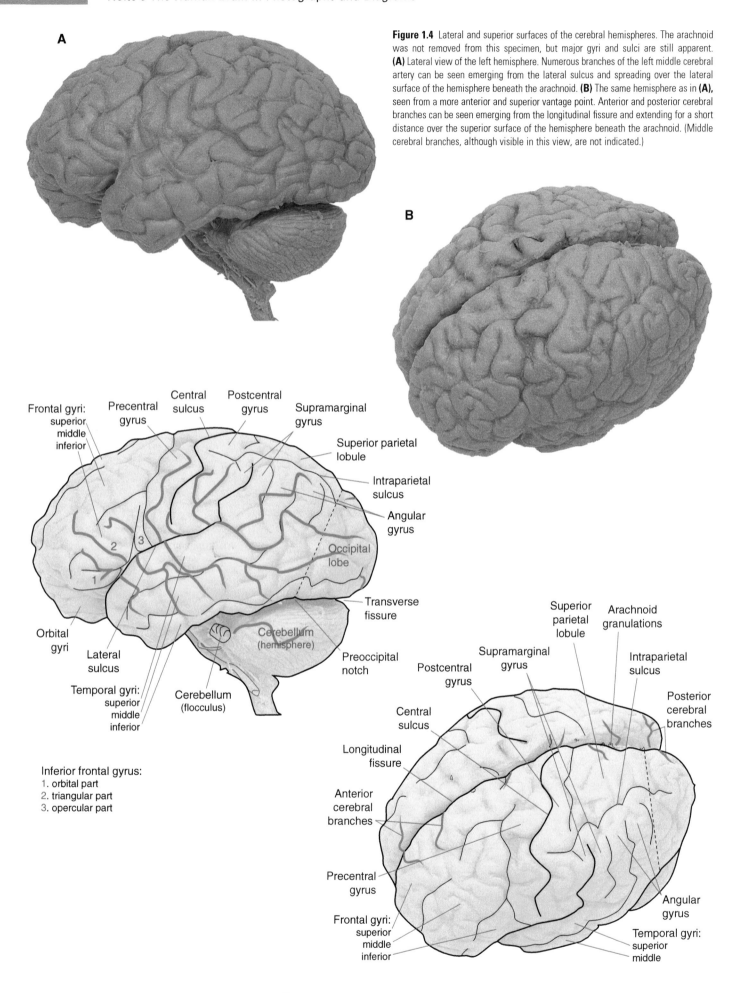

Figure 1.4 Lateral and superior surfaces of the cerebral hemispheres. The arachnoid was not removed from this specimen, but major gyri and sulci are still apparent. **(A)** Lateral view of the left hemisphere. Numerous branches of the left middle cerebral artery can be seen emerging from the lateral sulcus and spreading over the lateral surface of the hemisphere beneath the arachnoid. **(B)** The same hemisphere as in **(A)**, seen from a more anterior and superior vantage point. Anterior and posterior cerebral branches can be seen emerging from the longitudinal fissure and extending for a short distance over the superior surface of the hemisphere beneath the arachnoid. (Middle cerebral branches, although visible in this view, are not indicated.)

Inferior frontal gyrus:
1. orbital part
2. triangular part
3. opercular part

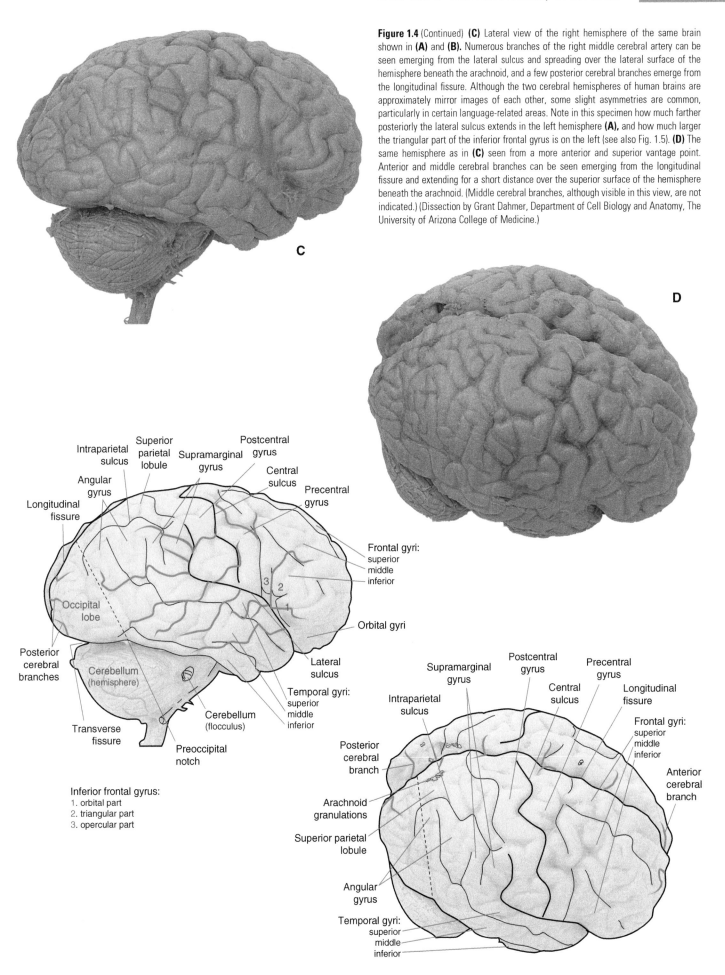

Figure 1.4 (Continued) **(C)** Lateral view of the right hemisphere of the same brain shown in **(A)** and **(B)**. Numerous branches of the right middle cerebral artery can be seen emerging from the lateral sulcus and spreading over the lateral surface of the hemisphere beneath the arachnoid, and a few posterior cerebral branches emerge from the longitudinal fissure. Although the two cerebral hemispheres of human brains are approximately mirror images of each other, some slight asymmetries are common, particularly in certain language-related areas. Note in this specimen how much farther posteriorly the lateral sulcus extends in the left hemisphere **(A),** and how much larger the triangular part of the inferior frontal gyrus is on the left (see also Fig. 1.5). **(D)** The same hemisphere as in **(C)** seen from a more anterior and superior vantage point. Anterior and middle cerebral branches can be seen emerging from the longitudinal fissure and extending for a short distance over the superior surface of the hemisphere beneath the arachnoid. (Middle cerebral branches, although visible in this view, are not indicated.) (Dissection by Grant Dahmer, Department of Cell Biology and Anatomy, The University of Arizona College of Medicine.)

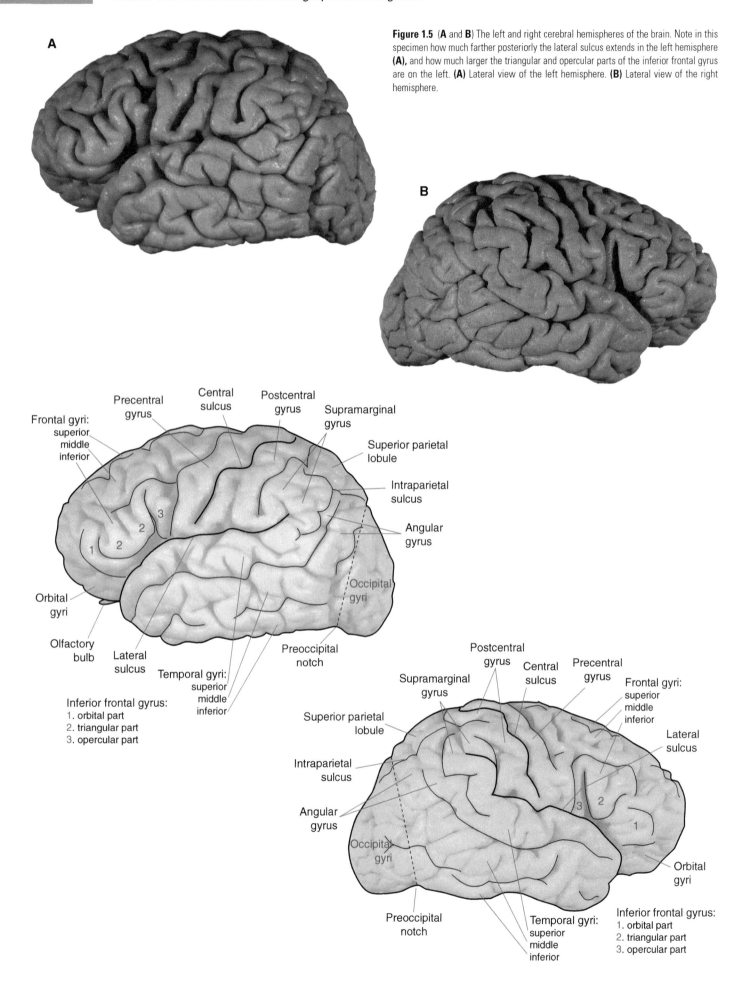

Figure 1.5 (**A** and **B**) The left and right cerebral hemispheres of the brain. Note in this specimen how much farther posteriorly the lateral sulcus extends in the left hemisphere (**A**), and how much larger the triangular and opercular parts of the inferior frontal gyrus are on the left. (**A**) Lateral view of the left hemisphere. (**B**) Lateral view of the right hemisphere.

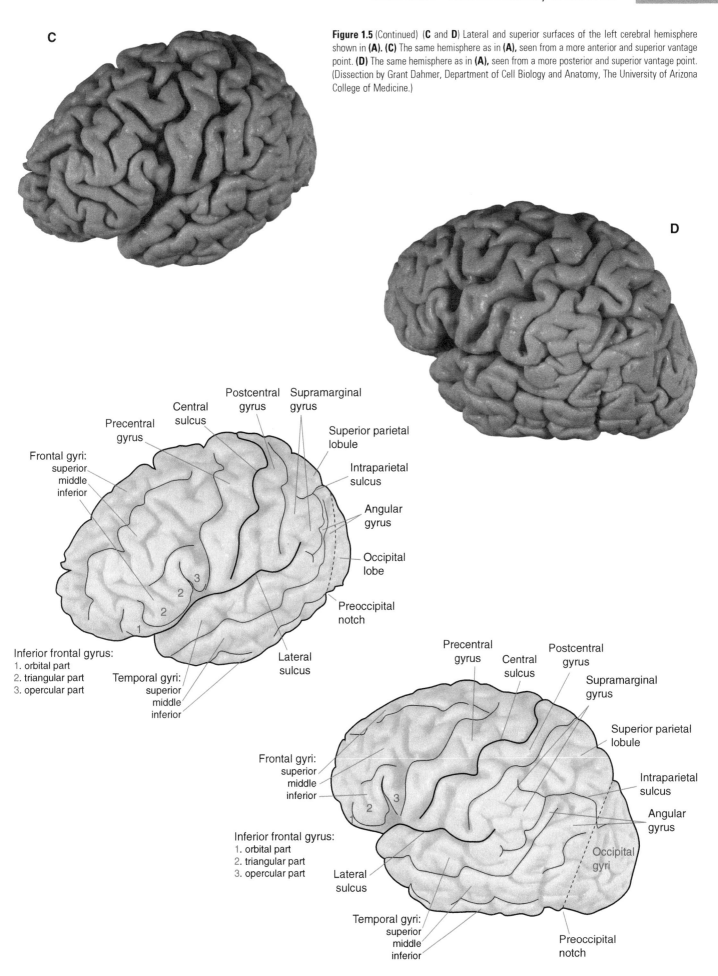

Figure 1.5 (Continued) (**C** and **D**) Lateral and superior surfaces of the left cerebral hemisphere shown in (**A**). (**C**) The same hemisphere as in (**A**), seen from a more anterior and superior vantage point. (**D**) The same hemisphere as in (**A**), seen from a more posterior and superior vantage point. (Dissection by Grant Dahmer, Department of Cell Biology and Anatomy, The University of Arizona College of Medicine.)

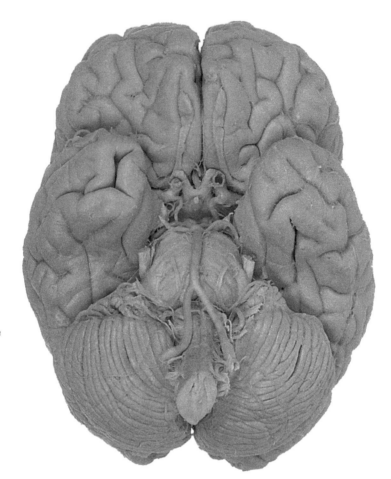

Figure 1.6 (A) Inferior surface of the human brain.

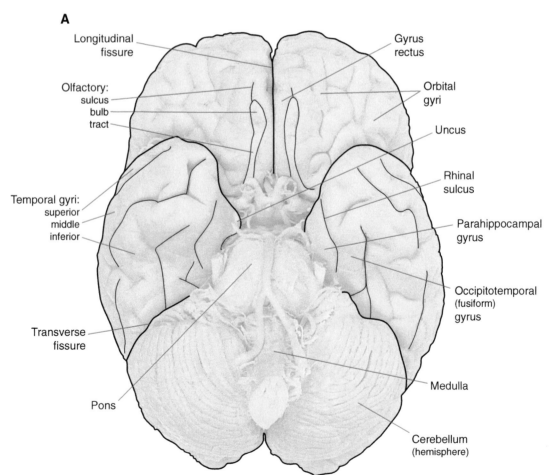

A

Longitudinal fissure

Gyrus rectus

Olfactory:
sulcus
bulb
tract

Orbital gyri

Uncus

Rhinal sulcus

Temporal gyri:
superior
middle
inferior

Parahippocampal gyrus

Occipitotemporal (fusiform) gyrus

Transverse fissure

Medulla

Pons

Cerebellum (hemisphere)

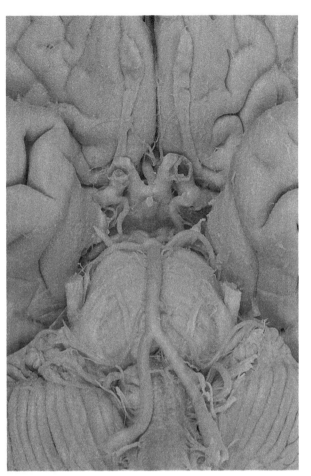

Figure 1.6 (Continued) **(B)** The brainstem and the base of the forebrain at a closer view. (The large left posterior communicating artery is a common variant of the circle of Willis.) (Dissection by Grant Dahmer, Department of Cell Biology and Anatomy, The University of Arizona College of Medicine.)

B

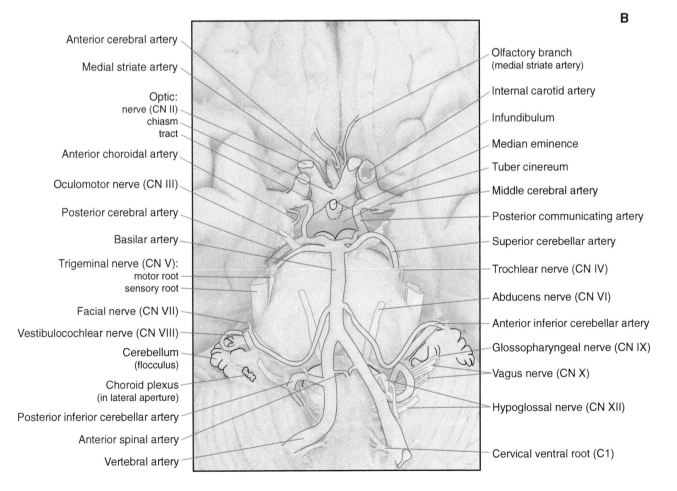

Anterior cerebral artery

Medial striate artery

Optic:
nerve (CN II)
chiasm
tract

Anterior choroidal artery

Oculomotor nerve (CN III)

Posterior cerebral artery

Basilar artery

Trigeminal nerve (CN V):
motor root
sensory root

Facial nerve (CN VII)

Vestibulocochlear nerve (CN VIII)

Cerebellum
(flocculus)

Choroid plexus
(in lateral aperture)

Posterior inferior cerebellar artery

Anterior spinal artery

Vertebral artery

Olfactory branch
(medial striate artery)

Internal carotid artery

Infundibulum

Median eminence

Tuber cinereum

Middle cerebral artery

Posterior communicating artery

Superior cerebellar artery

Trochlear nerve (CN IV)

Abducens nerve (CN VI)

Anterior inferior cerebellar artery

Glossopharyngeal nerve (CN IX)

Vagus nerve (CN X)

Hypoglossal nerve (CN XII)

Cervical ventral root (C1)

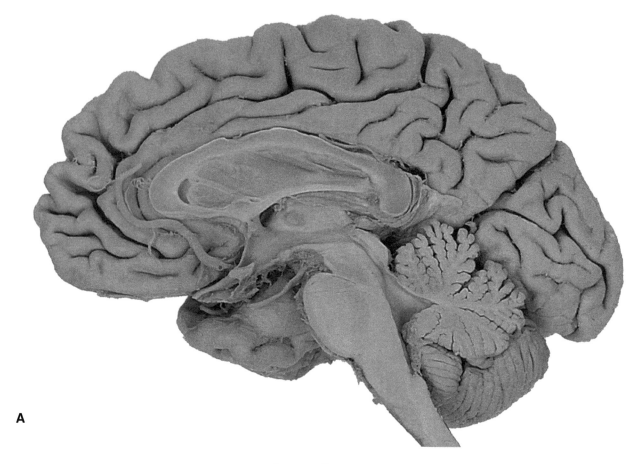

A

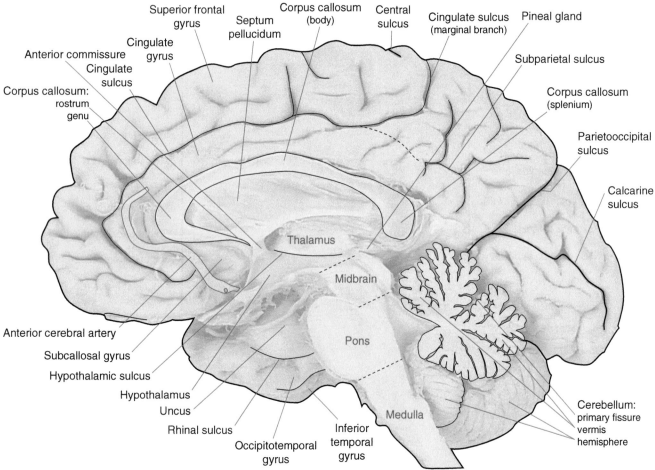

Figure 1.7 (A) Medial surface of the right half of a sagittally hemisected brain. The *dashed line* interconnecting the cingulate and subparietal sulci is meant to indicate that in some brains these two sulci are continuous.

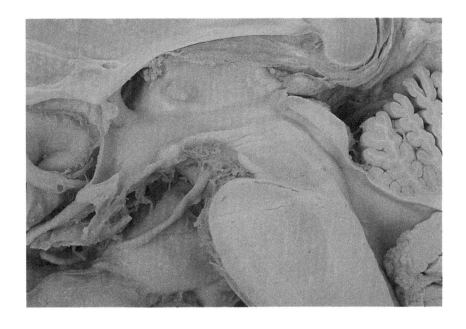

B

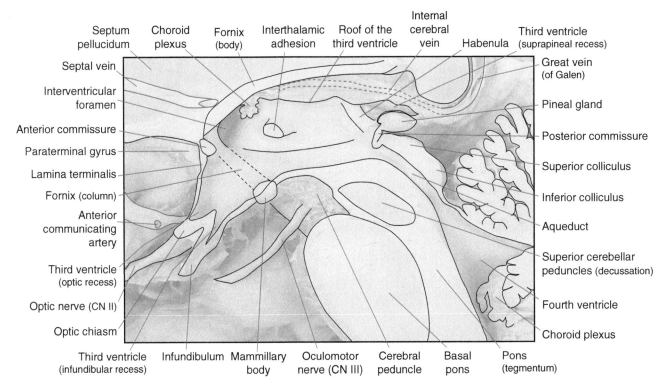

Septum pellucidum
Choroid plexus
Fornix (body)
Interthalamic adhesion
Roof of the third ventricle
Internal cerebral vein
Habenula
Third ventricle (suprapineal recess)

Septal vein
Interventricular foramen
Anterior commissure
Paraterminal gyrus
Lamina terminalis
Fornix (column)
Anterior communicating artery
Third ventricle (optic recess)
Optic nerve (CN II)
Optic chiasm

Great vein (of Galen)
Pineal gland
Posterior commissure
Superior colliculus
Inferior colliculus
Aqueduct
Superior cerebellar peduncles (decussation)
Fourth ventricle
Choroid plexus

Third ventricle (infundibular recess)
Infundibulum
Mammillary body
Oculomotor nerve (CN III)
Cerebral peduncle
Basal pons
Pons (tegmentum)

Figure 1.7 (Continued) **(B)** The diencephalon and part of the brainstem. (Dissection by Grant Dahmer, Department of Cell Biology and Anatomy, The University of Arizona College of Medicine.)

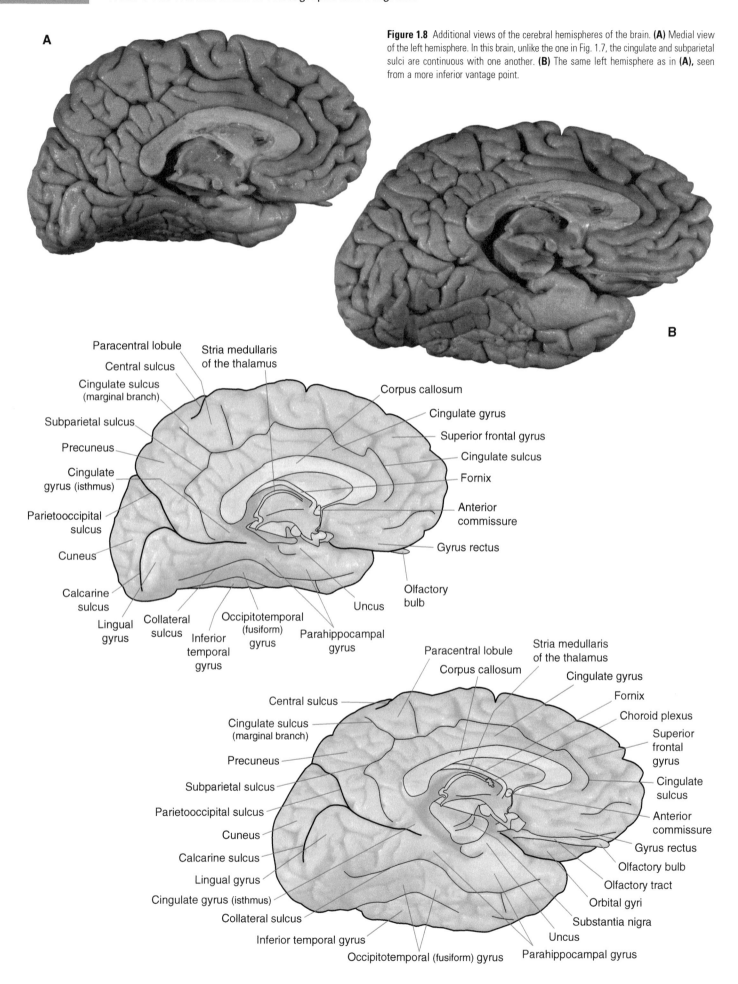

A

B

Figure 1.8 Additional views of the cerebral hemispheres of the brain. **(A)** Medial view of the left hemisphere. In this brain, unlike the one in Fig. 1.7, the cingulate and subparietal sulci are continuous with one another. **(B)** The same left hemisphere as in **(A)**, seen from a more inferior vantage point.

Paracentral lobule
Central sulcus
Cingulate sulcus (marginal branch)
Subparietal sulcus
Precuneus
Cingulate gyrus (isthmus)
Parietooccipital sulcus
Cuneus
Calcarine sulcus
Lingual gyrus
Collateral sulcus
Inferior temporal gyrus
Occipitotemporal (fusiform) gyrus
Parahippocampal gyrus
Uncus
Stria medullaris of the thalamus
Corpus callosum
Cingulate gyrus
Superior frontal gyrus
Cingulate sulcus
Fornix
Anterior commissure
Gyrus rectus
Olfactory bulb

Paracentral lobule
Corpus callosum
Central sulcus
Cingulate sulcus (marginal branch)
Precuneus
Subparietal sulcus
Parietooccipital sulcus
Cuneus
Calcarine sulcus
Lingual gyrus
Cingulate gyrus (isthmus)
Collateral sulcus
Inferior temporal gyrus
Occipitotemporal (fusiform) gyrus
Parahippocampal gyrus
Stria medullaris of the thalamus
Cingulate gyrus
Fornix
Choroid plexus
Superior frontal gyrus
Cingulate sulcus
Anterior commissure
Gyrus rectus
Olfactory bulb
Olfactory tract
Orbital gyri
Substantia nigra
Uncus

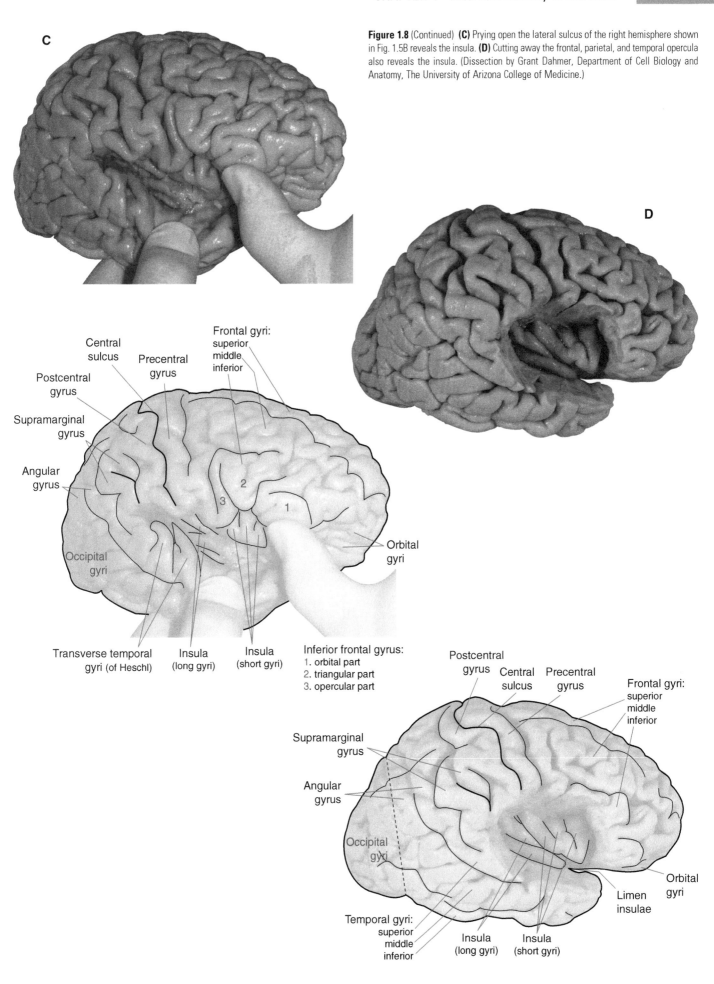

C

D

Figure 1.8 (Continued) **(C)** Prying open the lateral sulcus of the right hemisphere shown in Fig. 1.5B reveals the insula. **(D)** Cutting away the frontal, parietal, and temporal opercula also reveals the insula. (Dissection by Grant Dahmer, Department of Cell Biology and Anatomy, The University of Arizona College of Medicine.)

Central sulcus

Precentral gyrus

Frontal gyri:
superior
middle
inferior

Postcentral gyrus

Supramarginal gyrus

Angular gyrus

Occipital gyri

Orbital gyri

Transverse temporal gyri (of Heschl)

Insula (long gyri)

Insula (short gyri)

Inferior frontal gyrus:
1. orbital part
2. triangular part
3. opercular part

Postcentral gyrus

Central sulcus

Precentral gyrus

Frontal gyri:
superior
middle
inferior

Supramarginal gyrus

Angular gyrus

Occipital gyri

Orbital gyri

Limen insulae

Temporal gyri:
superior
middle
inferior

Insula (long gyri)

Insula (short gyri)

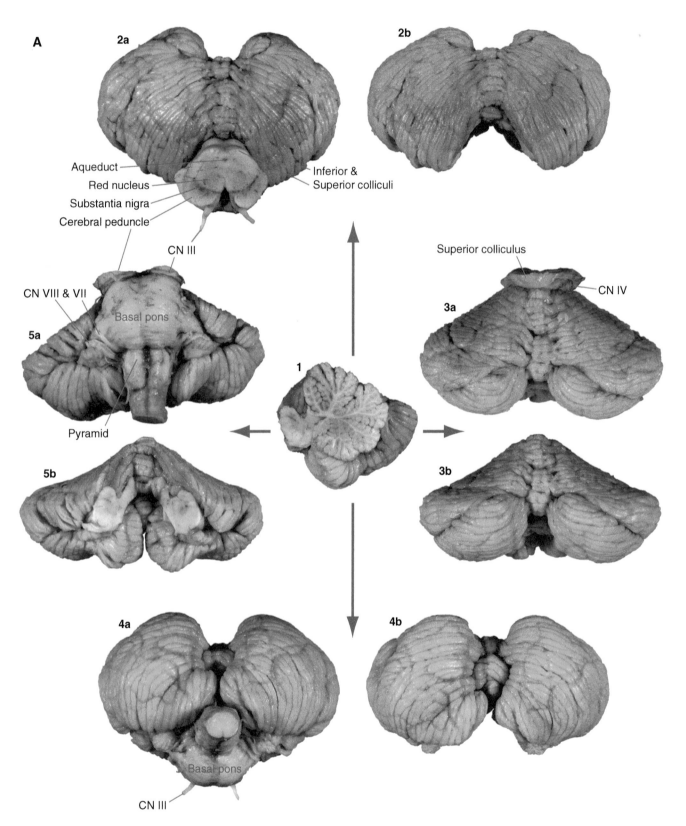

A

2a

2b

Aqueduct

Red nucleus

Substantia nigra

Cerebral peduncle

Inferior &
Superior colliculi

CN III

CN VIII & VII

Basal pons

5a

Superior colliculus

CN IV

3a

1

Pyramid

5b

3b

4a

4b

Basal pons

CN III

Figure 1.9 (A) The cerebellum from the same brain as in Fig. 1.3. Views of the superior *(2)*, posterior *(3)*, inferior *(4)*, and anterior *(5)* surfaces are shown, both before and after the brainstem was removed.

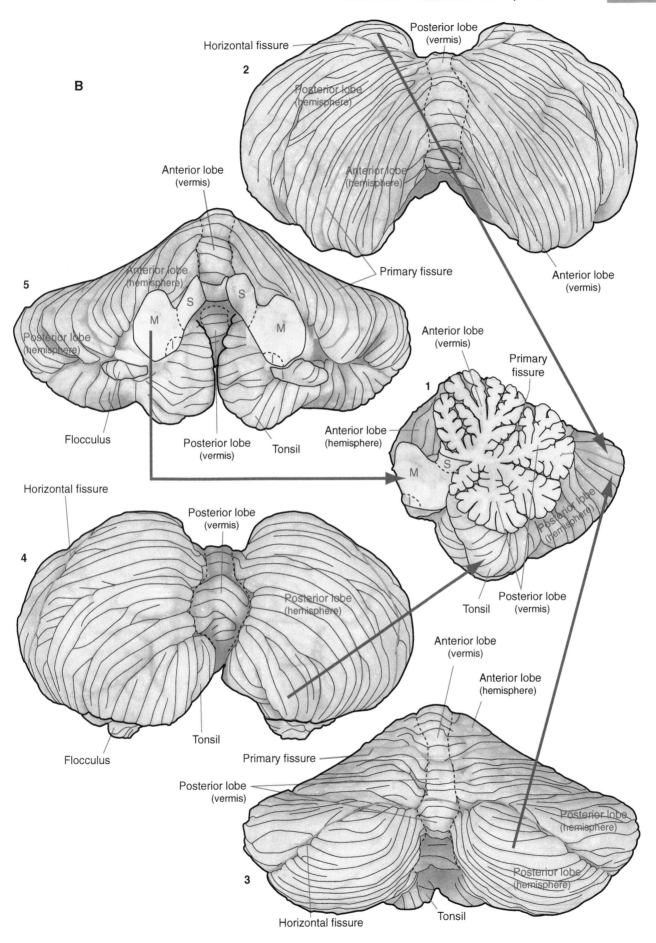

Figure 1.9 (Continued) **(B)** Major structures of the same cerebellum. *I*, *M*, and *S* indicate the inferior, middle, and superior cerebellar peduncles, respectively. (Dissection by Grant Dahmer, Department of Cell Biology and Anatomy, The University of Arizona College of Medicine.)

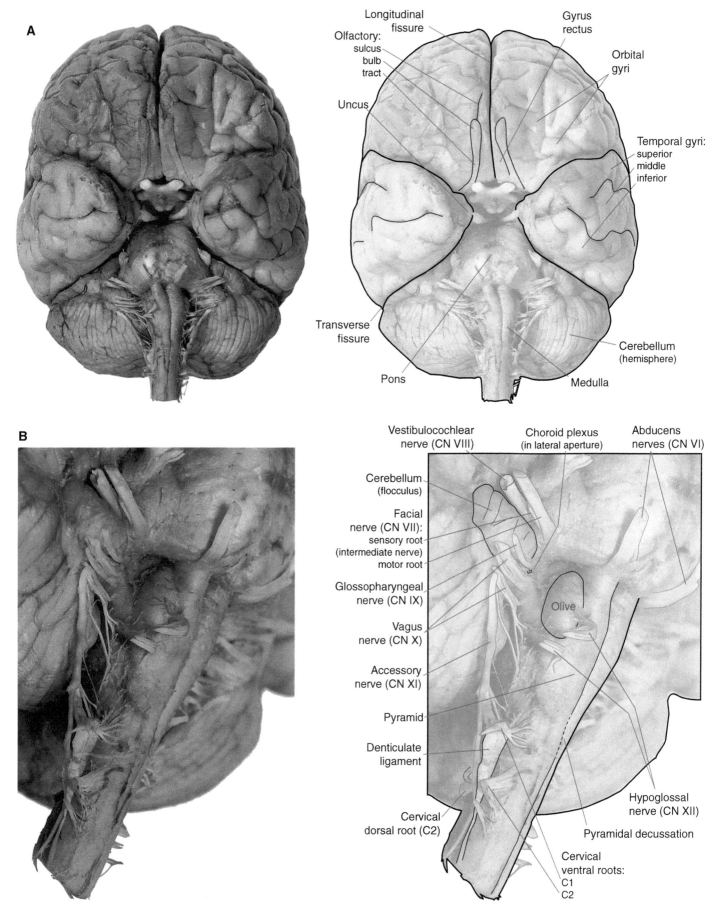

Figure 1.10 Inferior and lateral views of the cerebrum and brainstem, demonstrating the cranial nerves. **(A)** Inferior view. **(B)** Lateral and inferior view.

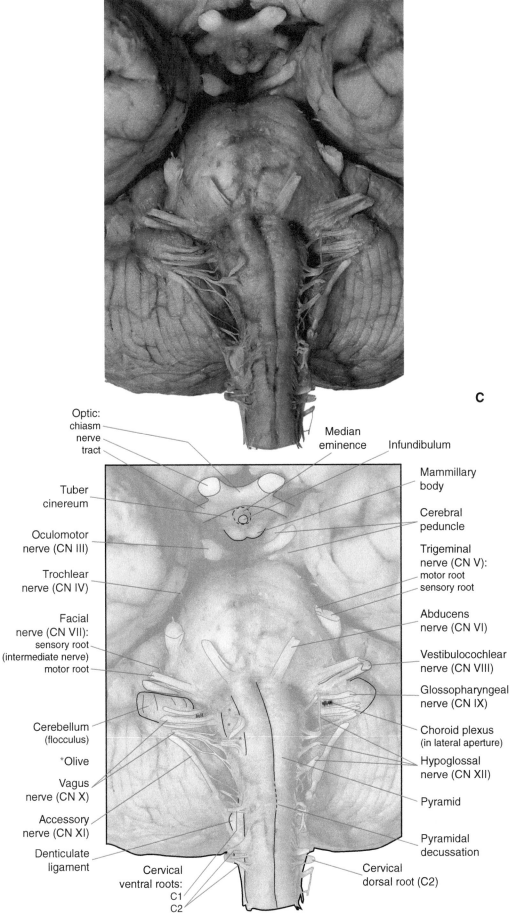

C

Optic:
chiasm
nerve
tract

Tuber
cinereum

Oculomotor
nerve (CN III)

Trochlear
nerve (CN IV)

Facial
nerve (CN VII):
sensory root
(intermediate nerve)
motor root

Cerebellum
(flocculus)

*Olive

Vagus
nerve (CN X)

Accessory
nerve (CN XI)

Denticulate
ligament

Cervical
ventral roots:
C1
C2

Median
eminence   Infundibulum

Mammillary
body

Cerebral
peduncle

Trigeminal
nerve (CN V):
motor root
sensory root

Abducens
nerve (CN VI)

Vestibulocochlear
nerve (CN VIII)

Glossopharyngeal
nerve (CN IX)

Choroid plexus
(in lateral aperture)

Hypoglossal
nerve (CN XII)

Pyramid

Pyramidal
decussation

Cervical
dorsal root (C2)

Figure 1.10 (Continued) **(C)** Inferior view. (Dissection by Dr. Norman Koelling, Department of Cell Biology and Anatomy, The University of Arizona College of Medicine.)

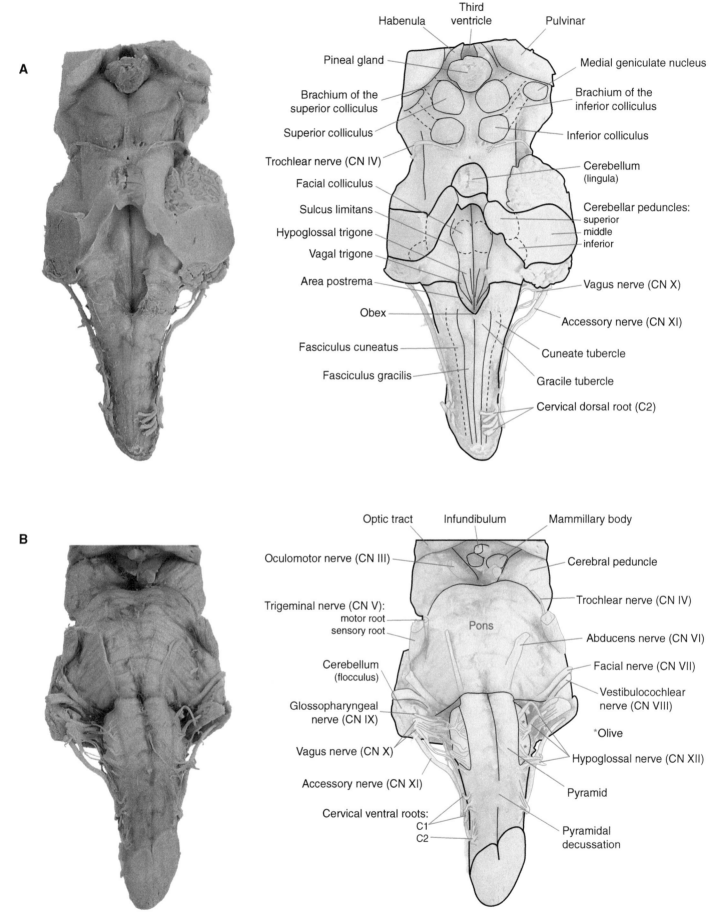

Figure 1.11 Four views of a brainstem. **(A)** The dorsal surface, looking down on the floor of the fourth ventricle. **(B)** The ventral surface.

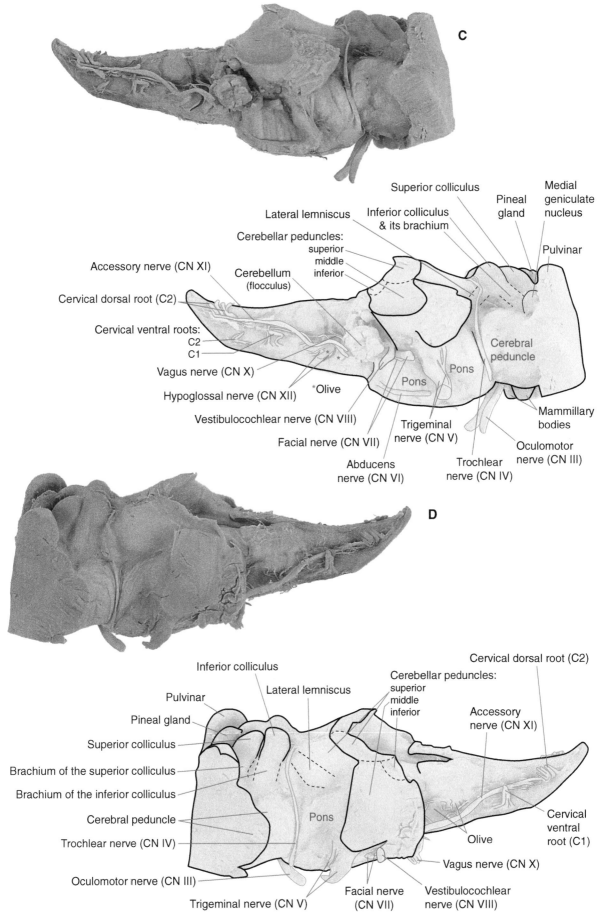

C

Superior colliculus
Medial geniculate nucleus
Pineal gland
Lateral lemniscus
Inferior colliculus & its brachium
Pulvinar
Cerebellar peduncles:
superior
middle
inferior
Accessory nerve (CN XI)
Cerebellum (flocculus)
Cervical dorsal root (C2)
Cerebral peduncle
Cervical ventral roots:
C2
C1
Pons
Pons
Vagus nerve (CN X)
Pons
Hypoglossal nerve (CN XII)
*Olive
Mammillary bodies
Vestibulocochlear nerve (CN VIII)
Facial nerve (CN VII)
Trigeminal nerve (CN V)
Oculomotor nerve (CN III)
Abducens nerve (CN VI)
Trochlear nerve (CN IV)

D

Inferior colliculus
Cervical dorsal root (C2)
Lateral lemniscus
Cerebellar peduncles:
superior
middle
inferior
Pulvinar
Accessory nerve (CN XI)
Pineal gland
Superior colliculus
Brachium of the superior colliculus
Brachium of the inferior colliculus
Cerebral peduncle
Pons
Cervical ventral root (C1)
Trochlear nerve (CN IV)
Olive
Oculomotor nerve (CN III)
Vagus nerve (CN X)
Facial nerve (CN VII)
Vestibulocochlear nerve (CN VIII)
Trigeminal nerve (CN V)

Figure 1.11 (Continued) **(C)** Right side. **(D)** Left side. (Dissection by Grant Dahmer, Department of Cell Biology and Anatomy, The University of Arizona College of Medicine.)

2

Transverse Sections of the Spinal Cord

The spinal cord is perhaps the most simply arranged part of the central nervous system (CNS). Its basic structure, indicated in a schematic drawing of the eighth cervical segment (Fig. 2.1), is the same at every level—a butterfly-shaped core of gray matter surrounded by white matter. An often indistinct **central canal** in the middle of the butterfly is the remnant of the lumen of the embryonic neural tube.

The extensions of the gray matter posteriorly and anteriorly are termed the **posterior** and **anterior** (**dorsal** and **ventral**) **horns**, respectively. The zone where the two horns meet is the **intermediate gray**. At every level, the posterior horn is capped by a zone of closely packed small neurons, the **substantia gelatinosa**. Beyond this, there are level-to-level variations in the configuration of the spinal gray (Fig. 2.2). For example, the motor neurons that innervate skeletal muscle are located in the anterior horns, so these horns expand laterally in lumbar and lower cervical segments to accommodate the many motor neurons required for the muscles of the lower and upper extremities. Other examples are pointed out in Fig. 2.2. When studied in microscopic detail, the spinal gray matter can be partitioned into a series of 10 layers **(Rexed laminae)**, as indicated on the right side of Fig. 2.1. Some of these laminae have clear functional significance. For example, lamina II corresponds to the substantia gelatinosa, which plays an important role in regulating sensations of pain and temperature.

Spinal white matter contains pathways ascending to or descending from higher levels of the nervous system, as well as nerve fibers interconnecting different levels of the spinal cord. The horns of the gray matter serve to divide the white matter into **posterior**, **lateral**, and **anterior funiculi**. In contrast to the level-to-level variations in the gray matter, the total amount of white matter increases steadily at progressively higher spinal levels (i.e., more white matter in the cervical area vs the sacral area). Moving rostrally, the ascending pathways enlarge as progressively more fibers are added to the funiculi; as fibers descend, they begin to stop at their corresponding levels of the spinal cord hence resulting in fewer fibers as they move caudally.

Information travels to and from the spinal gray matter in the **dorsal** and **ventral roots**. The dorsal roots convey the central processes of afferents with cell bodies in **dorsal root ganglia**. As the roots approach the spinal cord, they break up into **rootlets**, each of which sorts itself into a **medial division**, containing the large-diameter afferents, and a **lateral division**, containing the small-diameter afferents. This is the beginning of two great streams of somatosensory information that travel rostrally in the CNS. The large fibers, primarily carrying information about touch and position, send branches into multiple levels of the gray matter and may send a branch rostrally in the ipsilateral posterior funiculus (or **posterior column**). The small fibers, primarily carrying information about pain and temperature, traverse a distinctive area of the white matter **(Lissauer's tract)** and end more superficially in the gray matter of the posterior horn. Subsequent connections of both classes of afferents are reviewed in Chapter 8.

In the pages that follow (as in all chapters in this atlas), only the largest and best-known spinal structures and pathways are indicated. Many others are either known to exist in humans or inferred from animal studies. In many cases, however, their functional significance is not well understood.

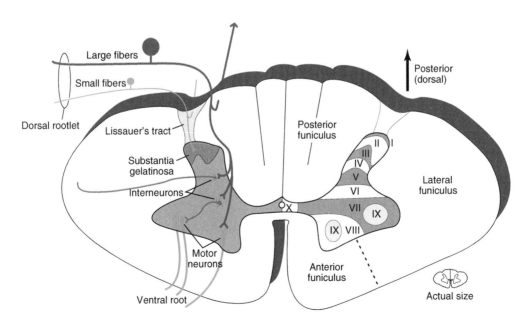

Figure 2.1 Schematic drawing of the spinal cord at the level of the eighth cervical segment. (Modified from Nolte J: *The Human Brain*, ed 6, Philadelphia, 2009, Elsevier.)

Figure 2.2 (A–H) Cross sections of a spinal cord at eight different levels, all shown at about the same magnification.

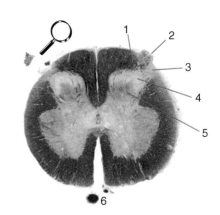

(A) The fourth sacral segment (S4). Several features common to all spinal levels can be seen. The substantia gelatinosa *(4)* caps the posterior horn *(5)*. Also, afferent fibers entering through dorsal rootlets *(2)* sort themselves into small-diameter fibers that move laterally and enter Lissauer's tract *(3)* and large-diameter fibers that enter more medially *(1)* at the edge of the posterior funiculus. (This sorting occurs at all spinal levels and can be seen in all of the sections in this series.) Little white matter is present in any of the funiculi because most fibers either have already left descending pathways or have not yet entered ascending pathways. The anterior spinal artery *(6)* is cut in cross section as it runs longitudinally near the anterior median fissure of the cord. Shown enlarged in Fig. 2.3.

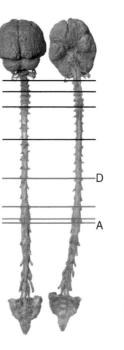

(B) The fifth lumbar segment (L5). This segment is in the lumbar enlargement (which extends from about L2 to S3) and has anterior horns that are enlarged, primarily in their lateral portions *(1)*, to accommodate motor neurons for leg and foot muscles. Motor neurons located more medially *(2)* in the anterior horn innervate more proximal muscles, in this case hip muscles.

(C) The second lumbar segment (L2). The posterior funiculus *(1)* is larger because ascending fibers carrying touch and position information from the lower limb have been added. The lateral funiculus is also larger, reflecting increased numbers of descending fibers in the lateral corticospinal tract *(2)* and ascending fibers in the spinothalamic tract *(4)*. This section is at the rostral end of the lumbar enlargement, so the anterior horn *(5)* no longer is enlarged laterally. Clarke's nucleus *(3)*, which extends from about T1 to L3 and contains the cells of origin of the posterior spinocerebellar tract, makes its appearance. The anterior white commissure *(6)*, the principal route through which axons can cross the midline in the spinal cord, is present at this and all other spinal levels. Shown enlarged in Fig. 2.4.

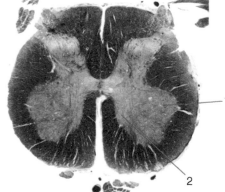

(D) The tenth thoracic segment (T10). The posterior *(1)* and anterior *(4)* horns are slender, corresponding to the relative dearth of sensory information arriving at this level and the relatively small number of motor neurons needed. Sympathetic preganglionic neurons form a lateral horn *(3)* containing the intermediolateral cell column, a characteristic feature of thoracic segments. Clarke's nucleus *(2)* is still apparent. Shown enlarged in Fig. 2.5.

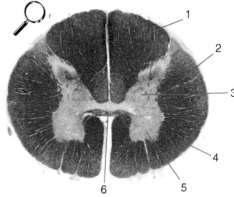

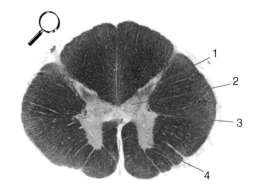

Figure 2.2 (Continued) Cross sections of a spinal cord.

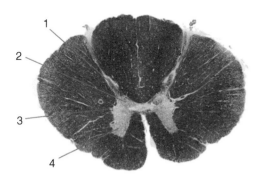

(E) The fifth thoracic segment (T5). The posterior *(1)* and anterior *(4)* horns are even more slender, reflecting the relative paucity of sensory information arriving from the trunk and the relatively small number of motor neurons required by trunk muscles. Clarke's nucleus *(2)*, though smaller, is still present, as is the lateral horn *(3)*.

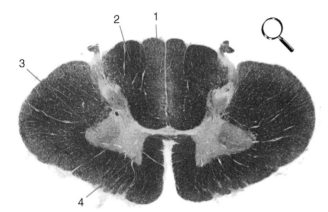

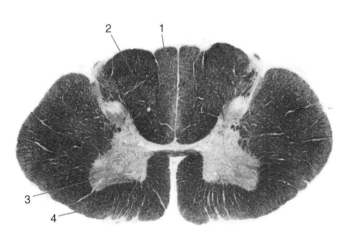

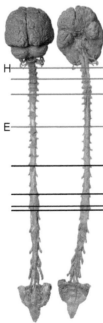

(F) The eighth cervical segment (C8), near the caudal end of the cervical enlargement (C5 to T1). The posterior funiculus is subdivided by a partial glial partition into fasciculus gracilis *(1)*, conveying touch and position information from the lower limb, and fasciculus cuneatus *(2)*, conveying touch and position information from the upper limb. The anterior horn is enlarged, primarily laterally *(3)*, to accommodate motor neurons for hand and forearm muscles. Motor neurons in more medial parts of the anterior horn *(4)* innervate more proximal muscles, such as the triceps. Shown enlarged in Fig. 2.6.

(G) The fifth cervical segment (C5), still in the cervical enlargement. As in the previous section, the posterior funiculus is subdivided into fasciculus gracilis *(1)* and fasciculus cuneatus *(2)*, and the anterior horn includes an expanded lateral region *(3*, here containing motor neurons for forearm muscles) and the more medial area *(4)* that is present at all spinal levels (and at this level innervates shoulder muscles).

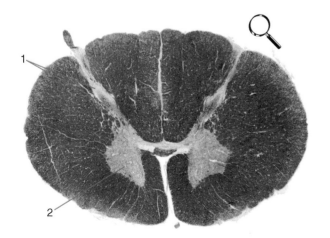

(H) The third cervical segment (C3), rostral to the cervical enlargement. The posterior horn *(1)* is more slender, reflecting the smaller amount of afferent input arriving from the neck. The anterior horn *(2)* is no longer enlarged laterally. The area of white matter, however, is larger than in any other section in this series, reflecting the near-maximal size of both ascending and descending pathways. Shown enlarged in Fig. 2.7.

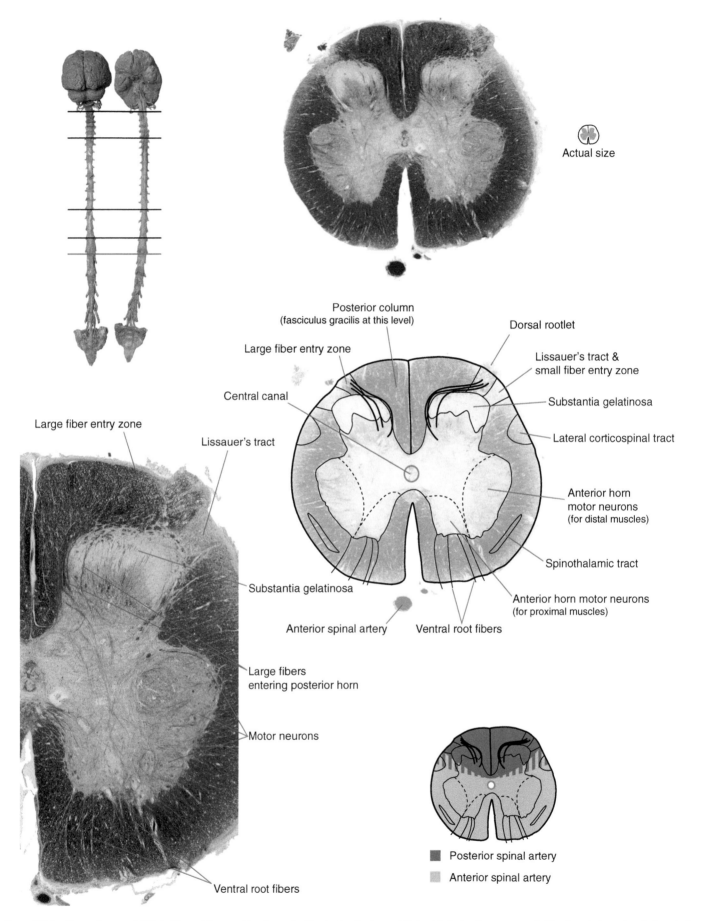

Actual size

Posterior column
(fasciculus gracilis at this level)

Dorsal rootlet

Large fiber entry zone

Lissauer's tract &
small fiber entry zone

Central canal

Substantia gelatinosa

Lateral corticospinal tract

Large fiber entry zone

Lissauer's tract

Anterior horn
motor neurons
(for distal muscles)

Substantia gelatinosa

Spinothalamic tract

Anterior spinal artery

Ventral root fibers

Anterior horn motor neurons
(for proximal muscles)

Large fibers
entering posterior horn

Motor neurons

Ventral root fibers

Posterior spinal artery

Anterior spinal artery

Figure 2.3 Fourth sacral segment (S4). In this and the remaining figures in this chapter, the lower right inset indicates the areas supplied by the anterior and posterior spinal arteries.

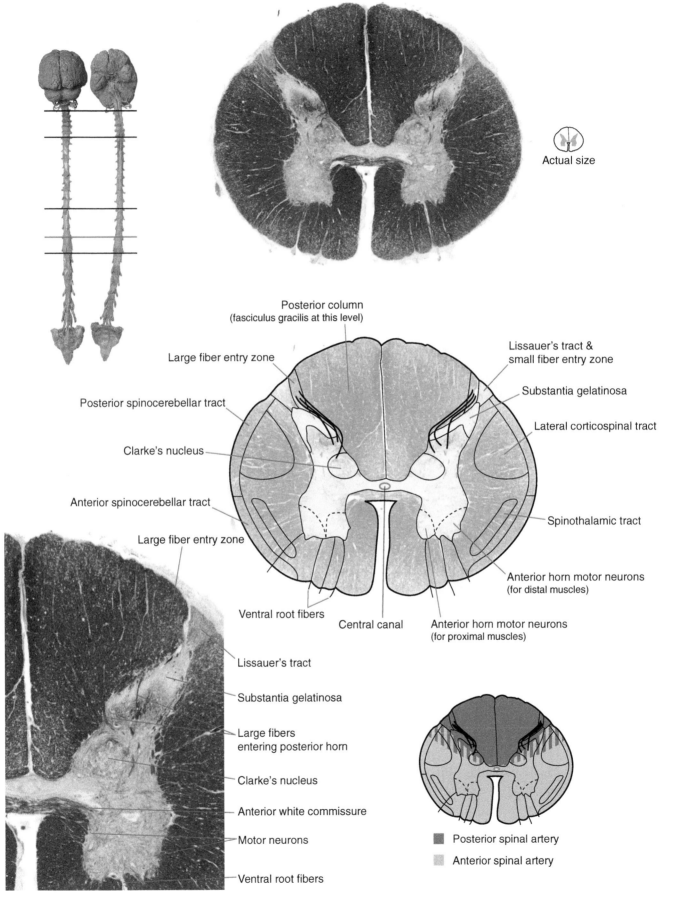

Actual size

Posterior column
(fasciculus gracilis at this level)

Large fiber entry zone

Lissauer's tract &
small fiber entry zone

Posterior spinocerebellar tract

Substantia gelatinosa

Lateral corticospinal tract

Clarke's nucleus

Anterior spinocerebellar tract

Spinothalamic tract

Large fiber entry zone

Anterior horn motor neurons
(for distal muscles)

Ventral root fibers

Central canal

Anterior horn motor neurons
(for proximal muscles)

Lissauer's tract

Substantia gelatinosa

Large fibers
entering posterior horn

Clarke's nucleus

Anterior white commissure

Motor neurons

Ventral root fibers

Posterior spinal artery

Anterior spinal artery

Figure 2.4 Second lumbar segment (L2).

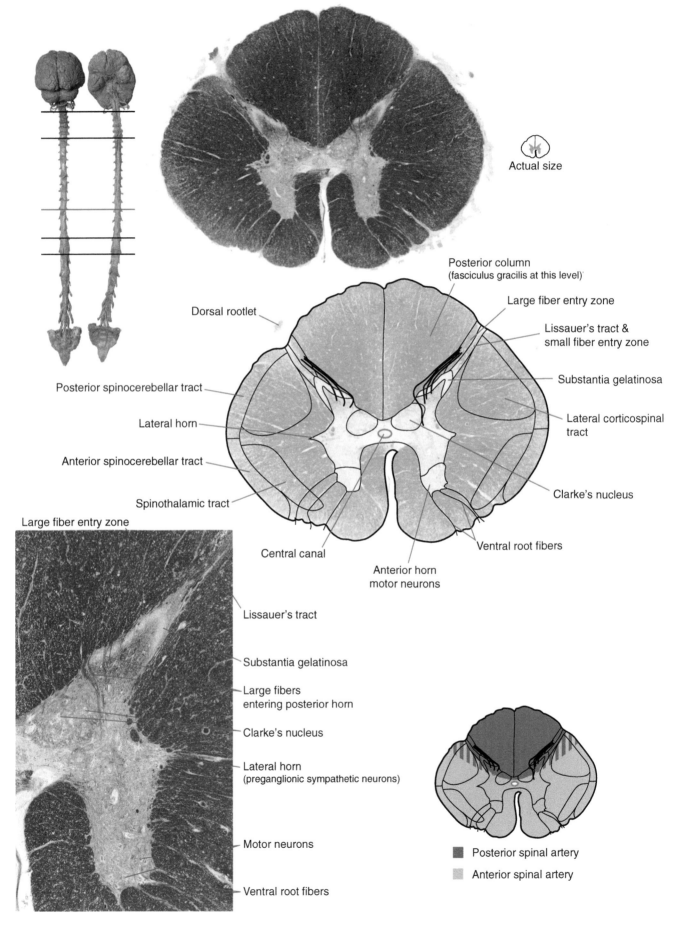

Actual size

Posterior column
(fasciculus gracilis at this level)

Dorsal rootlet

Large fiber entry zone

Lissauer's tract &
small fiber entry zone

Posterior spinocerebellar tract

Substantia gelatinosa

Lateral corticospinal
tract

Lateral horn

Anterior spinocerebellar tract

Clarke's nucleus

Spinothalamic tract

Ventral root fibers

Central canal

Anterior horn
motor neurons

Large fiber entry zone

Lissauer's tract

Substantia gelatinosa

Large fibers
entering posterior horn

Clarke's nucleus

Lateral horn
(preganglionic sympathetic neurons)

Motor neurons

Ventral root fibers

Posterior spinal artery

Anterior spinal artery

Figure 2.5 Tenth thoracic segment (T10).

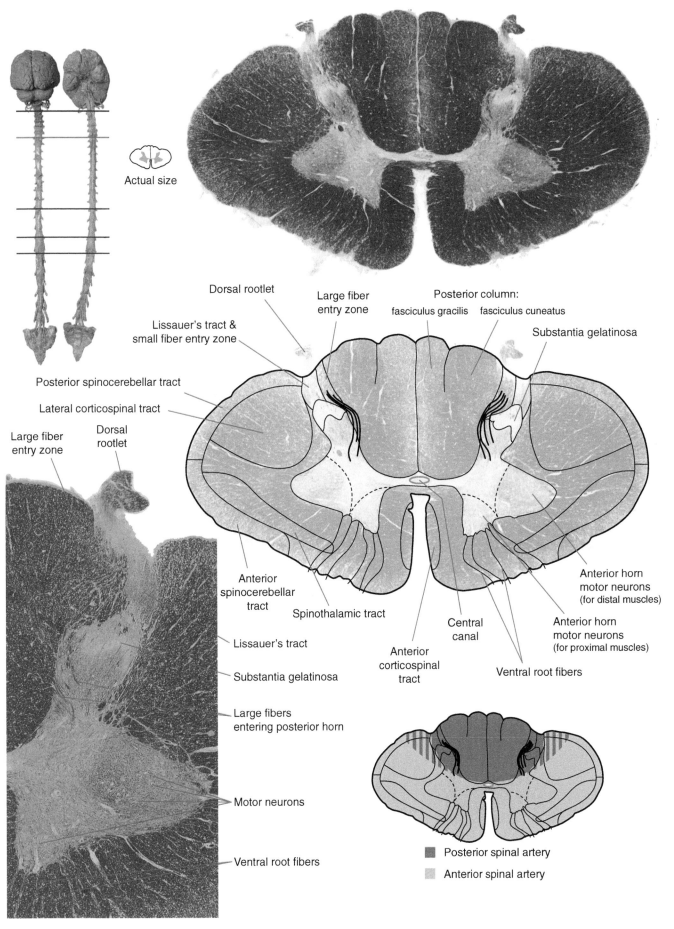

Actual size

Dorsal rootlet

Large fiber
entry zone

Posterior column:
fasciculus gracilis   fasciculus cuneatus

Lissauer's tract &
small fiber entry zone

Substantia gelatinosa

Posterior spinocerebellar tract

Lateral corticospinal tract

Large fiber
entry zone

Dorsal
rootlet

Anterior
spinocerebellar
tract

Spinothalamic tract

Anterior horn
motor neurons
(for distal muscles)

Anterior horn
motor neurons
(for proximal muscles)

Lissauer's tract

Substantia gelatinosa

Anterior
corticospinal
tract

Central
canal

Ventral root fibers

Large fibers
entering posterior horn

Motor neurons

Ventral root fibers

Posterior spinal artery

Anterior spinal artery

Figure 2.6 Eighth cervical segment (C8).

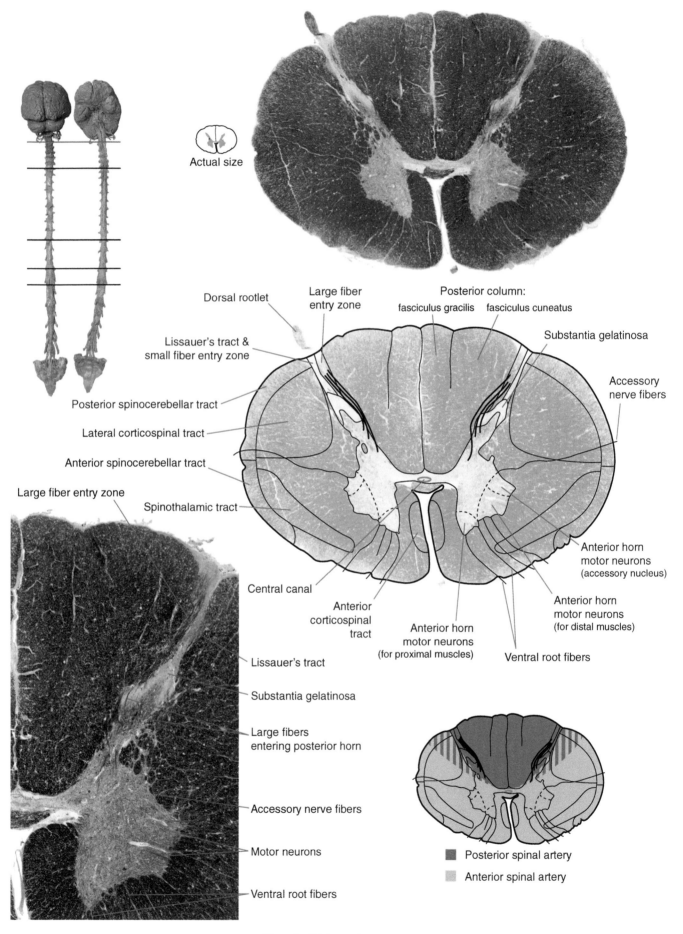

Actual size

Dorsal rootlet

Large fiber entry zone

Posterior column:
fasciculus gracilis   fasciculus cuneatus

Lissauer's tract & small fiber entry zone

Substantia gelatinosa

Posterior spinocerebellar tract

Accessory nerve fibers

Lateral corticospinal tract

Anterior spinocerebellar tract

Large fiber entry zone

Spinothalamic tract

Anterior horn motor neurons (accessory nucleus)

Anterior horn motor neurons (for distal muscles)

Central canal

Anterior corticospinal tract

Anterior horn motor neurons (for proximal muscles)

Ventral root fibers

Lissauer's tract

Substantia gelatinosa

Large fibers entering posterior horn

Accessory nerve fibers

Motor neurons

Ventral root fibers

Posterior spinal artery

Anterior spinal artery

Figure 2.7 Third cervical segment (C3).

3

Transverse Sections of the Brainstem

The brainstem contains the continuations of the long tracts seen in the spinal cord together with nuclei and tracts associated with **cranial nerves** and the cerebellum. These various tracts and nuclei surround, traverse, or are embedded in the **reticular formation** (named for its anatomical appearance—the Latin word *reticulum* means "network"), which forms a central core at all brainstem levels.

This chapter considers the level-to-level arrangements of structures as seen in transverse sections of the brainstem; many of the same structures are revisited in Chapter 8 as parts of functional systems. The sections were made by Pam Eller and stained, as were the spinal cord sections in the previous chapter, by the Klüver-Barrera method, using luxol fast blue for myelin and a neutral red counterstain (which, despite its name, is a basic stain with an affinity for nucleic acids). The result is blue-violet staining of white matter and red staining of large neurons with prominent Nissl substance (e.g., **hypoglossal motor neurons** in Fig. 3.10) and of areas tightly packed with small neurons (e.g., the **granular layer** of **cerebellar cortex** in Fig. 3.10). A parasagittal section of the brainstem (Fig. 3.1) is used as a reference view throughout the chapter. It includes some of the features characteristic of each

brainstem level (Fig. 3.2), such as the **superior** and **inferior colliculi** of the **midbrain**, the **basal pons**, and a **medullary pyramid**.

The three major longitudinal pathways (lateral corticospinal tract, posterior columns, and spinothalamic tract) that were followed through the spinal cord in Chapter 2 extend into the brainstem in consistent ways, as indicated in Fig. 3.3. Corticospinal fibers travel in the most ventral part of the brainstem, traversing the **cerebral peduncle**, **basal pons**, and **medullary pyramid**. At the spinomedullary junction, most of the fibers in each pyramid cross the midline (in the **pyramidal decussation**) and form the lateral corticospinal tract. Each posterior column terminates in the **posterior column nuclei** (**nucleus gracilis** and **nucleus cuneatus**) of the **medulla**. Afferent fibers from these nuclei decussate in the medulla to form the **medial lemniscus**, which travels rostrally and ends in the thalamus. The medial lemniscus starts out near the midline and then moves progressively more laterally as it proceeds rostrally through the brainstem (Fig. 3.4), rotating nearly 180 degrees in the process. The spinothalamic tract at all levels of the brainstem is at or near the lateral edge of the reticular formation. Cranial nerve nuclei are also arranged in reasonably consistent ways, as indicated schematically in Fig. 3.3 and in more detail in subsequent figures.

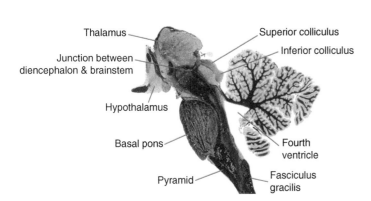

Figure 3.1 Parasagittal section of the brainstem and diencephalon.

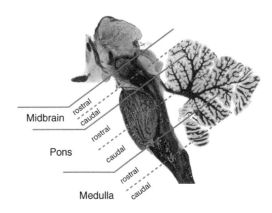

Figure 3.2 Levels of the brainstem.

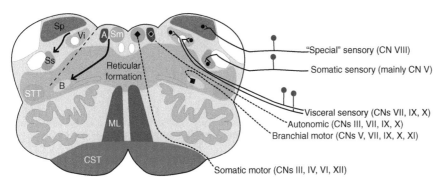

Figure 3.3 Arrangement of cranial nerve nuclei in the rostral medulla. The left side of the figure indicates how visceral sensory (*Vi*), somatic sensory (*Ss*), and "special" sensory (*Sp*) (e.g., vestibular) nuclei are located lateral to the nuclei containing preganglionic autonomic neurons (*A*), somatic motor neurons (*Sm*), and motor neurons for muscles of branchial arch origin (*B*) (e.g., muscles of the larynx and pharynx). The cranial nerves containing each of these components are indicated on the right. (Not all of the nerves indicated actually emerge from the rostral medulla; they are included here for summary purposes.) *CST*, Corticospinal tract; *ML*, medial lemniscus; *STT*, spinothalamic tract.

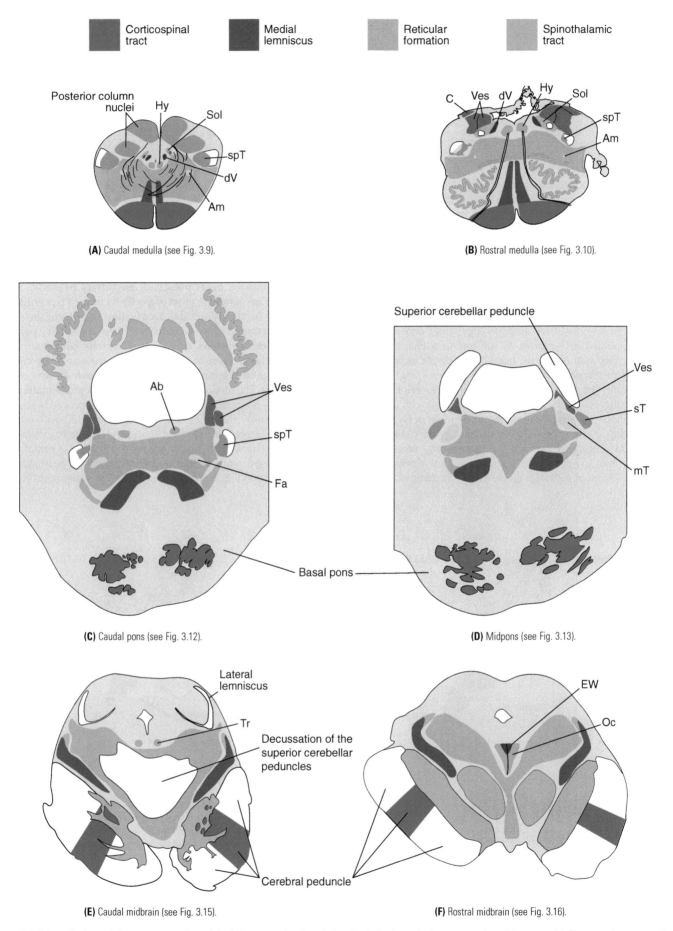

Figure 3.4 Schematic views of six transverse sections of the brainstem, each enlarged about 3×, indicating major long tracts and cranial nerve nuclei. These are the same sections shown photographically in Figs. 3.9, 3.10, 3.12, 3.13, 3.15, and 3.16, and they correspond to planes of section indicated in Fig. 3.6. Abbreviations as in Fig. 3.6.

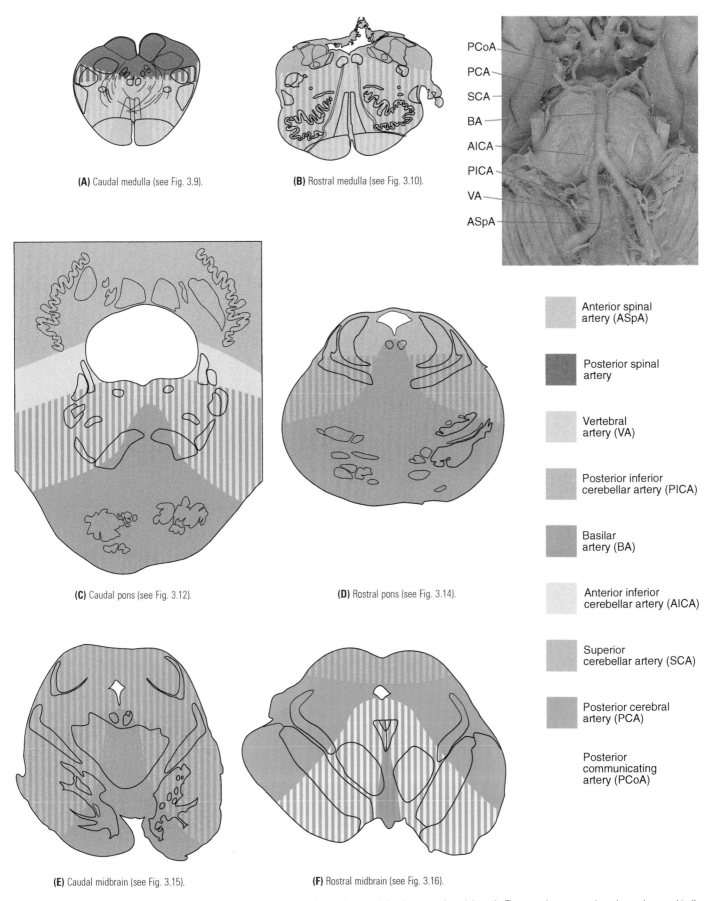

(A) Caudal medulla (see Fig. 3.9).

(B) Rostral medulla (see Fig. 3.10).

PCoA
PCA
SCA
BA
AICA
PICA
VA
ASpA

(C) Caudal pons (see Fig. 3.12).

(D) Rostral pons (see Fig. 3.14).

Anterior spinal artery (ASpA)

Posterior spinal artery

Vertebral artery (VA)

Posterior inferior cerebellar artery (PICA)

Basilar artery (BA)

Anterior inferior cerebellar artery (AICA)

Superior cerebellar artery (SCA)

Posterior cerebral artery (PCA)

Posterior communicating artery (PCoA)

(E) Caudal midbrain (see Fig. 3.15).

(F) Rostral midbrain (see Fig. 3.16).

Figure 3.5 Schematic views of six transverse sections of the brainstem, each enlarged about 3×, indicating areas of arterial supply. These are the same sections shown photographically in Figs. 3.9, 3.10, 3.12, and 3.14 through 3.16, and they correspond to planes of section indicated in Fig. 3.6. At each level, the brainstem supply is a series of wedge-shaped territories with anterolateral areas fed by midline arteries (e.g., vertebral, basilar) and posterolateral areas fed by circumferential branches (e.g., PICA, posterior cerebral).

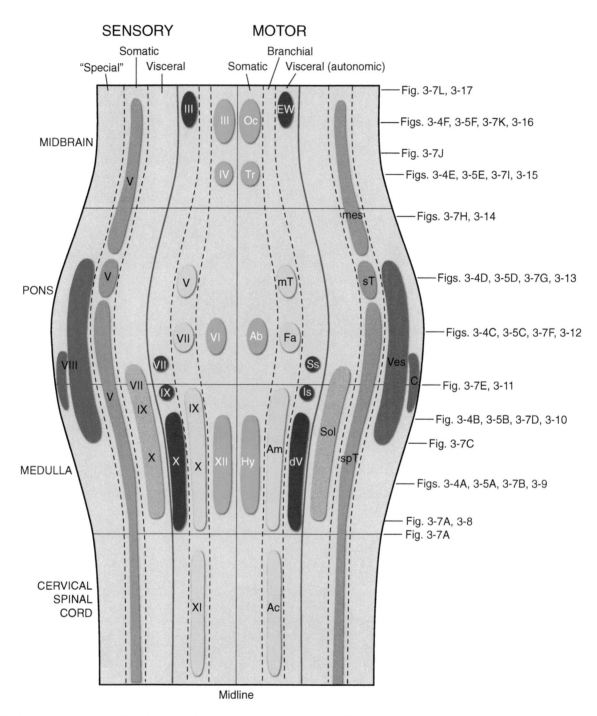

Figure 3.6 The longitudinal arrangement of functional types of cranial nerve nuclei in the brainstem. The cranial nerves involved with each type of function are indicated on the left side of the diagram, and the actual nuclei are indicated on the right side. The *dark blue line* on each side represents the sulcus limitans, which (ideally, at least) separates motor nuclei medial to it from sensory nuclei lateral to it. Abbreviations for nuclei on the right side: *Ab*, Abducens nucleus; *Ac*, accessory nucleus; *Am*, nucleus ambiguus; *C*, cochlear nuclei; *dV*, dorsal motor nucleus of the vagus; *EW*, Edinger-Westphal nucleus (a subdivision of the oculomotor nucleus); *Fa*, facial nucleus; *Hy*, hypoglossal nucleus; *Is*, inferior salivary nucleus; *mes*, mesencephalic nucleus of the trigeminal; *mT*, motor nucleus of the trigeminal; *Oc*, oculomotor nucleus; *Sol*, nucleus of the solitary tract; *spT*, spinal nucleus of the trigeminal; *Ss*, superior salivary nucleus; *sT*, main sensory nucleus of the trigeminal; *Tr*, trochlear nucleus; *Ves*, vestibular nuclei. All of these nuclei (except the salivary nuclei) are indicated in one or more of the cross sections along the right side of the figure. (Modified from Nieuwenhuys R, Voogd J, van Huijzen C: *The human central nervous system: a synopsis and atlas*, ed 3, New York, 1988, Springer-Verlag.)

Figure 3.7 (A–L) Cross sections of a brainstem at 13 different levels, all shown at about the same magnification.

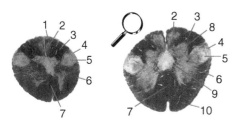

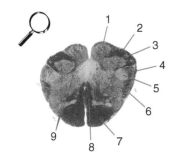

(A) Spinomedullary junction. Fasciculus cuneatus *(3)* proceeds rostrally toward nucleus cuneatus *(8*, not yet present in the section on the left), and fasciculus gracilis *(1)* begins to terminate in nucleus gracilis *(2)*. In the more rostral section on the right, internal arcuate fibers *(9)* leave the posterior column nuclei to cross the midline and form the medial lemniscus. The spinal trigeminal tract *(4)*, at this level containing trigeminal pain and temperature afferents, and the spinal trigeminal nucleus *(5)*, where these afferents terminate, replace Lissauer's tract and the posterior horn of the spinal cord. The spinothalamic tract *(6)* is located anterolaterally, much as it was in the spinal cord. Corticospinal fibers that descended through the internal capsule, cerebral peduncle, basal pons, and medullary pyramid *(10)* now cross the midline in the pyramidal decussation *(7)*. The section on the right is shown enlarged in Fig. 3.8.

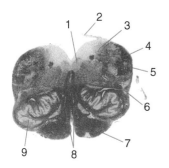

(B) Caudal medulla. Fasciculus gracilis has ended in nucleus gracilis *(1)*, and fasciculus cuneatus *(2)* ends in nucleus cuneatus *(3)*. Efferents from these posterior column nuclei cross the midline as internal arcuate fibers *(9)* and form the medial lemniscus *(8)*. The spinothalamic tract *(6)* is in its typical location in the lateral part of the reticular formation, and the corticospinal tract traverses the pyramids *(7)*. Trigeminal primary afferent fibers descend through the spinal trigeminal tract *(4)* to termination sites in the spinal trigeminal nucleus *(5)*. Shown enlarged in Fig. 3.9.

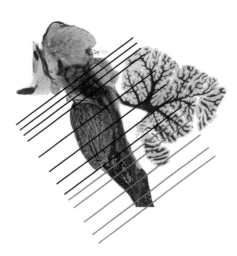

(C) Rostral medulla. The central canal of the spinal cord and caudal medulla has given way to the fourth ventricle; part of its roof can be seen *(2)*. Structures associated with cranial nerves appear in the floor of the fourth ventricle, including the hypoglossal nucleus *(1)*, vestibular nuclei *(3)*, and the solitary tract *(5)* surrounded by its nucleus. Efferents from the inferior olivary nucleus *(9)* cross the midline (again, as internal arcuate fibers) and join the contralateral inferior cerebellar peduncle *(4)*. The locations of the spinothalamic tract *(6)*, medial lemniscus *(8)*, and corticospinal tract *(7)* are unchanged.

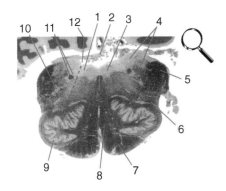

(D) Rostral medulla. A plane *(dashed line)* descending from the sulcus limitans *(12)* separates cranial nerve nuclei into a more medial group of motor nuclei and a more lateral group of sensory nuclei. Motor nuclei at this level include the hypoglossal nucleus *(3)* and the dorsal motor nucleus of the vagus *(1*, adjacent to the sulcus limitans). More laterally are vestibular nuclei *(4)*, the spinal trigeminal nucleus *(10)*, and the solitary tract and its nucleus *(11*, adjacent to the sulcus limitans). The locations of the medial lemniscus *(8)*, spinothalamic tract *(6)*, and corticospinal tract *(7*, in the pyramid) are unchanged. The inferior cerebellar peduncle *(5)* is substantially larger because efferents from the contralateral inferior olivary nucleus *(9)* have accumulated in it. Choroid plexus *(2)* can be seen in the roof of the fourth ventricle. Shown enlarged in Fig. 3.10.

Illustration continued on following page

Figure 3.7 (Continued) Cross sections of a brainstem at 13 different levels, all shown at about the same magnification.

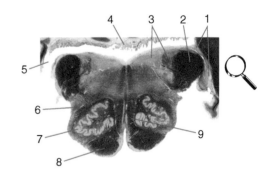

(E) Pontomedullary junction. The fourth ventricle extends laterally, leading off into the lateral recess *(5)*; choroid plexus *(4)* is visible in the roof of the ventricle. Vestibular *(3)* and cochlear *(1)* nuclei occupy the ventricular floor. The inferior cerebellar peduncle *(2)* has reached maximum size and is about to enter the cerebellum. The positions of the spinothalamic tract *(6)*, inferior olivary nucleus *(7)*, medial lemniscus *(9)*, and corticospinal tract *(8)* are unchanged. Shown enlarged in Fig. 3.11.

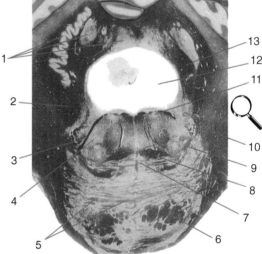

(F) Caudal pons. Now the floor of the fourth ventricle *(12)* is occupied by the abducens nucleus *(11)*, together with facial nerve fibers that emerge from the facial nucleus *(4)*, hook around the abducens nucleus as the genu of the facial nerve, and leave the brainstem as the root of the facial nerve *(3)*. The spinothalamic tract *(9)* is still located laterally in the reticular formation. The medial lemniscus *(8)* begins to move laterally and is traversed by crossing auditory fibers *(7)* of the trapezoid body. The corticospinal tract *(6)* is somewhat dispersed in the basal pons, surrounded by pontine nuclei and their transversely oriented efferents *(5)*, which cross the midline and form the middle cerebellar peduncle *(10)*. Deep cerebellar nuclei *(1)* appear in the roof of the fourth ventricle, and the superior cerebellar peduncle *(13)* begins to form adjacent to them. The inferior cerebellar peduncle *(2)* enters the cerebellum. Shown enlarged in Fig. 3.12.

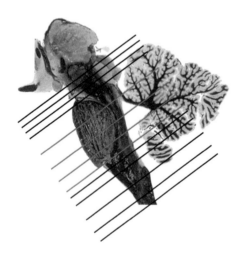

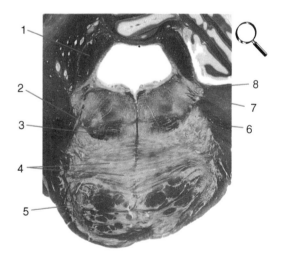

(G) Midpons, at the level of entry of the trigeminal nerve *(6)*. Many trigeminal fibers end in the main sensory nucleus of the trigeminal *(8)* or arise in the trigeminal motor nucleus *(7)*. The superior cerebellar peduncle *(1)*, carrying most of the output of the cerebellum, begins to enter the brainstem. The spinothalamic tract *(2)* is still located laterally in the reticular formation, the medial lemniscus *(3)* continues to move laterally, and the corticospinal tract *(5)* is still dispersed in the basal pons *(4)*. Shown enlarged in Fig. 3.13.

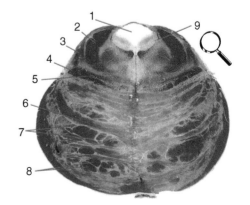

(H) Rostral pons, near the pons-midbrain junction. The fourth ventricle *(1)* narrows as it approaches the aqueduct. The superior cerebellar peduncle *(2)* moves deeper into the brainstem just before beginning to decussate. The medial lemniscus *(5)* is now a flattened band of fibers with the spinothalamic tract *(4)* laterally adjacent to it. The lateral lemniscus *(3)* conveys ascending auditory fibers to the midbrain. The corticospinal tract *(8)* is surrounded by pontine nuclei *(7)* and their transversely oriented efferents *(6)*. The locus ceruleus *(9)* is a small collection of pigmented neurons that provide most of the noradrenergic innervation of the CNS (see Fig. 8.38). Shown enlarged in Fig. 3.14.

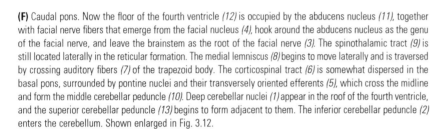

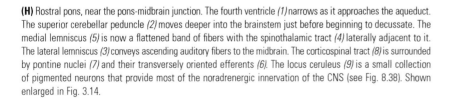

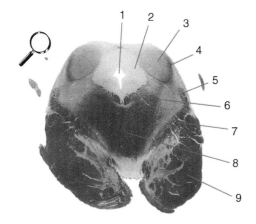

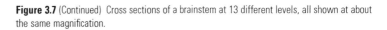

Figure 3.7 (Continued) Cross sections of a brainstem at 13 different levels, all shown at about the same magnification.

(I) Caudal midbrain. The lateral lemniscus *(4)* ends in the inferior colliculus *(3)*. The spinothalamic tract *(5)* and medial lemniscus *(7)* form a continuous band of fibers. The massive decussation of the superior cerebellar peduncles *(8)* occupies the center of the reticular formation. The basal pons gives way to a cerebral peduncle *(9)* on each side. The tiny trochlear nucleus *(6)* appears. At all midbrain levels, the cerebral aqueduct *(1)* is surrounded by periaqueductal gray matter *(2)*. Shown enlarged in Fig. 3.15.

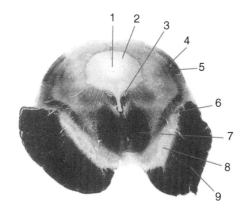

(J) Mid-midbrain. Characteristic midbrain features such as the aqueduct *(1)* and periaqueductal gray *(2)* can be seen, but no colliculi are present. The brachium of the inferior colliculus *(4)*, spinothalamic tract *(5)*, medial lemniscus *(6)*, and now-crossed superior cerebellar peduncle *(7)* are all on their way to the thalamus. The oculomotor nucleus *(3)*, substantia nigra *(8)*, and cerebral peduncle *(9)* appear—all harbingers of the rostral midbrain.

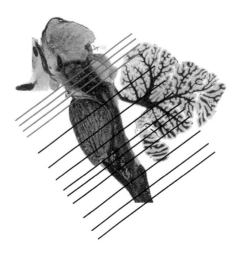

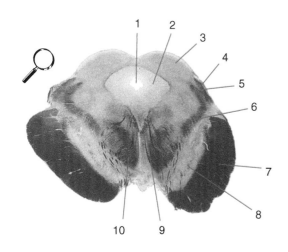

(K) Rostral midbrain. Now the superior colliculus *(3)* appears and the oculomotor nucleus *(9)* is fully formed. The auditory pathway continues in the brachium of the inferior colliculus *(4)*. The positions and appearance of the cerebral aqueduct *(1)*, periaqueductal gray *(2)*, spinothalamic tract *(5)*, medial lemniscus *(6)*, and cerebral peduncle *(7)* are little changed. Cerebellar efferents that reached the midbrain in the superior cerebellar peduncle *(10)* now begin to pass through or around the red nucleus. The substantia nigra *(8)* is more prominent. Shown enlarged in Fig. 3.16.

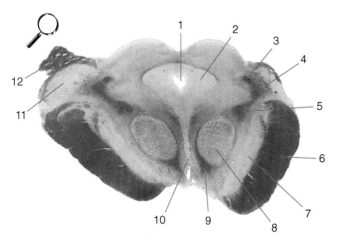

(L) Rostral midbrain, near the level of the midbrain-diencephalon junction. The cerebral aqueduct *(1)*, periaqueductal gray *(2)*, spinothalamic tract *(3)*, medial lemniscus *(5)*, cerebral peduncle *(6)*, and substantia nigra *(7)* are still evident. The brachium of the inferior colliculus *(4)* ends in the medial geniculate nucleus *(11)*, the first thalamic nucleus to appear in this plane of section. Cerebellar efferents *(9)* pass through and around the red nucleus *(8)* on their way to the thalamus. The ventral tegmental area *(10)* is a medial collection of neurons that provide the dopaminergic innervation of frontal cortex and limbic structures (see Fig. 8.39). Afferents from some retinal ganglion cells and visual cortex traverse the brachium of the superior colliculus *(12)* on their way to the superior colliculus. Shown enlarged in Fig. 3.17.

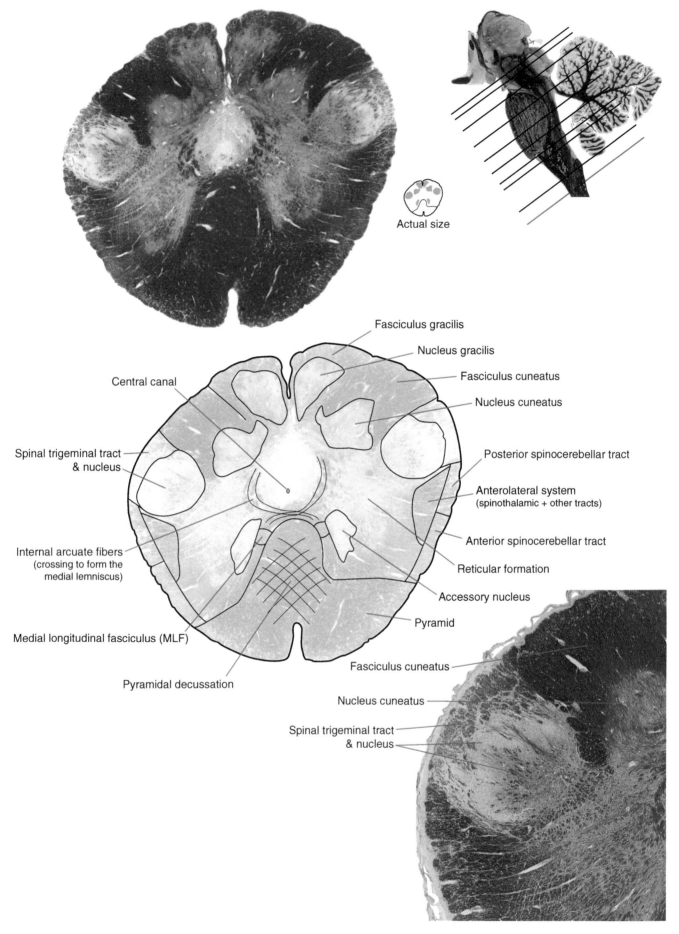

Actual size

Fasciculus gracilis

Nucleus gracilis

Fasciculus cuneatus

Nucleus cuneatus

Central canal

Spinal trigeminal tract
& nucleus

Posterior spinocerebellar tract

Anterolateral system
(spinothalamic + other tracts)

Anterior spinocerebellar tract

Reticular formation

Internal arcuate fibers
(crossing to form the
medial lemniscus)

Accessory nucleus

Pyramid

Medial longitudinal fasciculus (MLF)

Pyramidal decussation

Fasciculus cuneatus

Nucleus cuneatus

Spinal trigeminal tract
& nucleus

Figure 3.8 Caudal medulla, near the spinomedullary junction.

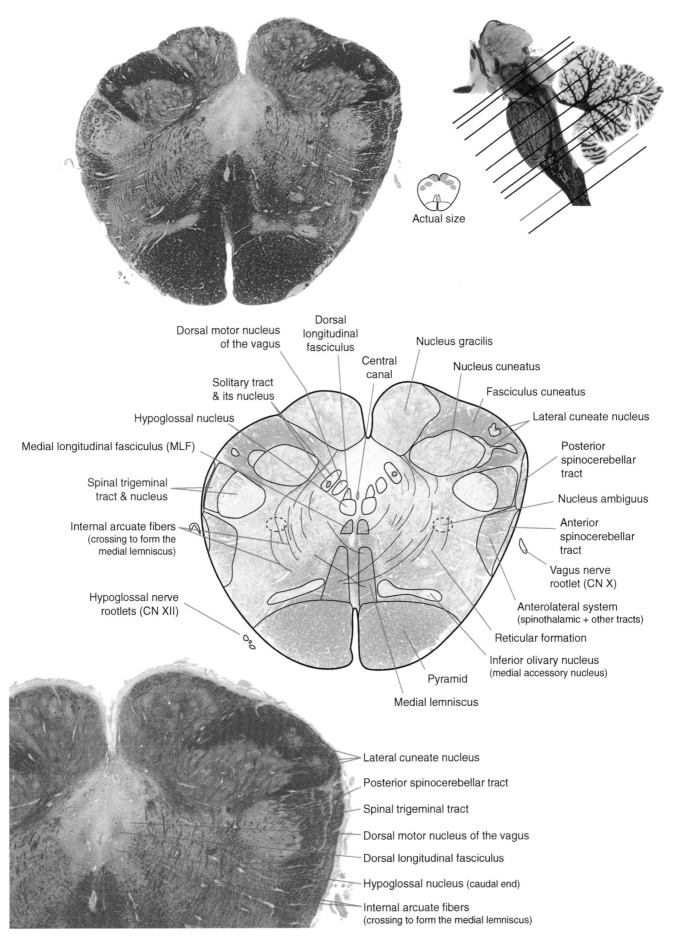

Actual size

Dorsal motor nucleus of the vagus

Dorsal longitudinal fasciculus

Central canal

Nucleus gracilis

Nucleus cuneatus

Fasciculus cuneatus

Solitary tract & its nucleus

Hypoglossal nucleus

Lateral cuneate nucleus

Medial longitudinal fasciculus (MLF)

Posterior spinocerebellar tract

Spinal trigeminal tract & nucleus

Nucleus ambiguus

Internal arcuate fibers (crossing to form the medial lemniscus)

Anterior spinocerebellar tract

Vagus nerve rootlet (CN X)

Hypoglossal nerve rootlets (CN XII)

Anterolateral system (spinothalamic + other tracts)

Reticular formation

Inferior olivary nucleus (medial accessory nucleus)

Pyramid

Medial lemniscus

Lateral cuneate nucleus

Posterior spinocerebellar tract

Spinal trigeminal tract

Dorsal motor nucleus of the vagus

Dorsal longitudinal fasciculus

Hypoglossal nucleus (caudal end)

Internal arcuate fibers (crossing to form the medial lemniscus)

Figure 3.9 Caudal medulla.

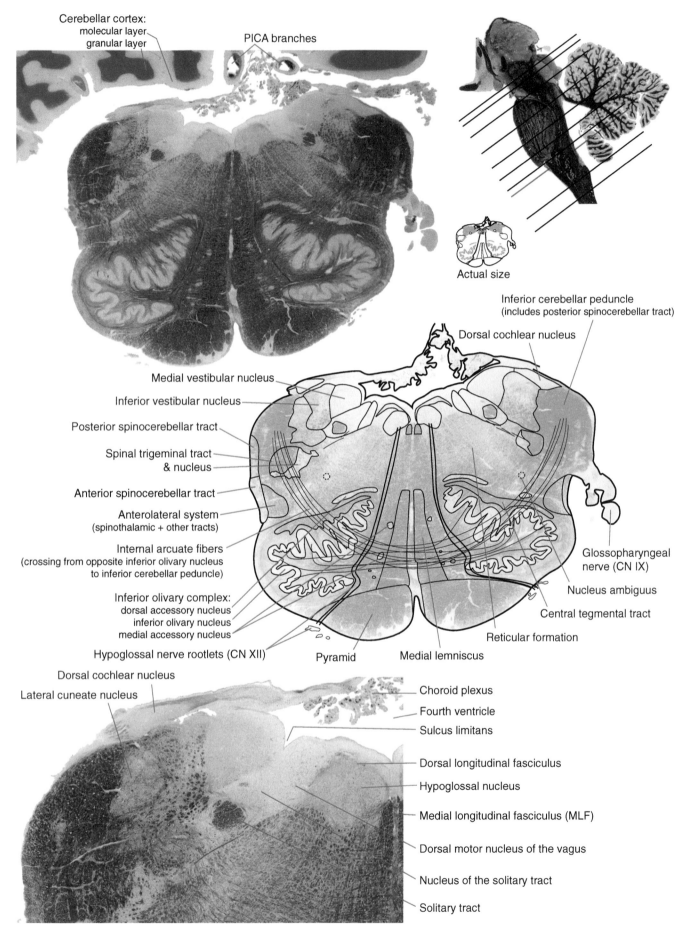

Cerebellar cortex:
molecular layer
granular layer

PICA branches

Actual size

Inferior cerebellar peduncle
(includes posterior spinocerebellar tract)

Dorsal cochlear nucleus

Medial vestibular nucleus

Inferior vestibular nucleus

Posterior spinocerebellar tract

Spinal trigeminal tract
& nucleus

Anterior spinocerebellar tract

Anterolateral system
(spinothalamic + other tracts)

Internal arcuate fibers
(crossing from opposite inferior olivary nucleus
to inferior cerebellar peduncle)

Inferior olivary complex:
dorsal accessory nucleus
inferior olivary nucleus
medial accessory nucleus

Hypoglossal nerve rootlets (CN XII)

Glossopharyngeal
nerve (CN IX)

Nucleus ambiguus

Central tegmental tract

Reticular formation

Pyramid

Medial lemniscus

Dorsal cochlear nucleus

Lateral cuneate nucleus

Choroid plexus

Fourth ventricle

Sulcus limitans

Dorsal longitudinal fasciculus

Hypoglossal nucleus

Medial longitudinal fasciculus (MLF)

Dorsal motor nucleus of the vagus

Nucleus of the solitary tract

Solitary tract

Figure 3.10 Rostral medulla. *PICA*, Posterior inferior cerebellar artery.

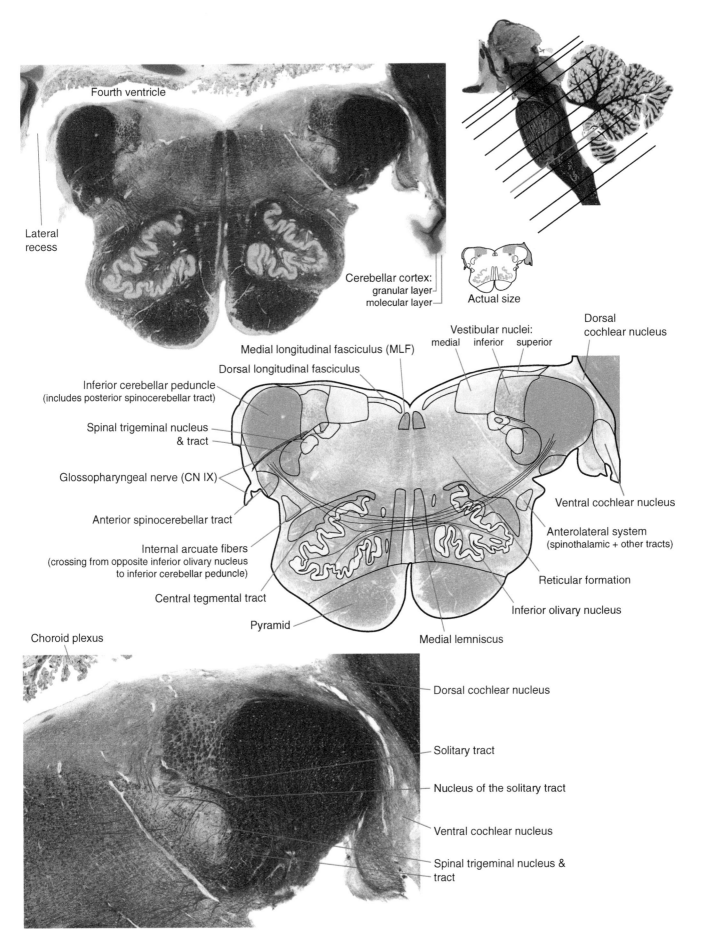

Fourth ventricle

Lateral recess

Cerebellar cortex:
granular layer
molecular layer

Actual size

Dorsal cochlear nucleus

Vestibular nuclei:
medial   inferior   superior

Medial longitudinal fasciculus (MLF)

Dorsal longitudinal fasciculus

Inferior cerebellar peduncle
(includes posterior spinocerebellar tract)

Spinal trigeminal nucleus
& tract

Glossopharyngeal nerve (CN IX)

Anterior spinocerebellar tract

Internal arcuate fibers
(crossing from opposite inferior olivary nucleus
to inferior cerebellar peduncle)

Central tegmental tract

Pyramid

Medial lemniscus

Ventral cochlear nucleus

Anterolateral system
(spinothalamic + other tracts)

Reticular formation

Inferior olivary nucleus

Choroid plexus

Dorsal cochlear nucleus

Solitary tract

Nucleus of the solitary tract

Ventral cochlear nucleus

Spinal trigeminal nucleus &
tract

Figure 3.11 Pontomedullary junction.

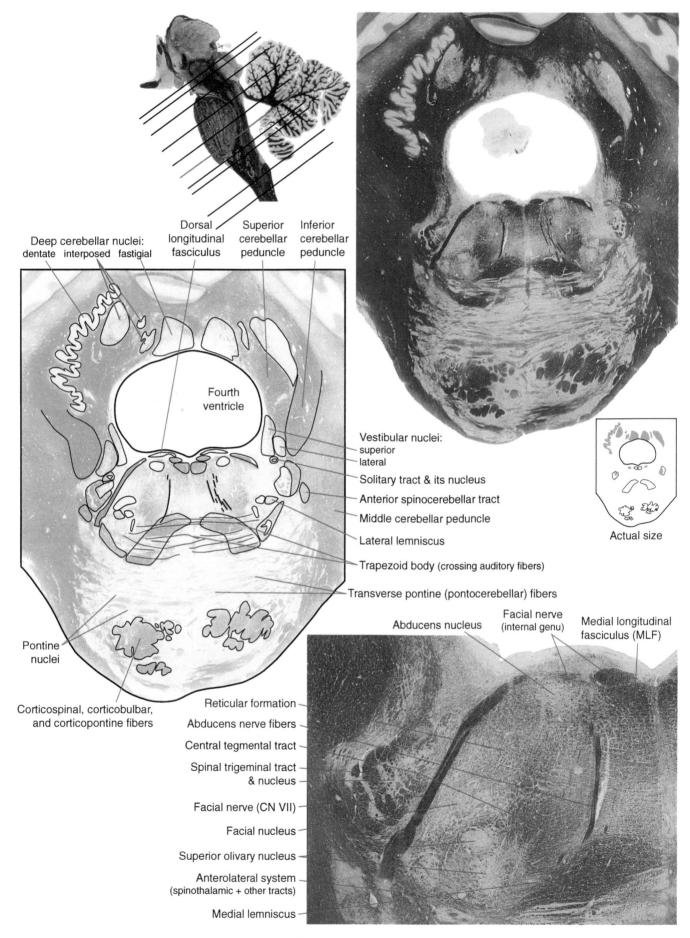

Deep cerebellar nuclei:
dentate   interposed   fastigial

Dorsal longitudinal fasciculus

Superior cerebellar peduncle

Inferior cerebellar peduncle

Fourth ventricle

Vestibular nuclei:
superior
lateral

Solitary tract & its nucleus

Anterior spinocerebellar tract

Middle cerebellar peduncle

Lateral lemniscus

Trapezoid body (crossing auditory fibers)

Transverse pontine (pontocerebellar) fibers

Actual size

Pontine nuclei

Corticospinal, corticobulbar, and corticopontine fibers

Abducens nucleus

Facial nerve (internal genu)

Medial longitudinal fasciculus (MLF)

Reticular formation

Abducens nerve fibers

Central tegmental tract

Spinal trigeminal tract & nucleus

Facial nerve (CN VII)

Facial nucleus

Superior olivary nucleus

Anterolateral system (spinothalamic + other tracts)

Medial lemniscus

Figure 3.12 Caudal pons.

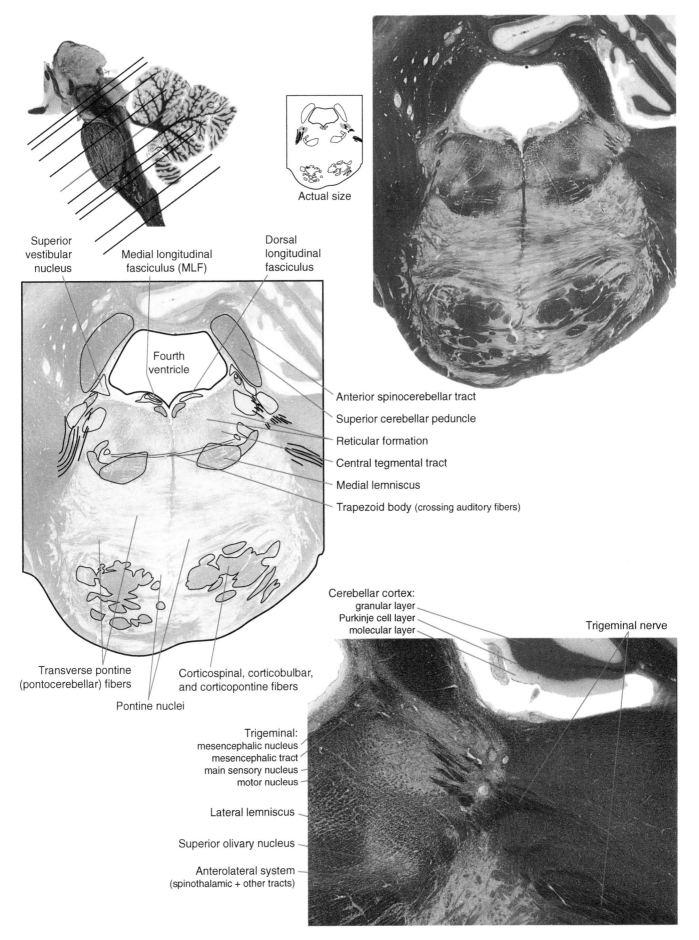

Actual size

Superior vestibular nucleus

Medial longitudinal fasciculus (MLF)

Dorsal longitudinal fasciculus

Fourth ventricle

Anterior spinocerebellar tract

Superior cerebellar peduncle

Reticular formation

Central tegmental tract

Medial lemniscus

Trapezoid body (crossing auditory fibers)

Transverse pontine (pontocerebellar) fibers

Corticospinal, corticobulbar, and corticopontine fibers

Pontine nuclei

Cerebellar cortex:
granular layer
Purkinje cell layer
molecular layer

Trigeminal nerve

Trigeminal:
mesencephalic nucleus
mesencephalic tract
main sensory nucleus
motor nucleus

Lateral lemniscus

Superior olivary nucleus

Anterolateral system (spinothalamic + other tracts)

Figure 3.13 Midpons.

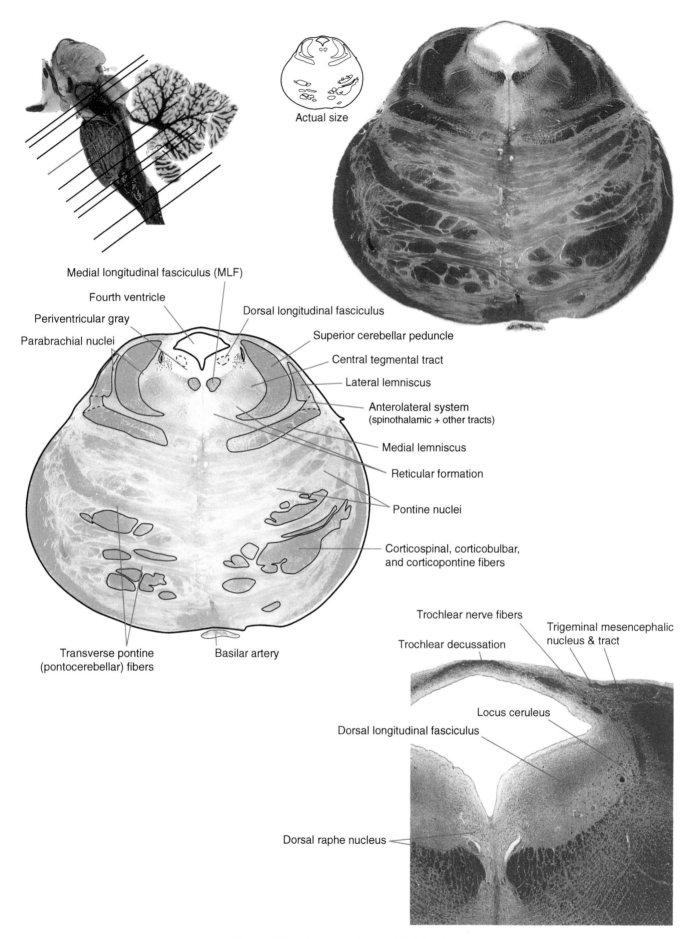

Actual size

Medial longitudinal fasciculus (MLF)

Fourth ventricle

Periventricular gray

Parabrachial nuclei

Dorsal longitudinal fasciculus

Superior cerebellar peduncle

Central tegmental tract

Lateral lemniscus

Anterolateral system
(spinothalamic + other tracts)

Medial lemniscus

Reticular formation

Pontine nuclei

Corticospinal, corticobulbar,
and corticopontine fibers

Transverse pontine
(pontocerebellar) fibers

Basilar artery

Trochlear nerve fibers

Trochlear decussation

Trigeminal mesencephalic
nucleus & tract

Locus ceruleus

Dorsal longitudinal fasciculus

Dorsal raphe nucleus

Figure 3.14 Rostral pons, near the pons-midbrain junction.

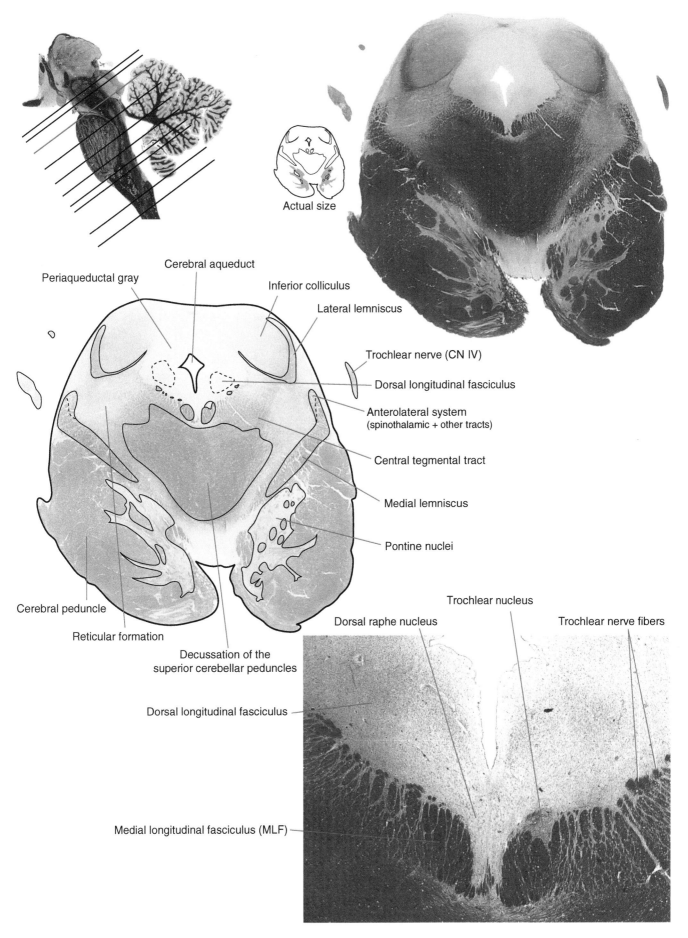

Actual size

Periaqueductal gray

Cerebral aqueduct

Inferior colliculus

Lateral lemniscus

Trochlear nerve (CN IV)

Dorsal longitudinal fasciculus

Anterolateral system
(spinothalamic + other tracts)

Central tegmental tract

Medial lemniscus

Pontine nuclei

Cerebral peduncle

Reticular formation

Decussation of the
superior cerebellar peduncles

Trochlear nucleus

Dorsal raphe nucleus

Trochlear nerve fibers

Dorsal longitudinal fasciculus

Medial longitudinal fasciculus (MLF)

Figure 3.15 Caudal midbrain.

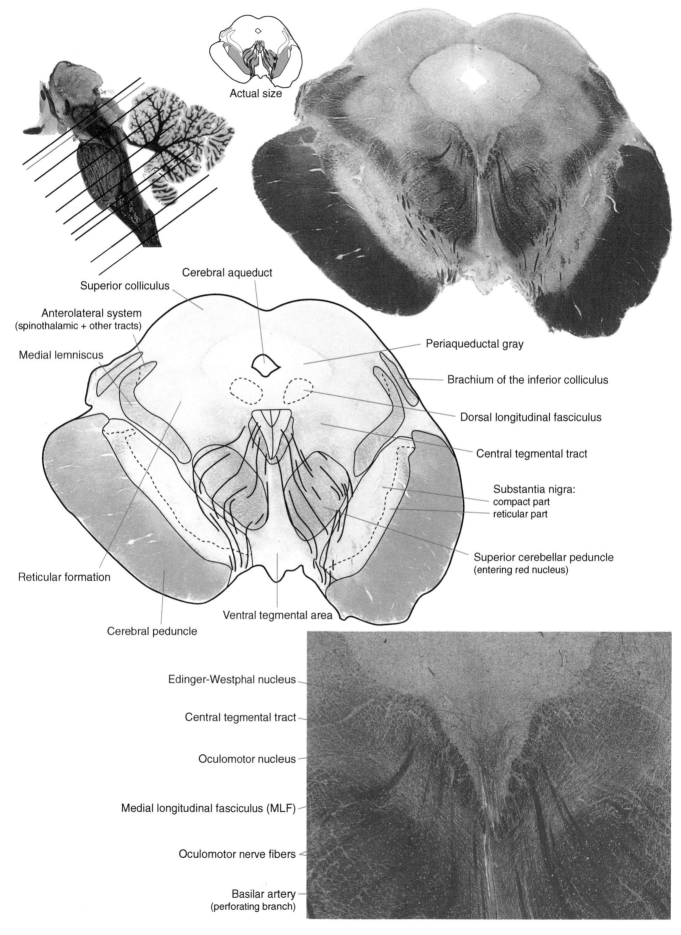

Actual size

Cerebral aqueduct

Superior colliculus

Anterolateral system
(spinothalamic + other tracts)

Medial lemniscus

Periaqueductal gray

Brachium of the inferior colliculus

Dorsal longitudinal fasciculus

Central tegmental tract

Substantia nigra:
compact part
reticular part

Superior cerebellar peduncle
(entering red nucleus)

Reticular formation

Ventral tegmental area

Cerebral peduncle

Edinger-Westphal nucleus

Central tegmental tract

Oculomotor nucleus

Medial longitudinal fasciculus (MLF)

Oculomotor nerve fibers

Basilar artery
(perforating branch)

Figure 3.16 Rostral midbrain.

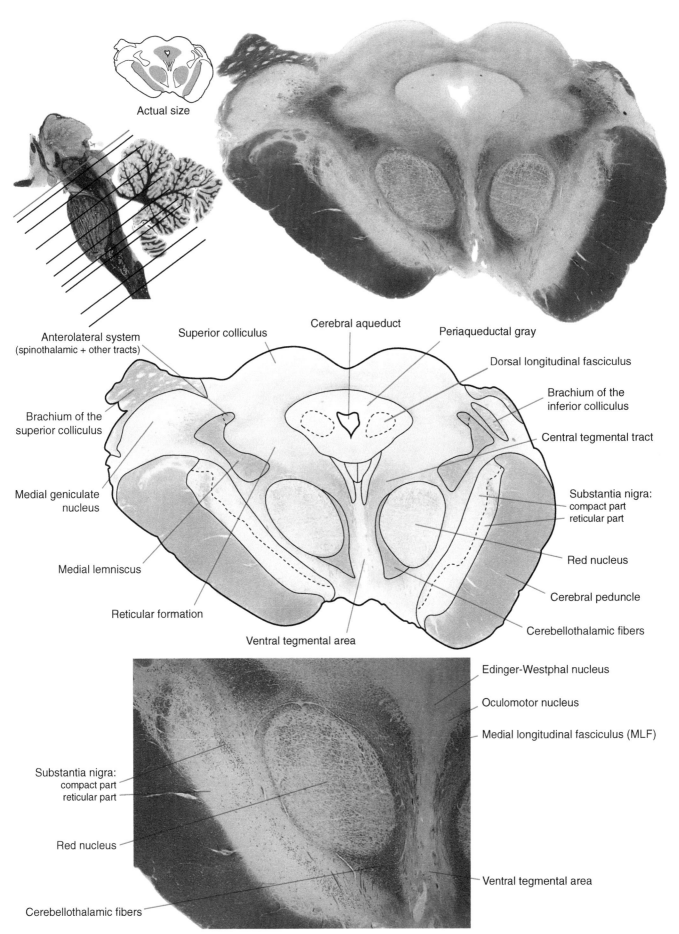

Actual size

Anterolateral system
(spinothalamic + other tracts)

Superior colliculus

Cerebral aqueduct

Periaqueductal gray

Dorsal longitudinal fasciculus

Brachium of the
inferior colliculus

Brachium of the
superior colliculus

Central tegmental tract

Medial geniculate
nucleus

Substantia nigra:
compact part
reticular part

Medial lemniscus

Red nucleus

Cerebral peduncle

Reticular formation

Cerebellothalamic fibers

Ventral tegmental area

Edinger-Westphal nucleus

Oculomotor nucleus

Medial longitudinal fasciculus (MLF)

Substantia nigra:
compact part
reticular part

Red nucleus

Ventral tegmental area

Cerebellothalamic fibers

Figure 3.17 Rostral midbrain, near the midbrain-diencephalon junction.

4

Building a Brain: Three-Dimensional Reconstructions

The interior of the **forebrain** is occupied by a series of structures that fit neatly together in three-dimensional space. As a consequence of the embryological development of the brain, some cerebral structures (e.g., **lateral ventricle**, **caudate nucleus**) curve around in a great C-shaped arc (Fig. 4.1), whereas others are more centrally located. One of the greatest impediments to understanding the interrelationships of cerebral structures in three dimensions is the typical presentation of the nervous system in a series of two-dimensional sections cut in various planes (as it is presented in much of this book).

As a partial solution to this dilemma, this chapter presents an overview of the arrangement of cerebral structures in the form of a series of computer-generated reconstructions kindly provided by Dr. John W. Sundsten and his colleagues (Department of Biological Structure, University of Washington School of Medicine). The images were made by cutting serial sections of a single human brain, digitizing outlines of structures of interest, and using these outlines to reconstruct (by computer) individual structures or groups of structures. Beginning with the reconstruction of the brainstem, cerebellum, and diencephalon shown in Fig. 4.2, major structures of the cerebral hemispheres are added sequentially in Fig. 4.3. Similar three-dimensional reconstructions are used in Chapters 5 through 7 to indicate the planes of sections through the forebrain.

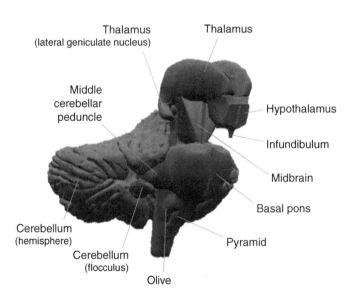

Figure 4.2 Three-dimensional reconstruction of the brainstem, cerebellum, and diencephalon. In an intact brain, the hypothalamus is continuous anteriorly with the preoptic and septal areas; in this reconstruction, the hypothalamus is shown ending abruptly at its approximate border with these structures. The midbrain is configured with a flattened anterior surface because the cerebral peduncle is not yet present; it will be added in Fig. 4.3E.

Figure 4.1 Three examples of C-shaped cerebral structures: **(A)** the caudate nucleus, **(B)** hippocampus/fornix system, **(C)** and lateral ventricle.

Figure 4.3 (A–H) Building a brain.

(A) The reconstruction of the brainstem, cerebellum, and diencephalon shown in Fig. 4.2. *CF*, Cerebellar flocculus (a specialized part of each cerebellar hemisphere); *CH*, cerebellar hemisphere; *Hy*, hypothalamus; *Mid*, midbrain.

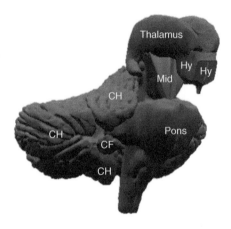

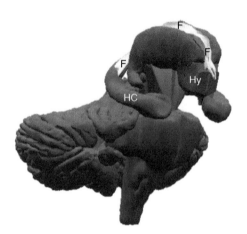

(B) The hippocampus *(HC)* is a special cortical area folded into the medial part of the limbic lobe, adjacent to the inferior horn of the lateral ventricle. The fornix *(F)* is a major output pathway from the hippocampus. It curves around in a C-shaped course (the Latin word *fornix* means "arch") and terminates primarily in the hypothalamus *(Hy)* and in the septal area anterior to it.

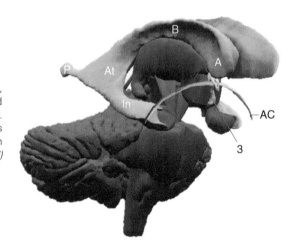

(C) The lateral ventricle is another C-shaped structure, curving from an anterior horn *(A)* in the frontal lobe, through a body *(B)*, and into an inferior horn *(In)* in the temporal lobe. A posterior horn *(P)* extends backward into the occipital lobe. The body, posterior horn, and inferior horn meet in the atrium *(At)* of the lateral ventricle. The body and anterior horn have a concave lateral wall; in reality, parts of the caudate nucleus occupy this depression (see Fig. 4.3D). The third ventricle *(3)* extends anteriorly beyond the truncated hypothalamus; in an intact brain, this anterior extension would be bordered by the preoptic area. The anterior commissure *(AC)* contains fibers interconnecting the temporal lobes.

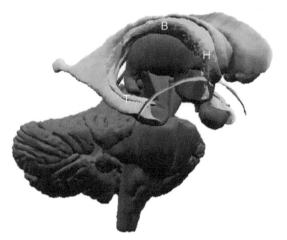

(D) The caudate nucleus, yet another C-shaped structure, curves through the hemisphere adjacent to the lateral ventricle. Its enlarged head *(H)* and body *(B)* account for the indented lateral wall of the anterior horn and body of the ventricle (see Fig. 4.3C). The attenuated tail *(T)* of the caudate nucleus forms part of the wall of the inferior horn of the ventricle.

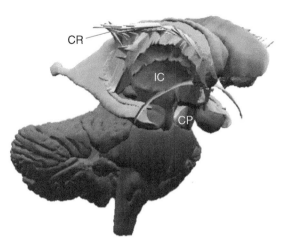

Figure 4.3 (Continued) Building a brain.

(E) The internal capsule *(IC)* is a thick band of fibers that covers the lateral aspect of the head of the caudate nucleus and the thalamus. It contains the vast majority of the fibers interconnecting the cerebral cortex and subcortical sites. Above the internal capsule, these fibers fan out within the cerebral hemisphere as the corona radiata *(CR)*. Many of the cortical efferent fibers in the internal capsule funnel down into the cerebral peduncle *(CP)*. The internal capsule also has a concave lateral surface; in this case the lenticular nucleus occupies the depression (see Fig. 4.3F).

(F) The lenticular nucleus, itself a combination of the putamen and the globus pallidus, occupies the depression in the internal capsule (see Fig. 4.3E). The putamen *(P*, the more lateral of the two) and the caudate nucleus *(C)* are actually continuous masses of gray matter. The area of continuity is called the nucleus accumbens *(A)*. The amygdala *(Am)* is a collection of nuclei underlying the medial surface of the limbic lobe at the anterior end of the hippocampus.

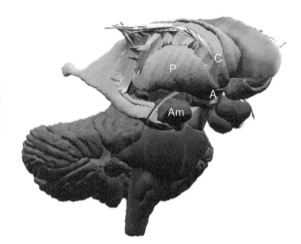

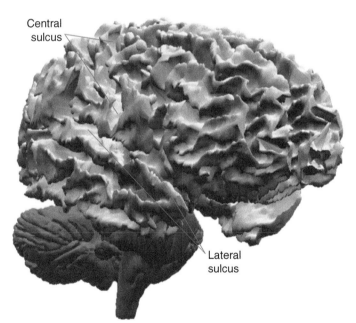

(G) The structures described thus far are enveloped in white matter, containing the billions of axons interconnecting different cortical areas or interconnecting the cortex and subcortical structures. This reconstruction shows the junction between the cerebral cortex and its underlying white matter.

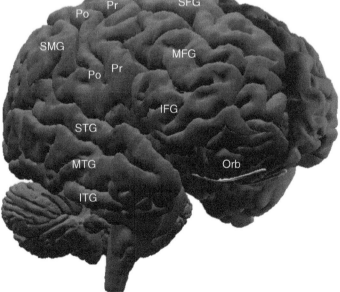

(H) Finally, a thin (1.5 to 4.5 mm) layer of cerebral cortex covers each hemisphere. *IFG*, Inferior frontal gyrus; *ITG*, inferior temporal gyrus; *MFG*, middle frontal gyrus; *MTG*, middle temporal gyrus; *Orb*, orbital gyri; *Po*, postcentral gyrus; *Pr*, precentral gyrus; *SFG*, superior frontal gyrus; *SMG*, supramarginal gyrus; *STG*, superior temporal gyrus.

Coronal Sections

This is the first of three chapters showing sections of entire human brains, in this case illustrating approximately coronal planes. Forebrain structures are emphasized, but parts of the brainstem and cerebellum are indicated as well. The organization of various functional systems in the forebrain (e.g., thalamus, hippocampus) and other parts of the central nervous system is presented in Chapter 8.

Drawings showing typical areas of arterial supply in each section are also provided in this and the next two chapters. We simplified these in two major ways. First, arterial territories are shown as sharply demarcated from each other, when in reality there is significant interdigitation and overlap. Second, perforating arteries arise from all the vessels of the circle of Willis, but we lumped together those from the posterior communicating and posterior cerebral arteries, and those from the anterior communicating and anterior cerebral arteries.

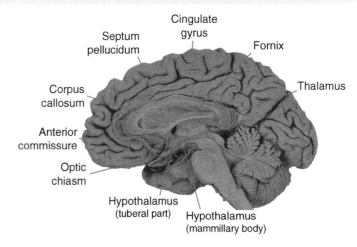

Figure 5.1 The hemisected brain from Fig. 1.7, used in much of this chapter to indicate planes of section.

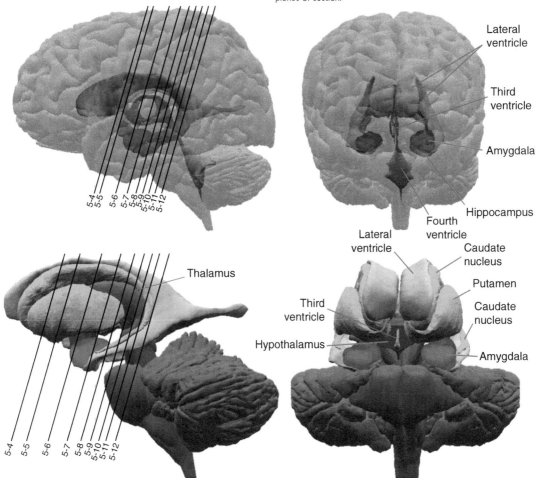

Figure 5.2 The planes of section shown in this chapter, indicated on three-dimensional reconstructions. (Courtesy Dr. John W. Sundsten, Department of Biological Structure, University of Washington School of Medicine.)

Figure 5.3 (A–X) Twenty-four coronal sections of a brain, arranged in an anterior-to-posterior sequence from the anterior edge of the corpus callosum to the beginning of the occipital lobe.

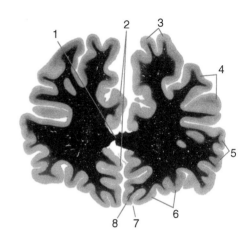

(A) Anterior end of the genu of the corpus callosum *(1)*. Convolutions that compose most of the frontal lobe are the superior *(3)*, middle *(4)*, and inferior *(5)* frontal gyri, orbital gyri *(6)*, and gyrus rectus *(8)*. The cingulate gyrus *(2)* is cut twice, once above and once below the genu of the corpus callosum. The olfactory sulcus *(7)*, which will be occupied by the olfactory tract at a slightly more posterior level, lies just lateral to gyrus rectus.

(B) The anterior horn of the lateral ventricle *(3)* appears. A septum pellucidum *(2)* forms the medial wall of each lateral ventricle. The corpus callosum is now cut in two places, once through its body *(1)* above the septum pellucidum and once *(4)* as the genu begins to taper into the rostrum below the septum pellucidum.

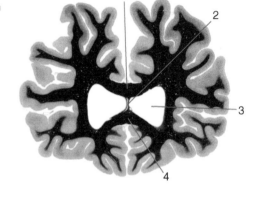

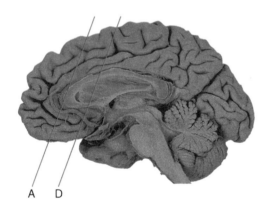

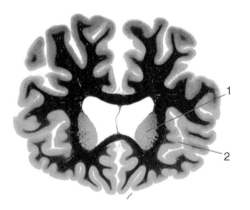

(C) The head of the caudate nucleus *(1)* appears in the lateral wall of the lateral ventricle. The anterior region of the insula *(2)* is also visible at this level, overlying the caudate nucleus.

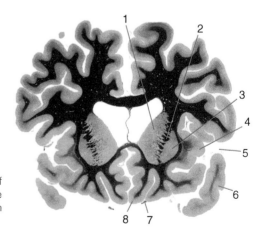

(D) The rostral end of the putamen *(3)* is separated from the head of the caudate nucleus *(1)* by the anterior limb of the internal capsule *(2)*. The putamen, the larger of the two parts of the lenticular nucleus, is overlain for its entire extent by the insula *(4)*. The olfactory tract *(7)* lies in the olfactory sulcus, just lateral to gyrus rectus *(8)*. The section passes through the tip of the temporal lobe *(6)*, separated from the frontal lobe by the lateral sulcus *(5)*.

Figure 5.3 (Continued) Coronal sections.

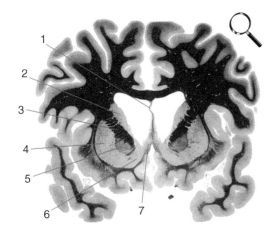

(E) The globus pallidus *(5)* makes its appearance medial to the putamen *(4)*; the two together compose the lenticular nucleus. Nucleus accumbens *(6)*, the region of continuity between the putamen and the head of the caudate nucleus *(2)*, is also apparent. The septum pellucidum *(1)* is continuous with the septal nuclei *(7)*. (The proximity of nucleus accumbens to the septal nuclei was reflected in its earlier but now outmoded name, *nucleus accumbens septi*—"the nucleus leaning against the septum.") The anterior limb of the internal capsule *(3)* still occupies the cleft between the lenticular nucleus and the head of the caudate nucleus. Shown enlarged in Fig. 5.4.

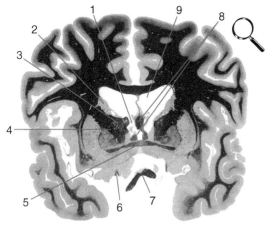

(F) The level of the interventricular foramen *(1)* and anterior commissure *(5)* is a transition point for many structures—for example, from the head to the body of the caudate nucleus *(2)* and from the anterior horn to the body of the lateral ventricle *(9)*. This section shaves off the anterior end of the thalamus *(3)*, passes through the genu of the internal capsule *(4)*, and cuts the fornix twice *(8)* as it curves ventrally toward the hypothalamus. The olfactory tract *(6)* joins the base of the forebrain, and the optic chiasm *(7)* appears. Shown enlarged in Fig. 5.5.

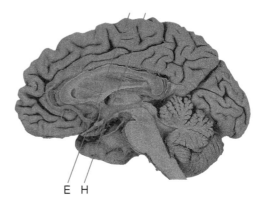

(G) Anterior diencephalon. Characteristic diencephalic features include the third ventricle *(12)*, hypothalamus *(8)* with its attached infundibulum *(7)*, and thalamic nuclei—anterior *(1)* and ventral anterior *(2)*. The external *(3)* and internal *(4)* segments of the globus pallidus are now apparent, as is the anterior end of the amygdala *(9)*. Fibers that will cross in the anterior commissure *(5)* accumulate beneath the lenticular nucleus. The fornix is cut twice, through the body *(13)* and column *(10)*. The optic tract *(6)* and posterior limb of the internal capsule *(11)* are also present.

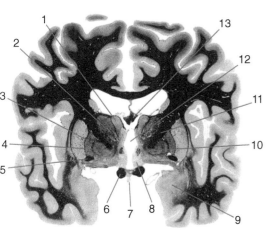

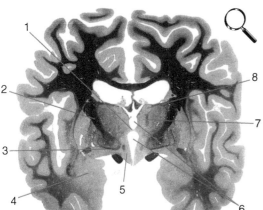

(H) The mammillothalamic tract *(7)* enters the anterior nucleus *(8)* of the thalamus. The two thalami fuse in the interthalamic adhesion *(1)* or massa intermedia, which bridges the third ventricle *(6)*. The ansa lenticularis *(3*, literally "the handle of the lenticular nucleus"*)* emerges from the inferior surface of the globus pallidus and hooks around the posterior limb of the internal capsule *(2)*. The amygdala *(4)* is larger, and the middle of the three zones of the hypothalamus (the tuberal zone, *5*) is present. Shown enlarged in Fig. 5.6.

Illustration continued on following page

Figure 5.3 (Continued) Coronal sections.

(I) Additional efferents from the globus pallidus penetrate the posterior limb of the internal capsule *(2)* as the lenticular fasciculus and collect on the other side *(1)* before entering the thalamus. The column of the fornix *(4)* continues through the hypothalamus, where it will soon end in the mammillary body. The surface of the temporal lobe includes the superior *(3)*, middle *(5)*, and inferior *(6)* temporal gyri and the occipitotemporal gyrus *(7)*, adjacent to the parahippocampal *(8)* gyrus. The amygdala *(9)* has reached nearly maximal size.

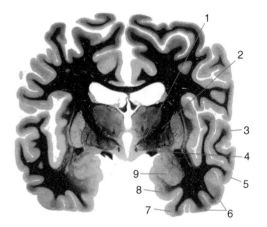

(J) Midthalamus. The dorsomedial *(2)* and ventrolateral *(3)* nuclei are prominent at this level. The optic tract *(6)* proceeds posteriorly toward its thalamic termination in the lateral geniculate nucleus. The column of the fornix is ending in the mammillary body *(10)*, which in turn gives rise to the mammillothalamic tract *(9)*. The lateral ventricle is another in a series of forebrain structures to be cut twice, here through the body *(1)* and through the inferior horn *(8)*, which has appeared adjacent to the amygdala *(7)*. Both the putamen *(4)* and the globus pallidus *(5)* begin to get smaller.

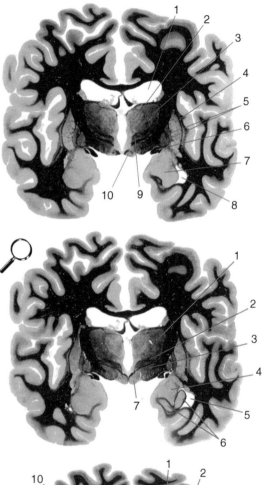

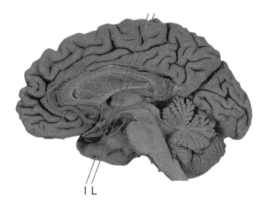

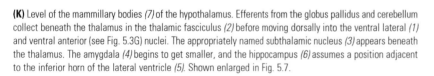

I L

(K) Level of the mammillary bodies *(7)* of the hypothalamus. Efferents from the globus pallidus and cerebellum collect beneath the thalamus in the thalamic fasciculus *(2)* before moving dorsally into the ventral lateral *(1)* and ventral anterior (see Fig. 5.3G) nuclei. The appropriately named subthalamic nucleus *(3)* appears beneath the thalamus. The amygdala *(4)* begins to get smaller, and the hippocampus *(6)* assumes a position adjacent to the inferior horn of the lateral ventricle *(5)*. Shown enlarged in Fig. 5.7.

(L) Brainstem structures begin to appear. The rostral end of the substantia nigra *(8)* is adjacent to the subthalamic nucleus *(9)*. Many fibers in the posterior limb of the internal capsule *(3)* continue into the cerebral peduncle *(7)*. Several structures are now cut twice, such as the body *(1)* and inferior horn *(6)* of the lateral ventricle and the body *(2)* and tail *(4)* of the caudate nucleus. The hippocampus *(5)* has almost completely replaced the amygdala on the right side of the section; the fornix *(10)*, the most prominent output bundle of the hippocampus, proceeds anteriorly in its characteristic trajectory medial to the lateral ventricle.

Figure 5.3 (Continued)

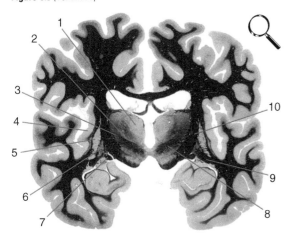

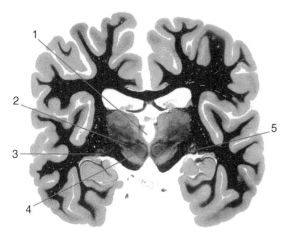

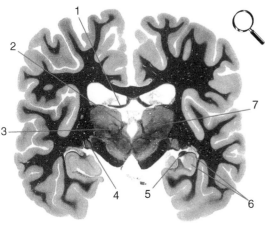

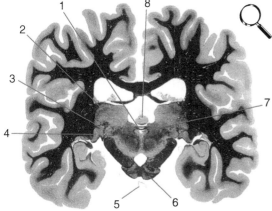

Coronal sections. **(M)** The dorsomedial *(1)*, ventral posteromedial *(2)*, and ventral posterolateral *(3)* nuclei now account for most of the thalamus. The putamen *(5)* and globus pallidus *(6)* continue to get smaller, as does the overlying insula *(4)*. Cerebellar efferents *(8)* proceed rostrally toward the ventral lateral nucleus of the thalamus (see Fig. 5.3K), and the optic tract *(7)* continues posteriorly toward the lateral geniculate nucleus. The posterior limb *(10)* and sublenticular part *(9)* of the internal capsule partially surround the lenticular nucleus. Shown enlarged in Fig. 5.8.

(N) Posterior to the lenticular nucleus, the third ventricle *(1)* is smaller as the plane of section gets closer to the cerebral aqueduct. Cerebellar efferents *(2)* that have passed through or around the red nucleus *(4)* collect beneath the thalamus. The optic tract *(3)* begins to terminate in the lateral geniculate nucleus *(5)* on the right side of the section.

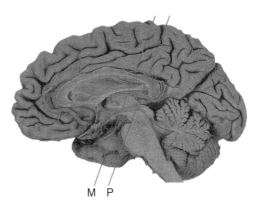

M   P

(O) Near the diencephalon-midbrain junction, the lateral geniculate nucleus *(4)* is present on both sides, and the largest of the thalamic intralaminar nuclei, the centromedian nucleus *(3)*, is apparent. The habenula *(2)* gives rise to the habenulointerpeduncular tract *(7)*. Fornix fibers are cut twice, this time where they are suspended from the corpus callosum as the posterior part of the body *(1)* and where they are still attached to the hippocampus *(6)* as the fimbria *(5)*. Shown enlarged in Fig. 5.9.

(P) Posterior commissure *(1)*, at the diencephalon-midbrain junction. The third ventricle has been replaced by the cerebral aqueduct *(7)*, and a bit of the basal pons *(6)* appears, accompanied by the basilar artery *(5)*. The only parts of the thalamus left are the pulvinar *(2)* and the medial *(3)* and lateral *(4)* geniculate nuclei. The pineal gland *(8)* is in the midline just above the posterior commissure. Shown enlarged in Fig. 5.10.

Illustration continued on following page

Figure 5.3 (Continued) Coronal sections.

(Q) Posterior thalamus. Only the pulvinar *(6)* and the medial geniculate nucleus *(9)* remain. The plane of section approaches the posterior edge of C-shaped telencephalic structures, so the two parts of twice-cut structures draw closer together—the crus of the fornix *(13)* and fimbria of the hippocampus *(12)*, the body *(5)* and tail *(7)* of the caudate nucleus, and the body *(4)* and inferior horn *(8)* of the lateral ventricle. Several brainstem structures are apparent, including the aqueduct *(2)* surrounded by periaqueductal gray *(3)*, the medial lemniscus *(10)*, and the now-crossed superior cerebellar peduncle *(11)*. The pineal gland *(1)* is still present above the most rostral part of the midbrain (the pretectal area). Shown enlarged in Fig. 5.11.

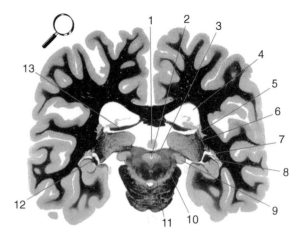

(R) Splenium of the corpus callosum *(1)*. The section passes tangentially through the posterior edge of the caudate nucleus *(8)*, through fibers of the fornix as they pass from the fimbria *(5)* into the crus *(3)*, and through the lateral ventricle as the body *(4)* joins the inferior horn *(6)*. The superior colliculus *(9)* and the decussation of the superior cerebellar peduncles *(7)* can be seen in the brainstem. A little piece of the pulvinar *(2)* is all that remains of the thalamus. Shown enlarged in Fig. 5.12.

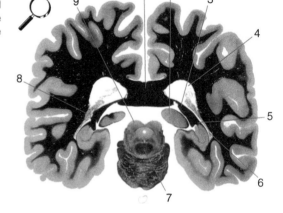

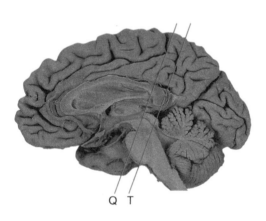

Q T

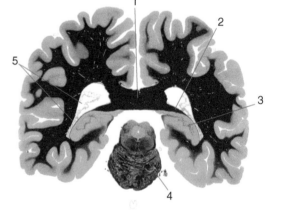

(S) Now the section passes tangentially through the posterior end of the hippocampus *(3)* as it curves up underneath the splenium of the corpus callosum *(1)* and through the crus *(2)* of the fornix, the atrium *(5)* of the lateral ventricle, and the decussation of the superior cerebellar peduncles *(4)*.

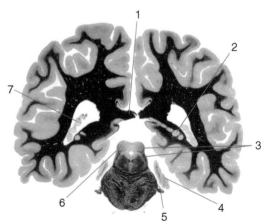

(T) Posterior edge of the splenium of the corpus callosum *(1)*. The section passes through an enlarged mass of choroid plexus (the glomus, *7)* that projects back into the posterior horn of the lateral ventricle, and through remnants of the hippocampus *(2)*. The cerebellar hemispheres *(4)* begin to appear, the lateral lemniscus *(3)* ends in the inferior colliculus *(6)*, and the trigeminal nerve *(5)* is attached to the pons.

Figure 5.3 (Continued) Coronal sections.

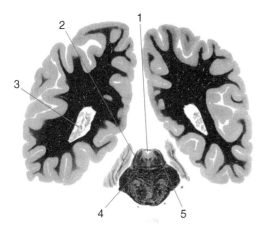

(U) Choroid plexus *(3)* still protrudes into the posterior horn of the lateral ventricle. The aqueduct *(1)* begins to enlarge into the rostral part of the fourth ventricle. The lateral *(2)* and medial *(4)* lemnisci and the superior cerebellar peduncle *(5)* are apparent in the pons.

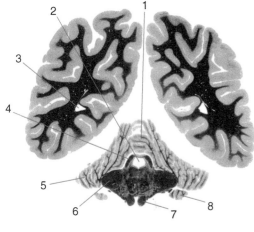

(V) Last bit of the posterior horn of the lateral ventricle *(3)*. The cerebellar vermis *(1)*, hemispheres *(5)*, and flocculus *(8*, actually part of each hemisphere) can now be distinguished. The aqueduct has opened into the fourth ventricle *(2)*, and the superior *(4)* and middle *(6)* cerebellar peduncles and the pyramid *(7)* are present.

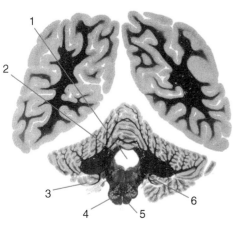

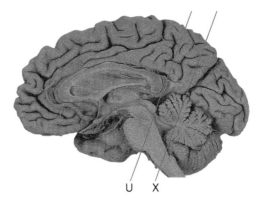

(W) Pons and medulla. The fourth ventricle *(1)* and pyramid *(5)* are large, and the inferior olivary nucleus *(4)* is now present. The superior cerebellar peduncle *(2)* leaves the cerebellum, and the inferior cerebellar peduncle *(6)* enters. The cerebellar flocculus *(3)* is still located adjacent to the pontomedullary junction.

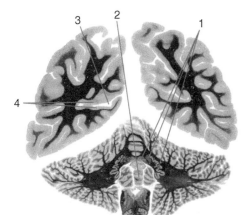

(X) Deep cerebellar nuclei *(1)* (termed dentate, interposed, and fastigial nuclei—laterally to medially) and nodulus *(2)*. The calcarine sulcus *(3)*, with visual cortex in its upper and lower banks *(4)*, deeply indents the medial surface of the occipital lobe.

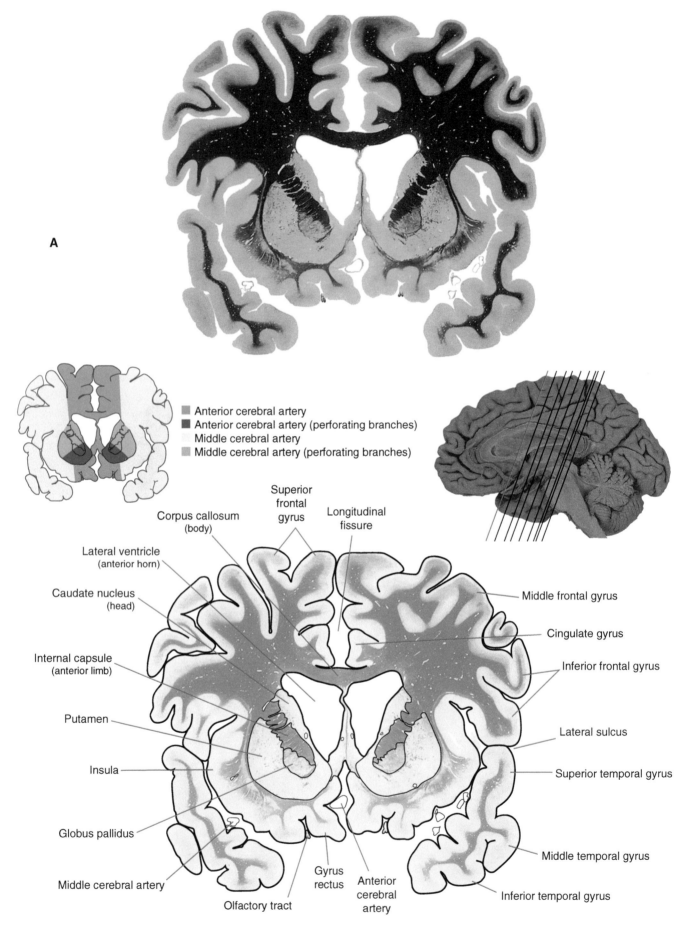

A

Anterior cerebral artery
Anterior cerebral artery (perforating branches)
Middle cerebral artery
Middle cerebral artery (perforating branches)

Corpus callosum
(body)

Superior
frontal
gyrus

Longitudinal
fissure

Lateral ventricle
(anterior horn)

Caudate nucleus
(head)

Middle frontal gyrus

Cingulate gyrus

Internal capsule
(anterior limb)

Inferior frontal gyrus

Putamen

Lateral sulcus

Insula

Superior temporal gyrus

Globus pallidus

Middle cerebral artery

Gyrus
rectus

Anterior
cerebral
artery

Middle temporal gyrus

Inferior temporal gyrus

Olfactory tract

Figure 5.4 (A) A coronal section at the level of the anterior limb of the internal capsule.

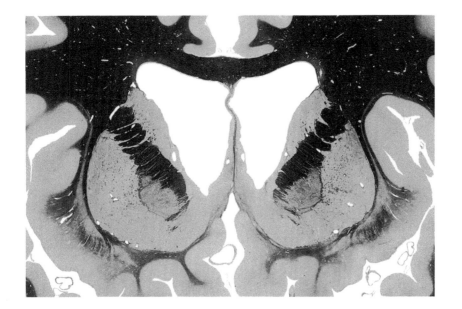

B

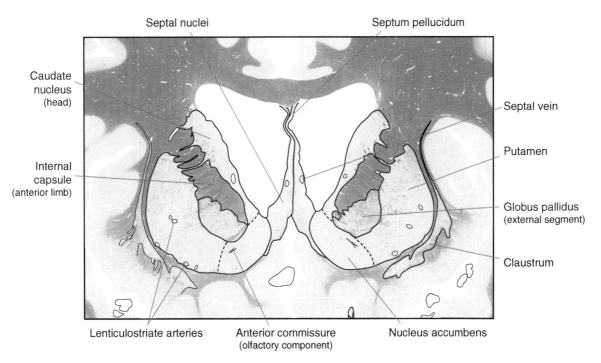

Septal nuclei   Septum pellucidum

Caudate
nucleus
(head)

Internal
capsule
(anterior limb)

Septal vein

Putamen

Globus pallidus
(external segment)

Claustrum

Lenticulostriate arteries   Anterior commissure   Nucleus accumbens
                                (olfactory component)

Figure 5.4 (Continued) **(B)** The central region of Fig. 5.4A, enlarged.

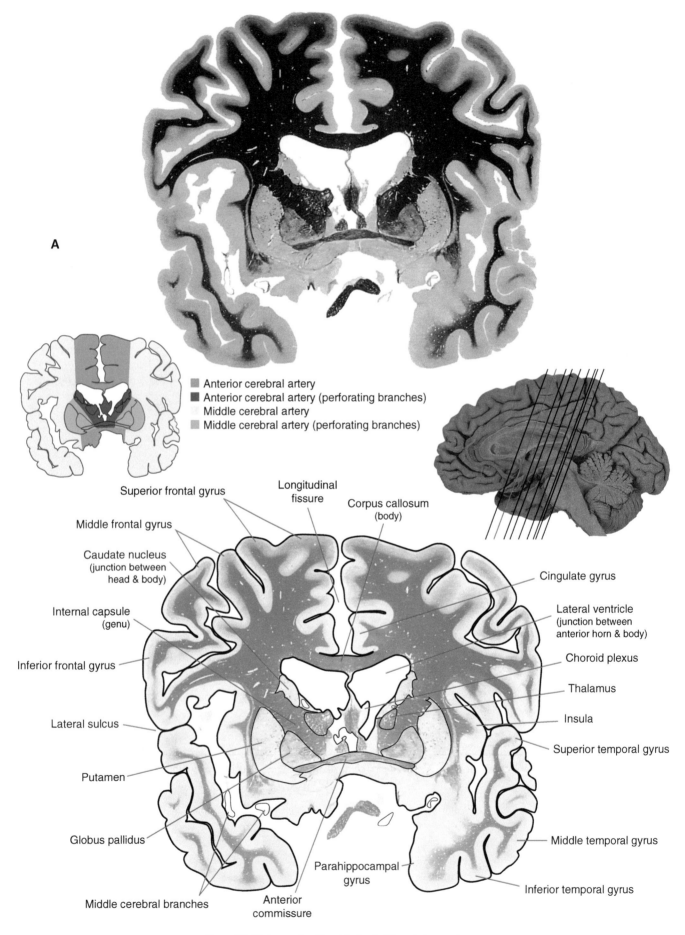

A

Anterior cerebral artery
Anterior cerebral artery (perforating branches)
Middle cerebral artery
Middle cerebral artery (perforating branches)

Superior frontal gyrus

Longitudinal fissure

Corpus callosum (body)

Middle frontal gyrus

Caudate nucleus (junction between head & body)

Cingulate gyrus

Internal capsule (genu)

Lateral ventricle (junction between anterior horn & body)

Inferior frontal gyrus

Choroid plexus

Thalamus

Lateral sulcus

Insula

Superior temporal gyrus

Putamen

Globus pallidus

Middle temporal gyrus

Parahippocampal gyrus

Inferior temporal gyrus

Middle cerebral branches

Anterior commissure

Figure 5.5 (A) A coronal section at the level of the anterior commissure.

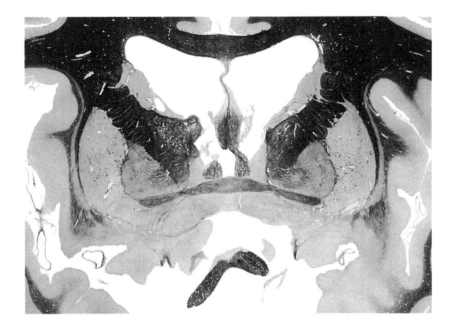

B

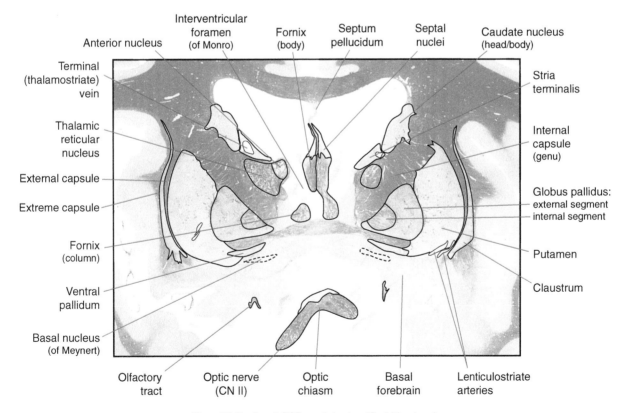

Interventricular
foramen
(of Monro)

Anterior nucleus

Terminal
(thalamostriate)
vein

Thalamic
reticular
nucleus

External capsule

Extreme capsule

Fornix
(column)

Ventral
pallidum

Basal nucleus
(of Meynert)

Fornix
(body)

Septum
pellucidum

Septal
nuclei

Caudate nucleus
(head/body)

Stria
terminalis

Internal
capsule
(genu)

Globus pallidus:
external segment
internal segment

Putamen

Claustrum

Olfactory
tract

Optic nerve
(CN II)

Optic
chiasm

Basal
forebrain

Lenticulostriate
arteries

Figure 5.5 (Continued) **(B)** The central region of Fig. 5.5A, enlarged.

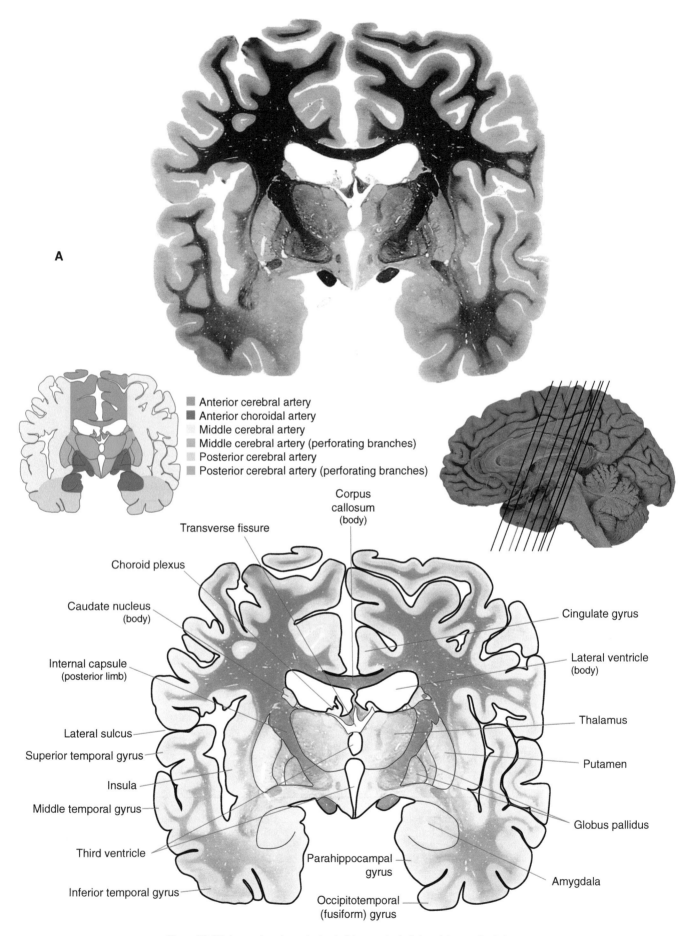

A

Anterior cerebral artery
Anterior choroidal artery
Middle cerebral artery
Middle cerebral artery (perforating branches)
Posterior cerebral artery
Posterior cerebral artery (perforating branches)

Corpus
callosum
(body)

Transverse fissure

Choroid plexus

Caudate nucleus
(body)

Cingulate gyrus

Internal capsule
(posterior limb)

Lateral ventricle
(body)

Lateral sulcus

Thalamus

Superior temporal gyrus

Putamen

Insula

Middle temporal gyrus

Third ventricle

Globus pallidus

Parahippocampal
gyrus

Amygdala

Inferior temporal gyrus

Occipitotemporal
(fusiform) gyrus

Figure 5.6 (A) A coronal section at the level of the ansa lenticularis and the anterior thalamus.

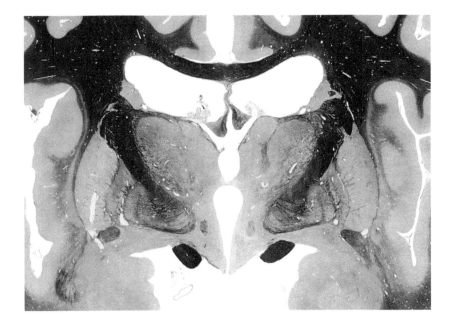

B

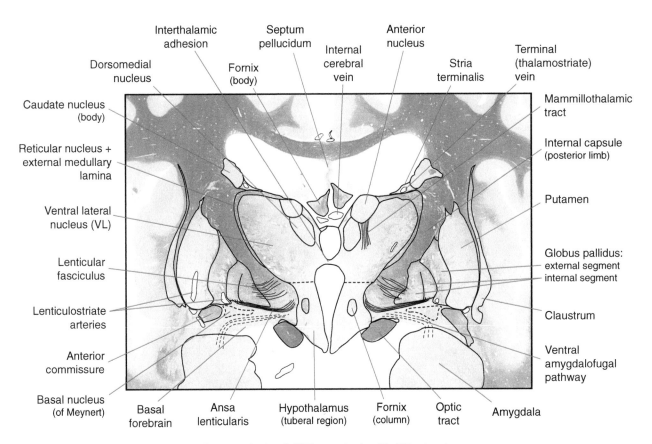

Figure 5.6 (Continued) **(B)** The central region of Fig. 5.6A, enlarged.

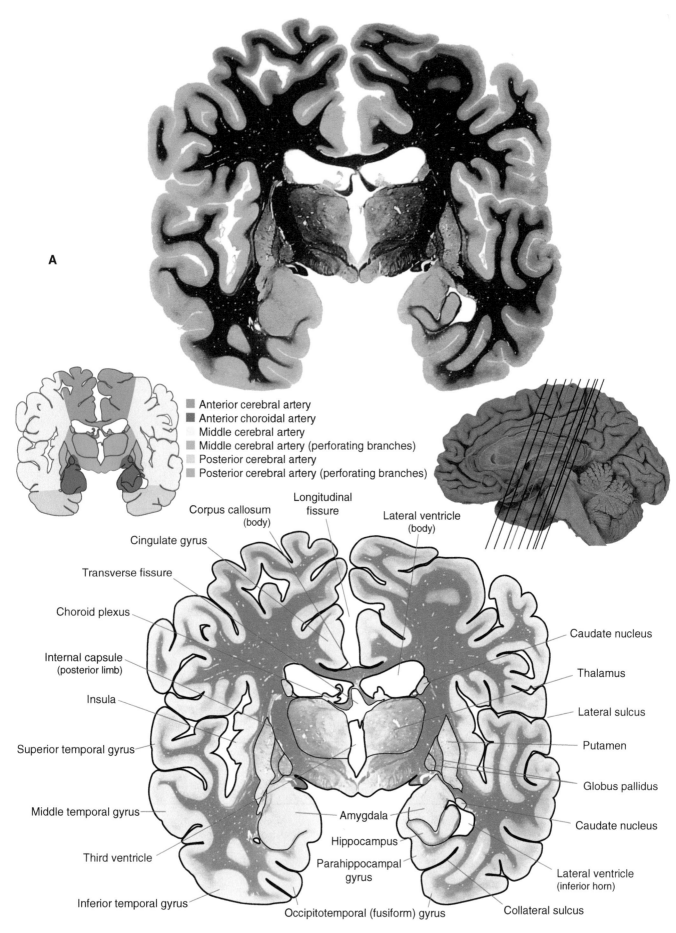

A

Anterior cerebral artery
Anterior choroidal artery
Middle cerebral artery
Middle cerebral artery (perforating branches)
Posterior cerebral artery
Posterior cerebral artery (perforating branches)

Corpus callosum (body)
Cingulate gyrus
Transverse fissure
Choroid plexus
Internal capsule (posterior limb)
Insula
Superior temporal gyrus
Middle temporal gyrus
Third ventricle
Inferior temporal gyrus

Longitudinal fissure
Lateral ventricle (body)

Caudate nucleus
Thalamus
Lateral sulcus
Putamen
Globus pallidus
Caudate nucleus
Lateral ventricle (inferior horn)

Amygdala
Hippocampus
Parahippocampal gyrus
Occipitotemporal (fusiform) gyrus
Collateral sulcus

Figure 5.7 (A) A coronal section at the level of the mammillary bodies.

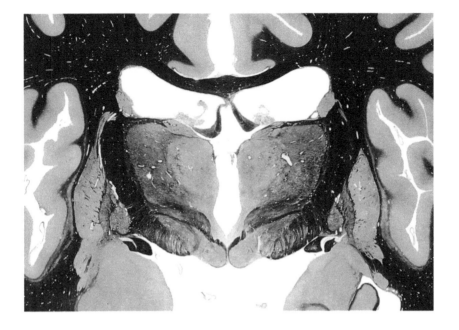

B

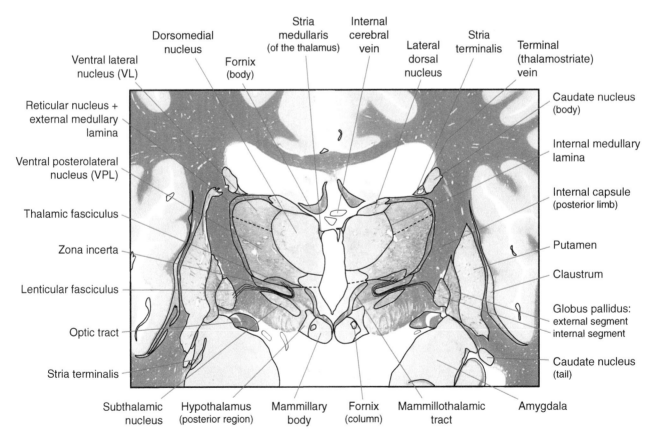

Figure 5.7 (Continued) **(B)** The central region of Fig. 5.7A, enlarged.

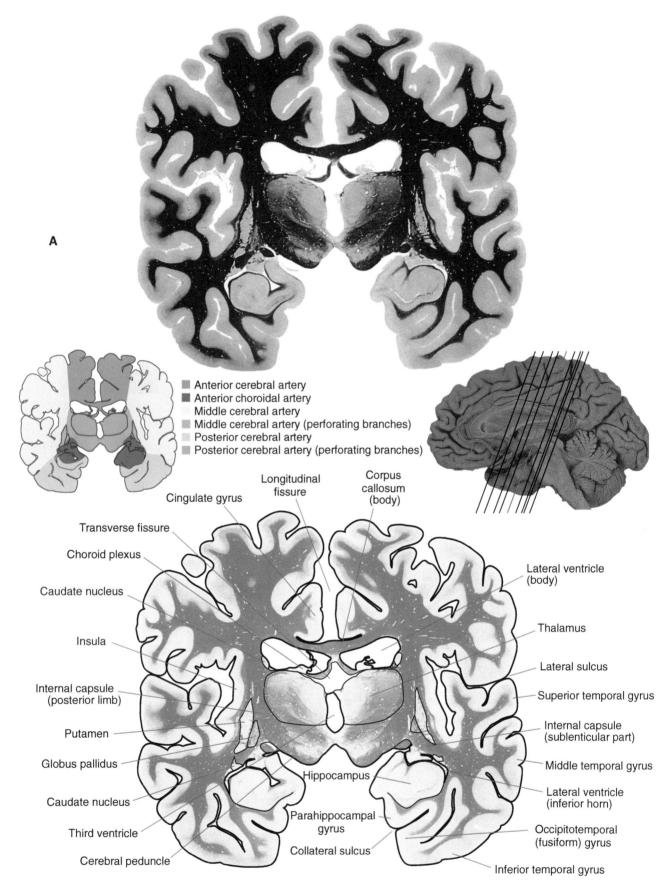

A

Anterior cerebral artery
Anterior choroidal artery
Middle cerebral artery
Middle cerebral artery (perforating branches)
Posterior cerebral artery
Posterior cerebral artery (perforating branches)

Cingulate gyrus
Longitudinal fissure
Corpus callosum (body)
Transverse fissure
Choroid plexus
Caudate nucleus
Lateral ventricle (body)
Insula
Thalamus
Internal capsule (posterior limb)
Lateral sulcus
Superior temporal gyrus
Putamen
Internal capsule (sublenticular part)
Globus pallidus
Middle temporal gyrus
Hippocampus
Lateral ventricle (inferior horn)
Caudate nucleus
Parahippocampal gyrus
Third ventricle
Occipitotemporal (fusiform) gyrus
Cerebral peduncle
Collateral sulcus
Inferior temporal gyrus

Figure 5.8 (A) A coronal section at the level of the anterior end of the hippocampus.

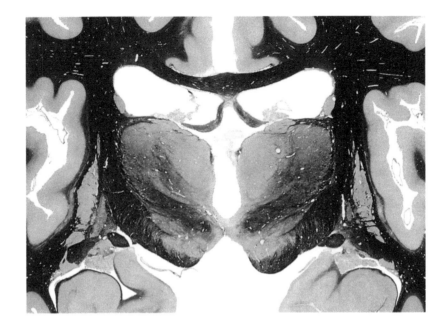

B

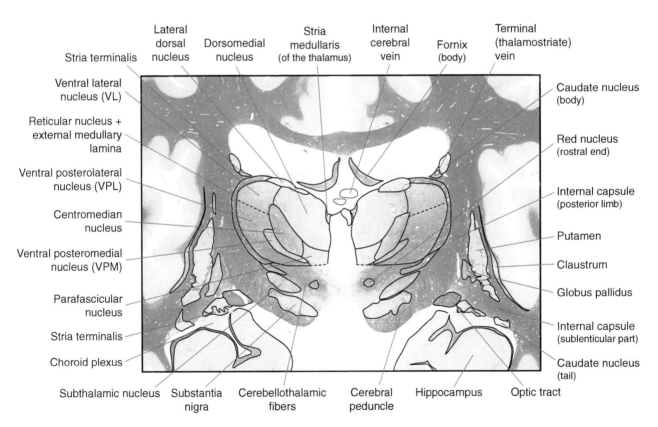

Stria terminalis

Ventral lateral
nucleus (VL)

Reticular nucleus +
external medullary
lamina

Ventral posterolateral
nucleus (VPL)

Centromedian
nucleus

Ventral posteromedial
nucleus (VPM)

Parafascicular
nucleus

Stria terminalis

Choroid plexus

Lateral
dorsal
nucleus

Dorsomedial
nucleus

Stria
medullaris
(of the thalamus)

Internal
cerebral
vein

Fornix
(body)

Terminal
(thalamostriate)
vein

Caudate nucleus
(body)

Red nucleus
(rostral end)

Internal capsule
(posterior limb)

Putamen

Claustrum

Globus pallidus

Internal capsule
(sublenticular part)

Caudate nucleus
(tail)

Subthalamic nucleus

Substantia
nigra

Cerebellothalamic
fibers

Cerebral
peduncle

Hippocampus

Optic tract

Figure 5.8 (Continued) **(B)** The central region of Fig. 5.8A, enlarged.

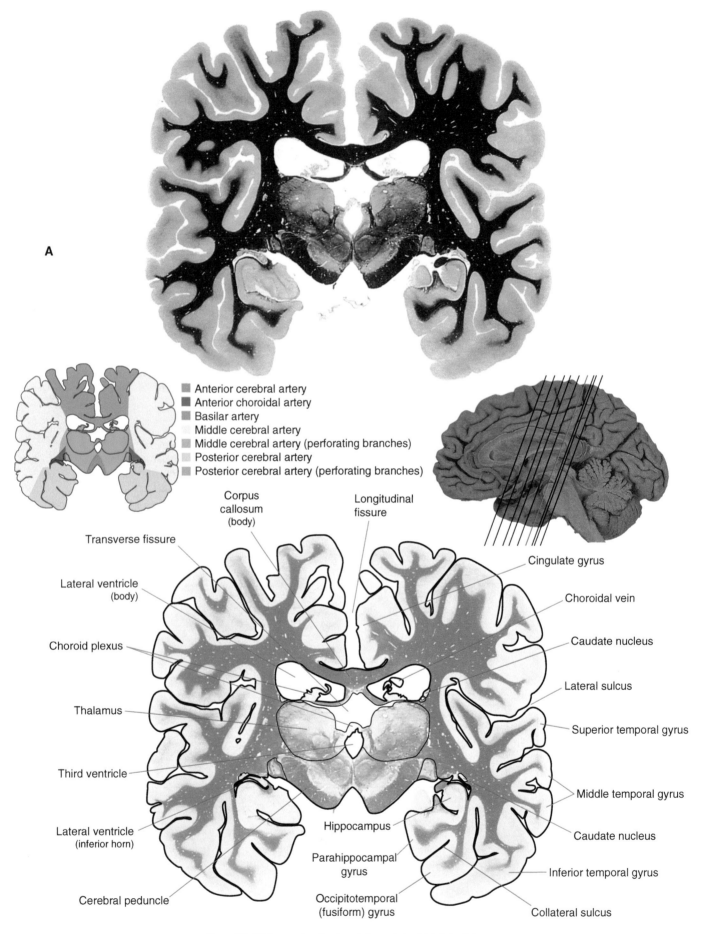

A

Anterior cerebral artery
Anterior choroidal artery
Basilar artery
Middle cerebral artery
Middle cerebral artery (perforating branches)
Posterior cerebral artery
Posterior cerebral artery (perforating branches)

Corpus callosum (body)

Longitudinal fissure

Transverse fissure

Lateral ventricle (body)

Choroid plexus

Thalamus

Third ventricle

Lateral ventricle (inferior horn)

Cerebral peduncle

Cingulate gyrus

Choroidal vein

Caudate nucleus

Lateral sulcus

Superior temporal gyrus

Middle temporal gyrus

Caudate nucleus

Inferior temporal gyrus

Collateral sulcus

Hippocampus

Parahippocampal gyrus

Occipitotemporal (fusiform) gyrus

Figure 5.9 (A) A coronal section through the posterior third of the thalamus.

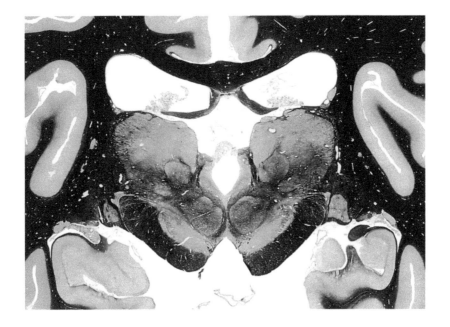

B

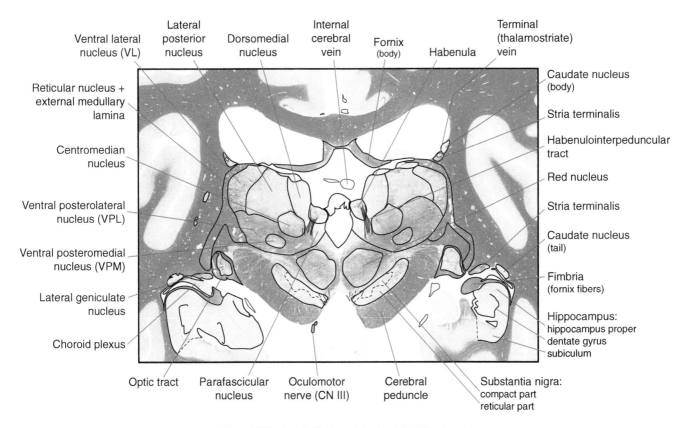

Ventral lateral nucleus (VL)

Lateral posterior nucleus

Dorsomedial nucleus

Internal cerebral vein

Fornix (body)

Habenula

Terminal (thalamostriate) vein

Reticular nucleus + external medullary lamina

Centromedian nucleus

Ventral posterolateral nucleus (VPL)

Ventral posteromedial nucleus (VPM)

Lateral geniculate nucleus

Choroid plexus

Caudate nucleus (body)

Stria terminalis

Habenulointerpeduncular tract

Red nucleus

Stria terminalis

Caudate nucleus (tail)

Fimbria (fornix fibers)

Hippocampus: hippocampus proper dentate gyrus subiculum

Optic tract

Parafascicular nucleus

Oculomotor nerve (CN III)

Cerebral peduncle

Substantia nigra: compact part reticular part

Figure 5.9 (Continued) **(B)** The central region of Fig. 5.9A, enlarged.

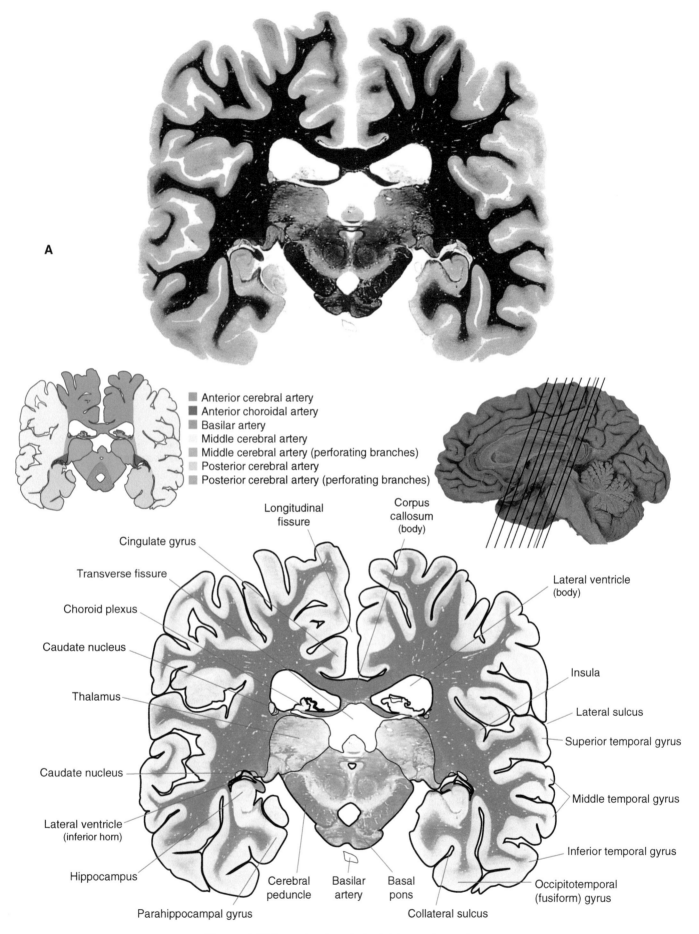

A

Anterior cerebral artery
Anterior choroidal artery
Basilar artery
Middle cerebral artery
Middle cerebral artery (perforating branches)
Posterior cerebral artery
Posterior cerebral artery (perforating branches)

Longitudinal fissure

Corpus callosum (body)

Cingulate gyrus

Transverse fissure

Choroid plexus

Caudate nucleus

Thalamus

Caudate nucleus

Lateral ventricle (inferior horn)

Hippocampus

Parahippocampal gyrus

Cerebral peduncle

Basilar artery

Basal pons

Collateral sulcus

Lateral ventricle (body)

Insula

Lateral sulcus

Superior temporal gyrus

Middle temporal gyrus

Inferior temporal gyrus

Occipitotemporal (fusiform) gyrus

Figure 5.10 (A) A coronal section at the level of the posterior commissure.

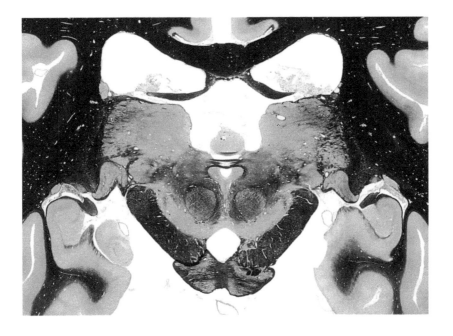

B

Caudate nucleus
(body)

External medullary
lamina

Reticular nucleus

Medial geniculate
nucleus

Lateral geniculate
nucleus

Caudate nucleus
(tail)

Cerebral
aqueduct

Pulvinar

Pineal
gland

Internal
cerebral
vein

Fornix
(crus/body)

Posterior
commissure

Terminal
(thalamostriate)
vein

Stria terminalis

Pretectal area

Periaqueductal gray

Stria terminalis

Choroid plexus

Fimbria
(fornix fibers)

Hippocampus:
hippocampus proper
dentate gyrus
subiculum

Cerebral
peduncle

Oculomotor
nucleus

Ventral
tegmental
area

Substantia nigra:
compact part
reticular part

Figure 5.10 (Continued) **(B)** The central region of Fig. 5.10A, enlarged.

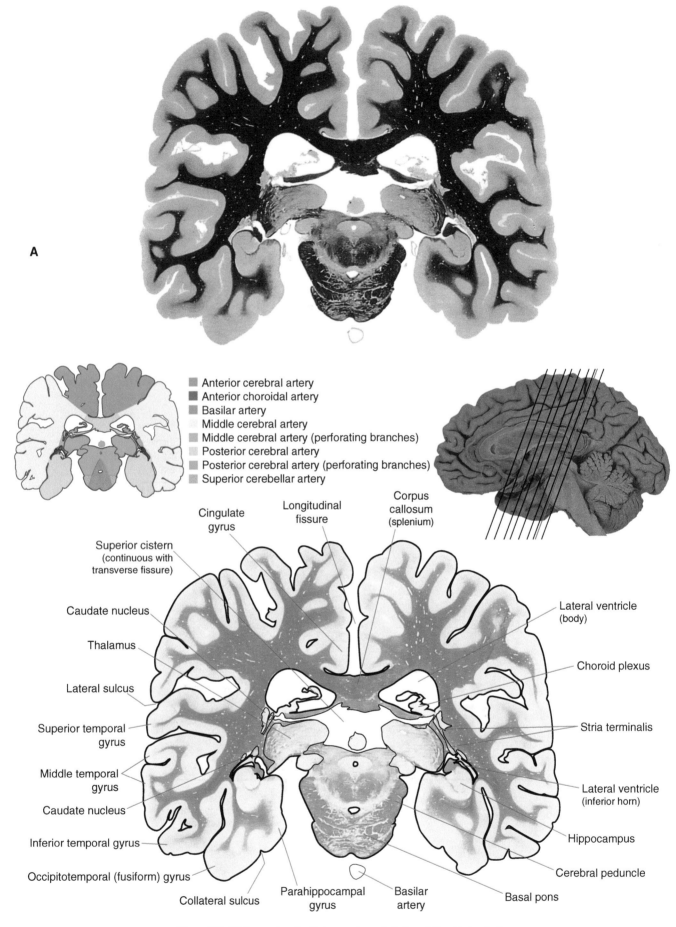

A

Anterior cerebral artery
Anterior choroidal artery
Basilar artery
Middle cerebral artery
Middle cerebral artery (perforating branches)
Posterior cerebral artery
Posterior cerebral artery (perforating branches)
Superior cerebellar artery

Cingulate gyrus

Longitudinal fissure

Corpus callosum (splenium)

Superior cistern (continuous with transverse fissure)

Caudate nucleus

Thalamus

Lateral sulcus

Superior temporal gyrus

Middle temporal gyrus

Caudate nucleus

Inferior temporal gyrus

Occipitotemporal (fusiform) gyrus

Collateral sulcus

Parahippocampal gyrus

Basilar artery

Lateral ventricle (body)

Choroid plexus

Stria terminalis

Lateral ventricle (inferior horn)

Hippocampus

Cerebral peduncle

Basal pons

Figure 5.11 (A) A coronal section that passes tangentially through the stria terminalis.

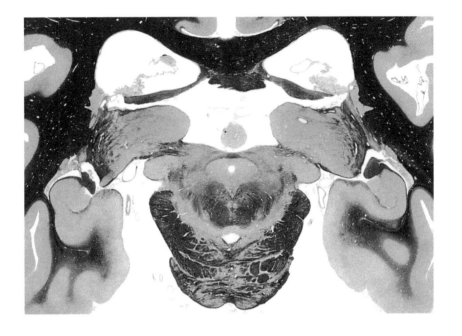

B

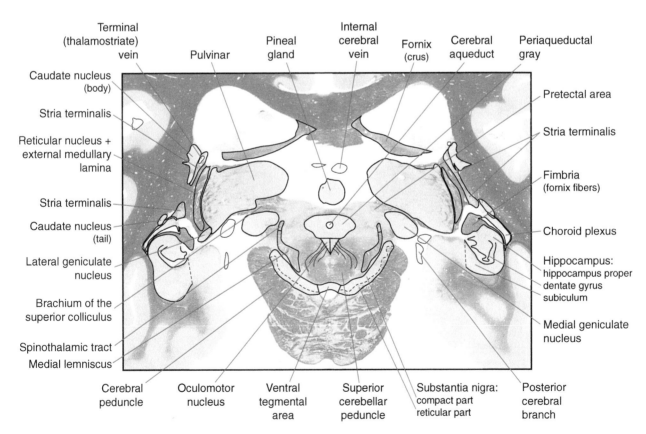

Terminal (thalamostriate) vein

Caudate nucleus (body)

Stria terminalis

Reticular nucleus + external medullary lamina

Stria terminalis

Caudate nucleus (tail)

Lateral geniculate nucleus

Brachium of the superior colliculus

Spinothalamic tract

Medial lemniscus

Pulvinar

Pineal gland

Internal cerebral vein

Fornix (crus)

Cerebral aqueduct

Periaqueductal gray

Pretectal area

Stria terminalis

Fimbria (fornix fibers)

Choroid plexus

Hippocampus: hippocampus proper dentate gyrus subiculum

Medial geniculate nucleus

Cerebral peduncle

Oculomotor nucleus

Ventral tegmental area

Superior cerebellar peduncle

Substantia nigra: compact part reticular part

Posterior cerebral branch

Figure 5.11 (Continued) **(B)** The central region of Fig. 5.11A, enlarged.

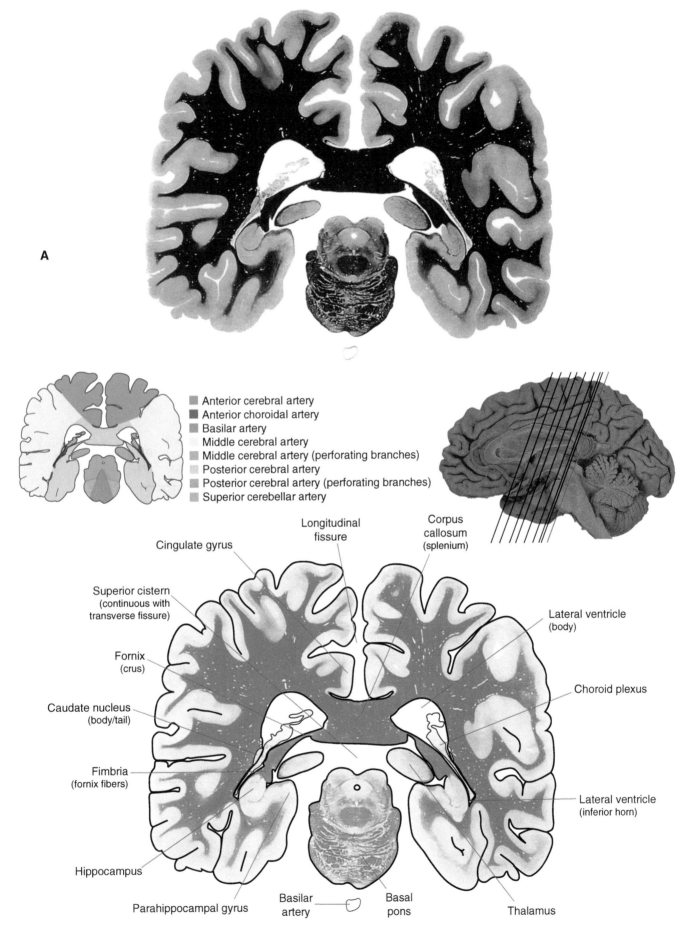

A

Anterior cerebral artery
Anterior choroidal artery
Basilar artery
Middle cerebral artery
Middle cerebral artery (perforating branches)
Posterior cerebral artery
Posterior cerebral artery (perforating branches)
Superior cerebellar artery

Cingulate gyrus

Longitudinal fissure

Corpus callosum (splenium)

Superior cistern (continuous with transverse fissure)

Lateral ventricle (body)

Fornix (crus)

Choroid plexus

Caudate nucleus (body/tail)

Fimbria (fornix fibers)

Lateral ventricle (inferior horn)

Hippocampus

Parahippocampal gyrus

Basilar artery

Basal pons

Thalamus

Figure 5.12 (A) A coronal section that passes tangentially through the fornix and caudate nucleus.

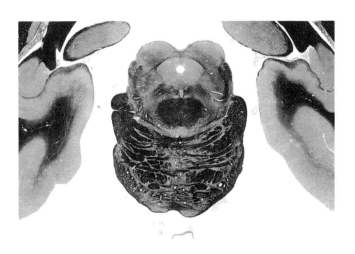

B

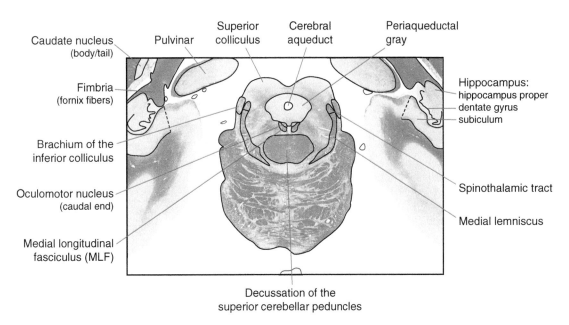

Caudate nucleus
(body/tail)

Pulvinar

Superior
colliculus

Cerebral
aqueduct

Periaqueductal
gray

Fimbria
(fornix fibers)

Hippocampus:
hippocampus proper
dentate gyrus
subiculum

Brachium of the
inferior colliculus

Oculomotor nucleus
(caudal end)

Spinothalamic tract

Medial lemniscus

Medial longitudinal
fasciculus (MLF)

Decussation of the
superior cerebellar peduncles

Figure 5.12 (Continued) **(B)** The central region of Fig. 5.12A, enlarged.

6

Axial Sections

This chapter, the second of three showing sections of entire human brains, illustrates axial planes approximating those used in computed tomography scans (see Chapter 9). Forebrain structures continue to be emphasized, but parts of the brainstem and cerebellum are indicated as well. The organization of various functional systems in the forebrain (e.g., thalamus, hippocampus) is presented in Chapter 8.

Colored diagrams showing typical areas of arterial supply in each section are provided in this and the preceding and following chapter. We simplified these in two major ways. First, arterial territories are shown as sharply demarcated from each other, when in reality there is significant interdigitation and overlap. Second, perforating arteries arise from all the vessels of the circle of Willis, but we lumped together those from the posterior communicating and posterior cerebral arteries, and those from the anterior communicating and anterior cerebral arteries.

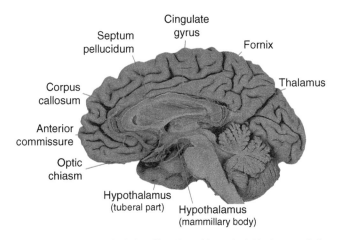

Figure 6.1 The hemisected brain from Fig. 1.7, used in much of this chapter to indicate planes of section.

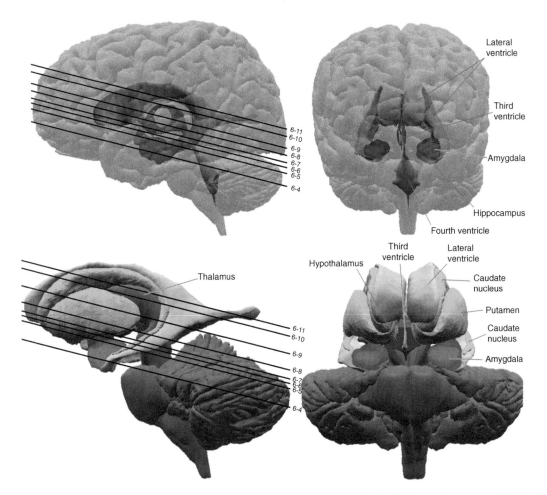

Figure 6.2 The planes of section shown in this chapter, indicated on three-dimensional reconstructions. (Courtesy Dr. John W. Sundsten, Department of Biological Structure, University of Washington School of Medicine.)

Figure 6.3 (A–X) Twenty-four axial sections of a brain, arranged in an inferior-to-superior sequence extending from the orbital surface of the frontal lobe to just above the corpus callosum. Anterior is toward the top, as in the conventional orientation of computed tomography (CT) and magnetic resonance (MR) images (Chapter 9); as a result the brainstem, when present, is inverted relative to its orientation in Chapter 3.

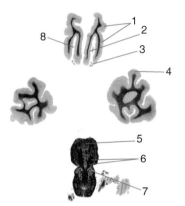

(A) The first section just reaches the orbital surface of the frontal lobe, including gyrus rectus *(2)* and the beginning of other parts of the orbital frontal cortex *(1)*, and passes through the olfactory sulcus *(8)* and olfactory tract *(3)*. The temporal pole *(4)* can also be seen. The brainstem is cut at an odd angle in these sections, with more rostral parts toward the top. This section passes through the basal pons *(5)* and the inferior olivary nucleus *(7)* of the medulla. The corticospinal tract *(6)* can be seen passing from the basal pons into the medullary pyramid.

(B) Gyrus rectus *(2)* is still present, joined by a little more of the orbital frontal cortex *(1)*. The section again passes through the basal pons *(4)* and the basilar artery *(3)* anterior to it, as well as parts of the rostral medulla. It includes the cerebellar flocculus *(5)*, the inferior cerebellar peduncle *(6)*, the vestibulocochlear *(8)* nerve, and choroid plexus *(7)* in the lateral aperture of the fourth ventricle.

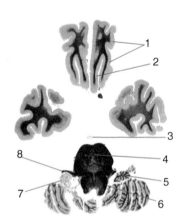

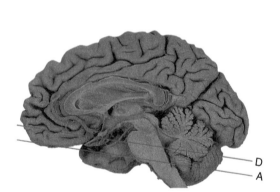

(C) The olfactory tract *(1)* has now reached the posterior end of the olfactory sulcus, near where it attaches to the base of the forebrain. The optic nerve *(2)* moves posteriorly toward the optic chiasm; the internal carotid artery *(3)* is just lateral to where the optic chiasm will soon be located. The inferior horn of the lateral ventricle *(5)* and adjacent amygdala *(4)* begin to appear in the temporal lobe. The inferior cerebellar peduncle *(6)* turns posteriorly toward the cerebellum.

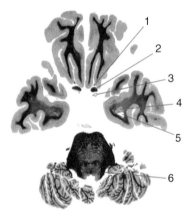

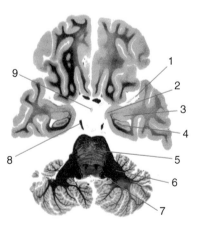

(D) The middle cerebral artery *(1)* moves laterally into the lateral sulcus. The amygdala *(3)* is larger, and the hippocampus *(4)* appears just posterior to it; both structures underlie the uncus *(2)*. The plane of section moves closer to the hypothalamus and passes through the infundibulum *(9)*. The middle cerebellar peduncle *(6)* connects the basal pons *(5)* to the cerebellum. The inferior cerebellar peduncle *(7)* has completed its posterior turn and is now cut in cross section as it moves into the cerebellum. The oculomotor nerve *(8)* moves anteriorly from its point of emergence from the brainstem.

Figure 6.3 (Continued) Axial sections.

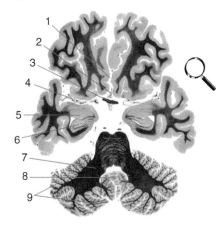

(E) The anterior cerebral artery *(2)* moves into the longitudinal fissure *(1)*, and the middle cerebral artery *(4)* continues on its course toward the insula. The optic nerves partially decussate in the optic chiasm *(3)*. The amygdala *(5)* and hippocampus *(6)* continue to increase in size. The cerebellar vermis *(8)* and hemispheres *(9)* can be distinguished, and the middle cerebellar peduncle *(7)* still connects the basal pons to the cerebellum. Shown enlarged in Fig. 6.4.

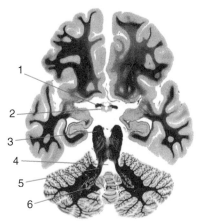

(F) The optic tract *(1)* begins to move posteriorly from the optic chiasm, and the plane of section reaches the tuberal zone of the hypothalamus *(2)*. The superior cerebellar peduncle *(5)* leaves the deep cerebellar nuclei (represented here by the dentate nucleus *[6]*), forms part of the wall of the fourth ventricle *(4)*, and enters the pons. The first part of the midbrain to appear in this plane of section is the cerebral peduncle *(3)*.

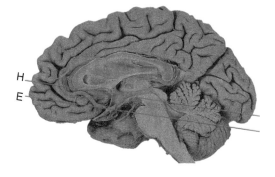

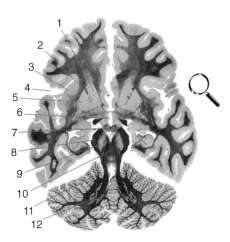

(G) The base of the forebrain, beginning to pass through the head of the caudate nucleus *(1)*, the putamen *(5)*, the nucleus accumbens *(6)*, and the anterior limb of the internal capsule *(2)*. The insula *(3)*, buried in the lateral sulcus *(4)*, overlies the putamen. The mammillary bodies *(8)* and other parts of the hypothalamus border the third ventricle *(7)*. The cerebral peduncle *(9)* and substantia nigra *(10)* are apparent in the midbrain. The superior cerebellar peduncle *(12)* leaves the dentate nucleus *(13)*, enters the brainstem, and decussates *(11)*. Shown enlarged in Fig. 6.5.

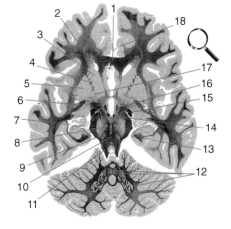

(H) The lateral ventricle is now cut twice, through the anterior *(2)* and inferior *(7)* horns, and the corpus callosum *(1)* makes its first appearance. The limbic lobe is also cut twice, through the cingulate *(18)* and parahippocampal *(13)* gyri. The head of the caudate nucleus *(3)*, the putamen *(5)*, the nucleus accumbens *(17)* and the anterior limb of the internal capsule *(4)* all increase in size. Fibers that will cross in the anterior commissure *(6)* begin to move toward the midline, and the optic tract *(15)* continues to move posteriorly. The column of the fornix *(16)* and the mammillothalamic tract *(14)* are transected just above each mammillary body. All of the deep cerebellar nuclei *(12)* are now apparent. The vast majority of efferents from these nuclei travel through the superior cerebellar peduncle *(11)* and decussate *(10)*, and then most of them *(9)* pass through or around the red nucleus *(8)*. Shown enlarged in Fig. 6.6.

Illustration continued on following page

Figure 6.3 (Continued) Axial sections.

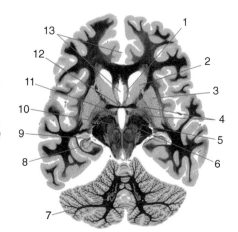

(I) The subcallosal gyrus *(1)*, the last bit of limbic cortex adjacent to the corpus callosum, borders the longitudinal fissure *(13)*. The head of the caudate nucleus *(2)* continues; both parts of the lenticular nucleus—the putamen *(3)* and the globus pallidus *(4)*—are now apparent, and the subthalamic nucleus *(6)* can be seen just across the internal capsule/cerebral peduncle *(5)* from the globus pallidus. Fornix fibers are cut twice, once through the fimbria *(9)* as it leaves the hippocampus *(8)* and again through the column of the fornix *(11)* as it approaches the mammillary body. The mammillothalamic tract *(10)* continues on its course toward the anterior nucleus of the thalamus. Fibers of the anterior commissure *(12)* cross the midline. The dentate nucleus *(7)* is the only deep cerebellar nucleus remaining.

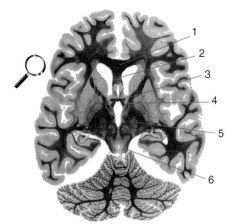

(J) The section passes tangentially through the corpus callosum as the genu *(1)* tapers into the rostrum *(2)*. The anterior commissure *(3)*, column of the fornix *(4)*, and subthalamic nucleus *(5)* are still visible, and the inferior colliculus *(6)* appears. Shown enlarged in Fig. 6.7.

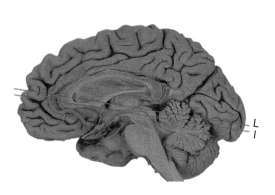

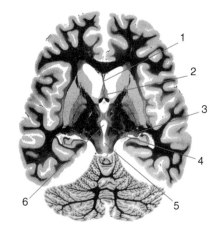

(K) The septum pellucidum *(1)*, merging with the septal nuclei *(2)*, succeeds the rostrum of the corpus callosum. The lateral *(3)* and medial *(4)* geniculate nuclei (the most inferior parts of the thalamus) can now be seen, and the continuity of the third ventricle *(6)* and the cerebral aqueduct *(5)* is apparent.

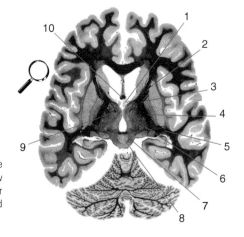

(L) Choroid plexus *(1)* passes through each interventricular foramen adjacent to the column of the fornix *(10)*. Four of the five parts of the internal capsule—the anterior limb *(2)*, genu *(3)*, posterior limb *(4)*, and retrolenticular part *(5)* —are now present, as is much more of the thalamus *(6)*. The mammillothalamic tract *(9)* continues on its path toward the anterior nucleus of the thalamus. The posterior commissure *(7)* crosses the midline near the periaqueductal gray *(8)*. Shown enlarged in Fig. 6.8.

Figure 6.3 (Continued) Axial sections.

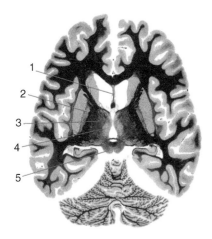

(M) The septum pellucidum *(1)* still separates the anterior horns of the two lateral ventricles from each other. The globus pallidus *(2)* gets smaller as the plane of section moves superiorly through the lenticular nucleus. Lateral *(3)* and medial *(4)* divisions of the thalamus can be distinguished because of differences in the numbers of myelinated fibers entering and leaving them. The superior colliculus *(5)* appears in the midbrain.

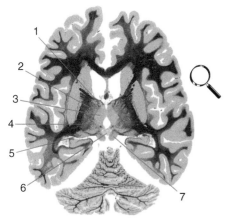

(N) Now more parts of the thalamus can be seen: the lateral *(2)* and medial *(3)* divisions, the anterior *(1)* and centromedian *(4)* nuclei, and the pulvinar *(5)*. (The mammillothalamic tract has terminated in the anterior nucleus and is no longer visible.) The pineal gland *(6)* protrudes posteriorly between the superior colliculi *(7)*. Shown enlarged in Fig. 6.9.

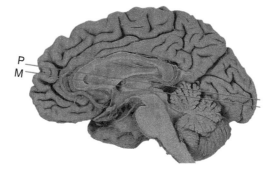

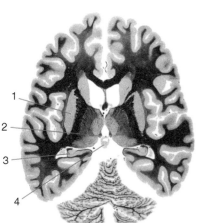

(O) The plane of section is above the globus pallidus, and now the putamen *(1)* begins to get smaller. The stria medullaris of the thalamus terminates in the habenula *(2)*. The hippocampus *(3)* and pineal gland *(4)* are still apparent.

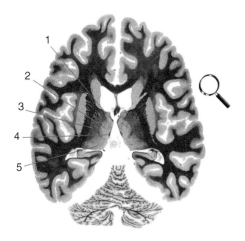

(P) In the thalamus, lateral *(3)* and medial *(2)* divisions, the anterior nucleus *(1)*, and the pulvinar *(5)* can still be distinguished. Fibers travel posteriorly in the stria medullaris *(4)* of the thalamus toward the habenula. Shown enlarged in Fig. 6.10.

Illustration continued on following page

Figure 6.3 (Continued) Axial sections.

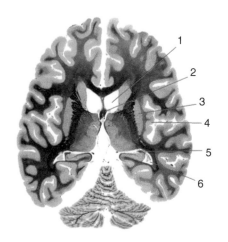

(Q) The putamen *(3)* continues to get smaller, as does the overlying insula *(4)*. As the plane of section moves upward through the cerebral hemisphere, the profiles of twice-cut structures, such as the lateral ventricle *(1, 6)* and fornix fibers *(2, 5)*, will draw progressively closer to each other until these C-shaped structures are finally cut tangentially (e.g., *T, V*).

(R) Near the top of the putamen *(3)* and internal capsule *(2)*. The fornix *(1)* is now cut obliquely as it begins to curve downward toward the interventricular foramen. Although the thalamus begins to get smaller, medial *(6)* and lateral *(5)* divisions, the anterior nucleus *(4)*, and the pulvinar *(7)* can still be distinguished.

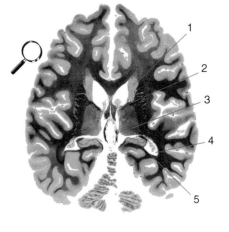

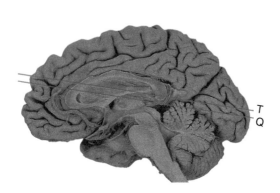

(S) Just below the splenium of the corpus callosum and completely above the putamen. The head of the caudate nucleus *(1)* begins to taper into the body of the caudate nucleus, and the posterior part of the hippocampus *(5)* has a distinctive pattern of folding (compare with *R*). The plane of section still passes through the inferior horn *(4)* but will soon enter the atrium and posterior horn of the lateral ventricle. The fornix *(2)* is cut obliquely once again. The internal cerebral vein *(3)* of each hemisphere travels posteriorly toward the great cerebral vein. Shown enlarged in Fig. 6.11.

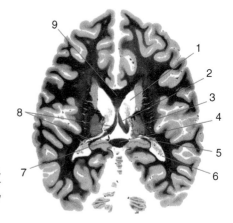

(T) The corpus callosum is now cut twice, through the body *(9)* and the splenium *(4)*. The thalamus *(3)* continues to dwindle, the distinctive appearance of the hippocampus *(7)* continues, and the two profiles of the lateral ventricle *(1, 6)* draw closer together. On the right side of the section, fornix fibers are still cut twice *(2, 5)*, but on the left side the section cuts tangentially through these fibers *(8)*, showing their entire course as they pass from the fimbria to the fornix.

Figure 6.3 (Continued) Axial sections.

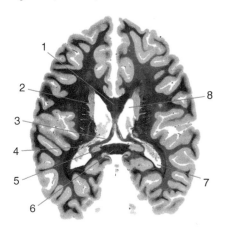

(U) The plane of section has nearly reached the top of several C-shaped forebrain structures. It passes tangentially through the fornix *(3)*, but still cuts the corpus callosum *(1, 6)*, caudate nucleus *(2, 4)*, and lateral ventricle *(7, 8)* twice. The last bit of the hippocampus *(5)* can be seen adjacent to the splenium of the corpus callosum *(6)*.

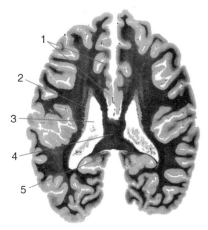

(V) A tangential section through the body of the caudate nucleus *(2)*, the lateral ventricle *(3)*, and the body of the corpus callosum *(4)*. The limbic lobe is still cut twice, once (nearly tangentially) through the cingulate gyrus *(1)* and again through the narrow isthmus *(5)* joining the cingulate and parahippocampal gyri.

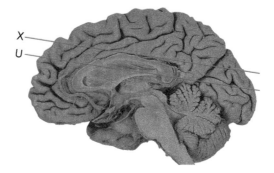

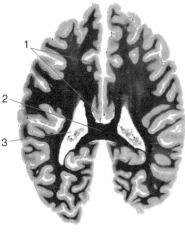

(W) A tangential cut through the corpus callosum *(2)*, lateral ventricle *(3)*, and a larger expanse of the cingulate gyrus *(1)*.

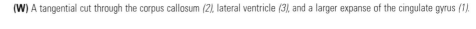

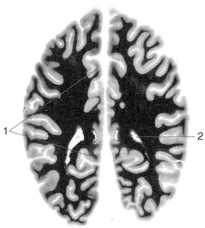

(X) Finally, a tangential cut through the cingulate gyrus *(1)* just above the corpus callosum and near the roof of the lateral ventricle *(2)*.

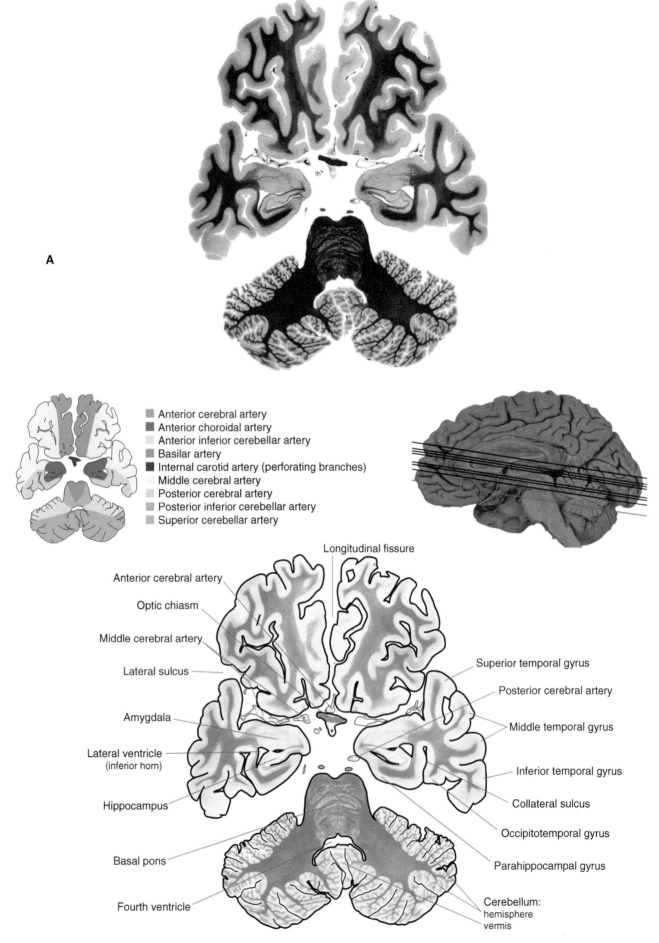

A

Anterior cerebral artery
Anterior choroidal artery
Anterior inferior cerebellar artery
Basilar artery
Internal carotid artery (perforating branches)
Middle cerebral artery
Posterior cerebral artery
Posterior inferior cerebellar artery
Superior cerebellar artery

Longitudinal fissure

Anterior cerebral artery

Optic chiasm

Middle cerebral artery

Lateral sulcus

Amygdala

Lateral ventricle
(inferior horn)

Hippocampus

Basal pons

Fourth ventricle

Superior temporal gyrus

Posterior cerebral artery

Middle temporal gyrus

Inferior temporal gyrus

Collateral sulcus

Occipitotemporal gyrus

Parahippocampal gyrus

Cerebellum:
hemisphere
vermis

Figure 6.4 (A) An axial section through the uncus and optic chiasm.

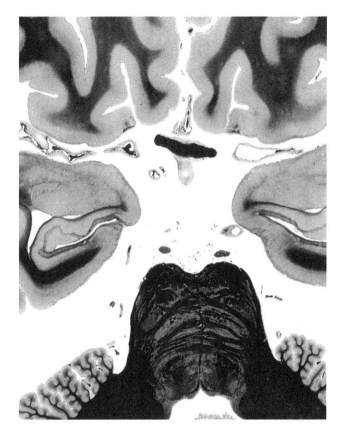

B

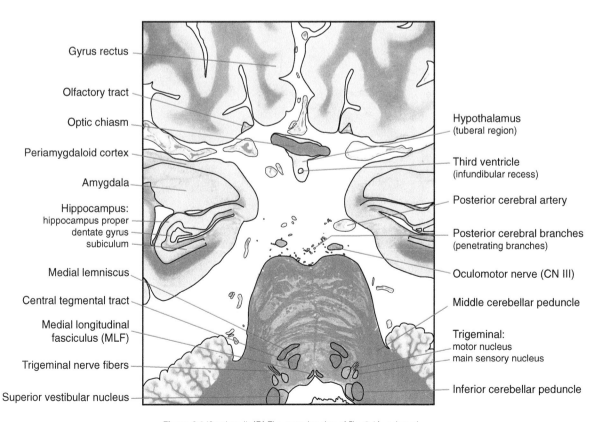

Gyrus rectus

Olfactory tract

Optic chiasm

Periamygdaloid cortex

Amygdala

Hippocampus:
hippocampus proper
dentate gyrus
subiculum

Medial lemniscus

Central tegmental tract

Medial longitudinal
fasciculus (MLF)

Trigeminal nerve fibers

Superior vestibular nucleus

Hypothalamus
(tuberal region)

Third ventricle
(infundibular recess)

Posterior cerebral artery

Posterior cerebral branches
(penetrating branches)

Oculomotor nerve (CN III)

Middle cerebellar peduncle

Trigeminal:
motor nucleus
main sensory nucleus

Inferior cerebellar peduncle

Figure 6.4 (Continued) **(B)** The central region of Fig. 6.4A, enlarged.

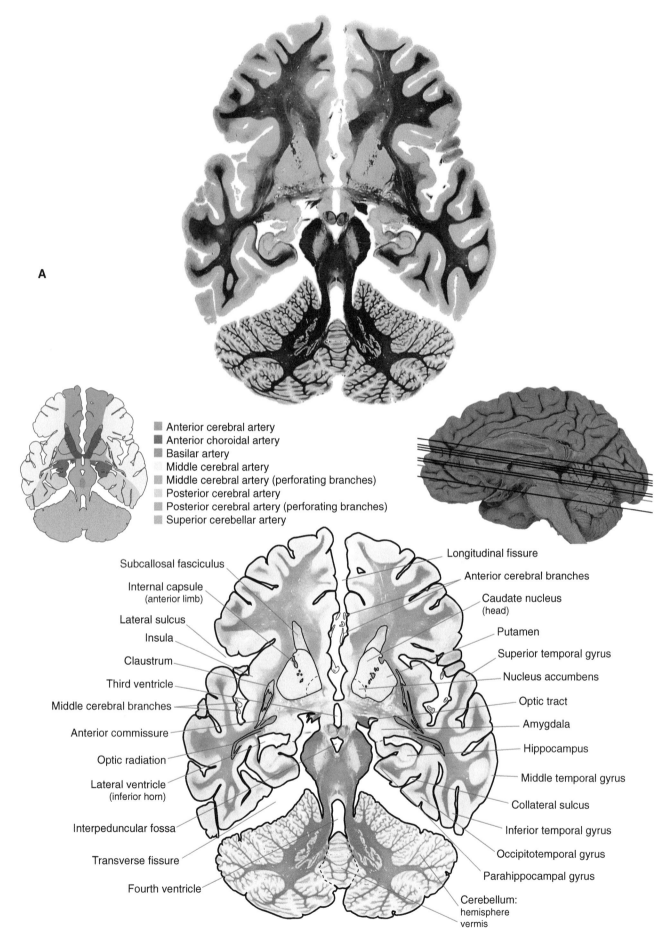

A

Anterior cerebral artery
Anterior choroidal artery
Basilar artery
Middle cerebral artery
Middle cerebral artery (perforating branches)
Posterior cerebral artery
Posterior cerebral artery (perforating branches)
Superior cerebellar artery

Subcallosal fasciculus

Internal capsule
(anterior limb)

Lateral sulcus

Insula

Claustrum

Third ventricle

Middle cerebral branches

Anterior commissure

Optic radiation

Lateral ventricle
(inferior horn)

Interpeduncular fossa

Transverse fissure

Fourth ventricle

Longitudinal fissure

Anterior cerebral branches

Caudate nucleus
(head)

Putamen

Superior temporal gyrus

Nucleus accumbens

Optic tract

Amygdala

Hippocampus

Middle temporal gyrus

Collateral sulcus

Inferior temporal gyrus

Occipitotemporal gyrus

Parahippocampal gyrus

Cerebellum:
hemisphere
vermis

Figure 6.5 (A) An axial section through the base of the diencephalon.

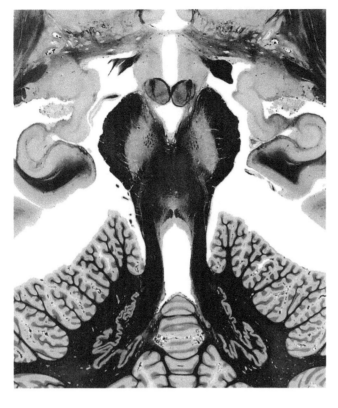

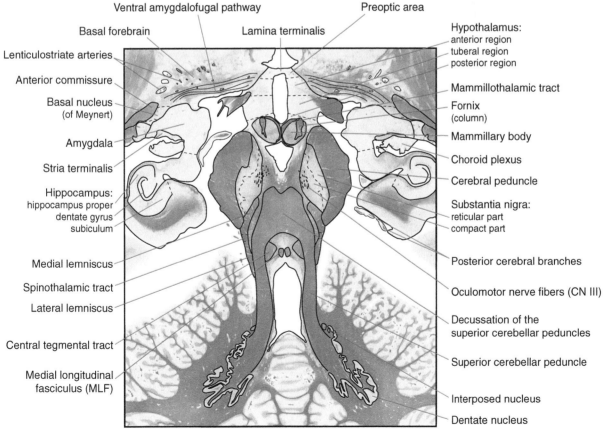

Ventral amygdalofugal pathway

Basal forebrain

Lenticulostriate arteries

Anterior commissure

Basal nucleus
(of Meynert)

Amygdala

Stria terminalis

Hippocampus:
hippocampus proper
dentate gyrus
subiculum

Medial lemniscus

Spinothalamic tract

Lateral lemniscus

Central tegmental tract

Medial longitudinal
fasciculus (MLF)

Lamina terminalis

Preoptic area

Hypothalamus:
anterior region
tuberal region
posterior region

Mammillothalamic tract

Fornix
(column)

Mammillary body

Choroid plexus

Cerebral peduncle

Substantia nigra:
reticular part
compact part

Posterior cerebral branches

Oculomotor nerve fibers (CN III)

Decussation of the
superior cerebellar peduncles

Superior cerebellar peduncle

Interposed nucleus

Dentate nucleus

Figure 6.5 (Continued) **(B)** The central region of Fig. 6.5A, enlarged.

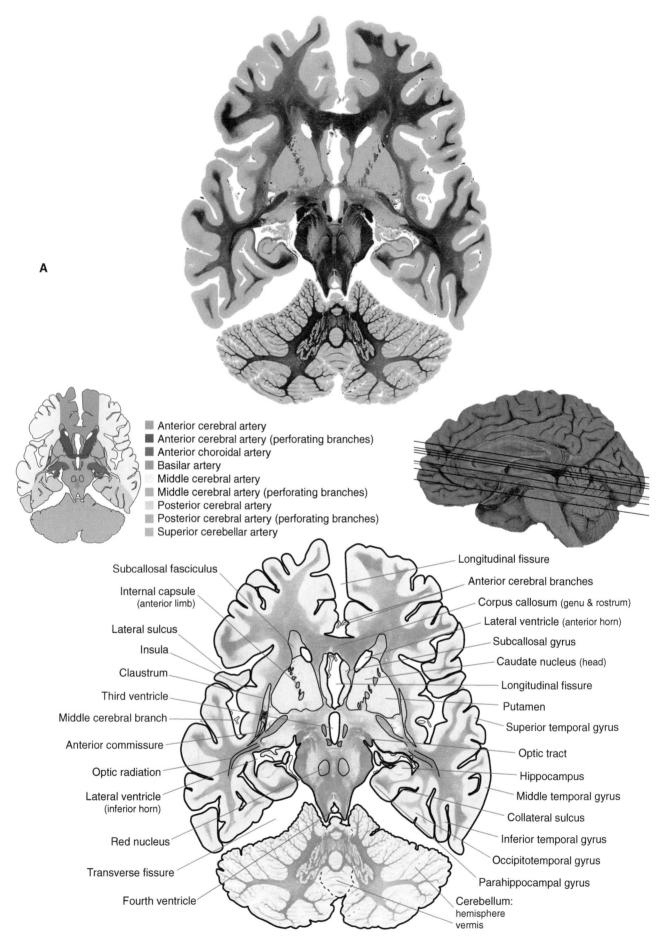

A

Anterior cerebral artery
Anterior cerebral artery (perforating branches)
Anterior choroidal artery
Basilar artery
Middle cerebral artery
Middle cerebral artery (perforating branches)
Posterior cerebral artery
Posterior cerebral artery (perforating branches)
Superior cerebellar artery

Subcallosal fasciculus
Internal capsule (anterior limb)
Lateral sulcus
Insula
Claustrum
Third ventricle
Middle cerebral branch
Anterior commissure
Optic radiation
Lateral ventricle (inferior horn)
Red nucleus
Transverse fissure
Fourth ventricle

Longitudinal fissure
Anterior cerebral branches
Corpus callosum (genu & rostrum)
Lateral ventricle (anterior horn)
Subcallosal gyrus
Caudate nucleus (head)
Longitudinal fissure
Putamen
Superior temporal gyrus
Optic tract
Hippocampus
Middle temporal gyrus
Collateral sulcus
Inferior temporal gyrus
Occipitotemporal gyrus
Parahippocampal gyrus
Cerebellum: hemisphere vermis

Figure 6.6 (A) An axial section through all the deep cerebellar nuclei.

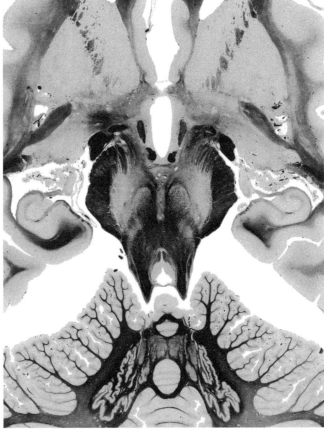

B

Globus pallidus

Basal forebrain

Ventral amygdalofugal pathway

Anterior commissure

Amygdala

Stria terminalis

Fimbria (fornix fibers)

Posterior cerebral artery

Cerebral peduncle

Red nucleus

Decussation of the
superior cerebellar peduncles

Central tegmental tract

Medial longitudinal fasciculus (MLF)

Superior cerebellar peduncle

Lamina terminalis

Preoptic area

Hypothalamus

Fornix (column)

Lenticulostriate arteries

Ansa lenticularis

Mammillothalamic tract

Choroid plexus

Hippocampus:
hippocampus proper
dentate gyrus
subiculum

Substantia nigra:
reticular part
compact part

Medial lemniscus

Spinothalamic tract

Lateral lemniscus

Fastigial nucleus

Interposed nucleus

Dentate nucleus

Figure 6.6 (Continued) **(B)** The central region of Fig. 6.6A, enlarged.

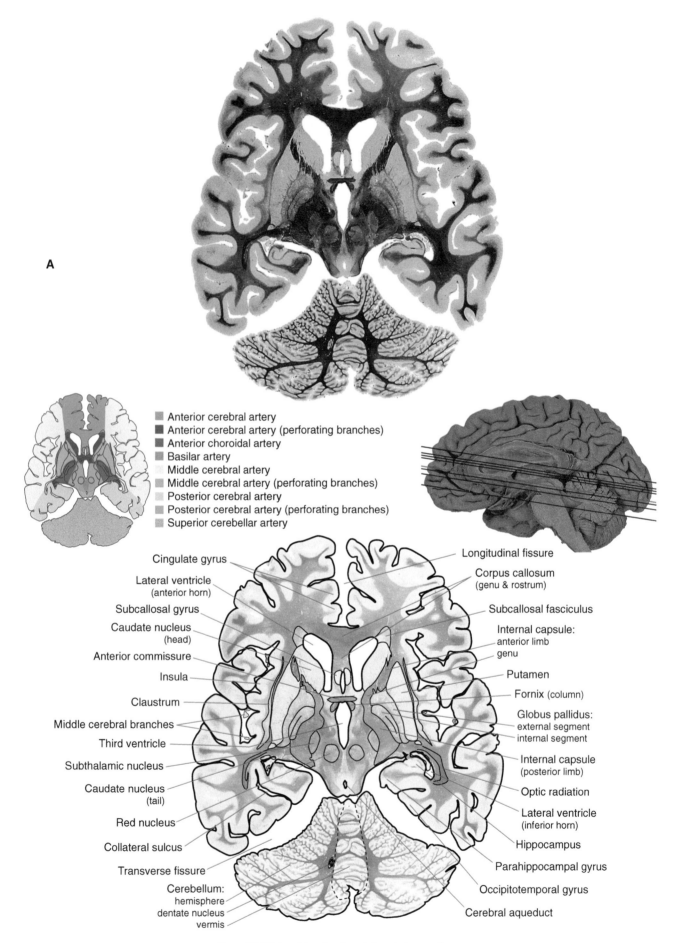

A

Anterior cerebral artery
Anterior cerebral artery (perforating branches)
Anterior choroidal artery
Basilar artery
Middle cerebral artery
Middle cerebral artery (perforating branches)
Posterior cerebral artery
Posterior cerebral artery (perforating branches)
Superior cerebellar artery

Cingulate gyrus
Lateral ventricle (anterior horn)
Subcallosal gyrus
Caudate nucleus (head)
Anterior commissure
Insula
Claustrum
Middle cerebral branches
Third ventricle
Subthalamic nucleus
Caudate nucleus (tail)
Red nucleus
Collateral sulcus
Transverse fissure
Cerebellum: hemisphere dentate nucleus vermis

Longitudinal fissure
Corpus callosum (genu & rostrum)
Subcallosal fasciculus
Internal capsule: anterior limb genu
Putamen
Fornix (column)
Globus pallidus: external segment internal segment
Internal capsule (posterior limb)
Optic radiation
Lateral ventricle (inferior horn)
Hippocampus
Parahippocampal gyrus
Occipitotemporal gyrus
Cerebral aqueduct

Figure 6.7 (A) An axial section through the anterior commissure.

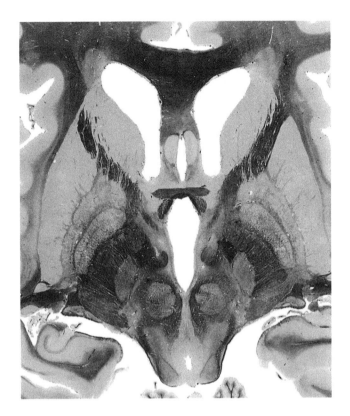

B

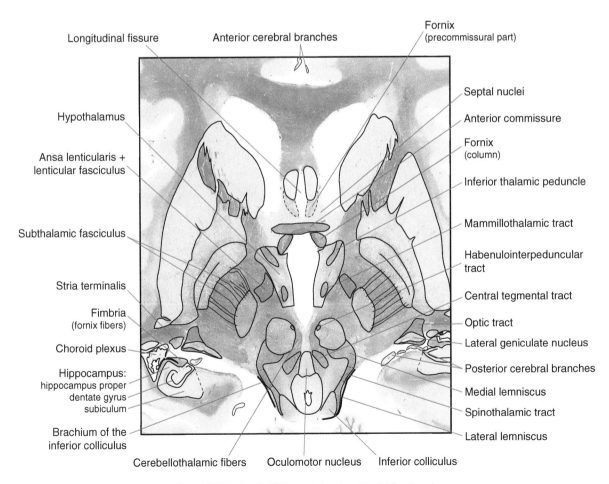

Longitudinal fissure

Anterior cerebral branches

Fornix
(precommissural part)

Hypothalamus

Ansa lenticularis +
lenticular fasciculus

Subthalamic fasciculus

Stria terminalis

Fimbria
(fornix fibers)

Choroid plexus

Hippocampus:
hippocampus proper
dentate gyrus
subiculum

Brachium of the
inferior colliculus

Septal nuclei

Anterior commissure

Fornix
(column)

Inferior thalamic peduncle

Mammillothalamic tract

Habenulointerpeduncular
tract

Central tegmental tract

Optic tract

Lateral geniculate nucleus

Posterior cerebral branches

Medial lemniscus

Spinothalamic tract

Lateral lemniscus

Cerebellothalamic fibers   Oculomotor nucleus   Inferior colliculus

Figure 6.7 (Continued) **(B)** The central region of Fig. 6.7A, enlarged.

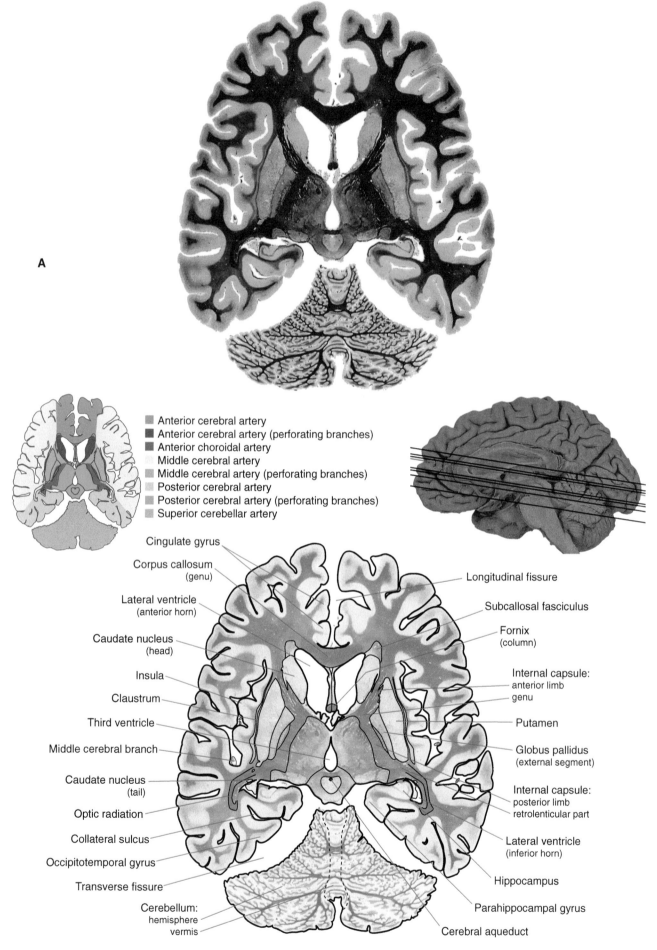

A

Anterior cerebral artery
Anterior cerebral artery (perforating branches)
Anterior choroidal artery
Middle cerebral artery
Middle cerebral artery (perforating branches)
Posterior cerebral artery
Posterior cerebral artery (perforating branches)
Superior cerebellar artery

Cingulate gyrus

Corpus callosum
(genu)

Lateral ventricle
(anterior horn)

Caudate nucleus
(head)

Insula

Claustrum

Third ventricle

Middle cerebral branch

Caudate nucleus
(tail)

Optic radiation

Collateral sulcus

Occipitotemporal gyrus

Transverse fissure

Cerebellum:
hemisphere
vermis

Longitudinal fissure

Subcallosal fasciculus

Fornix
(column)

Internal capsule:
anterior limb
genu

Putamen

Globus pallidus
(external segment)

Internal capsule:
posterior limb
retrolenticular part

Lateral ventricle
(inferior horn)

Hippocampus

Parahippocampal gyrus

Cerebral aqueduct

Figure 6.8 (A) An axial section through the interventricular foramen and posterior commissure.

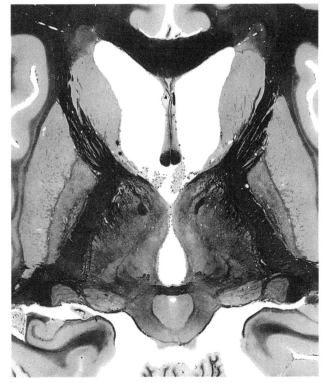

B

Septal vein

Anterior cerebral branches

Interventricular foramen
(of Monro)

Stria terminalis

Mammillothalamic tract

Thalamic nuclei:
CM, centromedian
DM, dorsomedial
LG, lateral geniculate
MG, medial geniculate
VA, ventral anterior
VL, ventral lateral
VPL, ventral posterolateral
VPM, ventral posteromedial

Stria terminalis

Fimbria
(fornix fibers)

Choroid plexus

Hippocampus:
hippocampus proper
dentate gyrus
subiculum

Septum pellucidum

Septal nuclei

Fornix
(column)

Terminal (thalamostriate) vein

Choroid plexus

Interthalamic adhesion

Reticular nucleus +
external medullary lamina

Parafascicular nucleus

Habenulointerpeduncular
tract

Pretectal area

Posterior commissure

Periaqueductal gray

Posterior cerebral branch

Brachium of the
inferior colliculus

Inferior colliculus

Superior colliculus

VA

VL

DM

VPL

VPM

CM

LG

MG

Figure 6.8 (Continued) **(B)** The central region of Fig. 6.8A, enlarged.

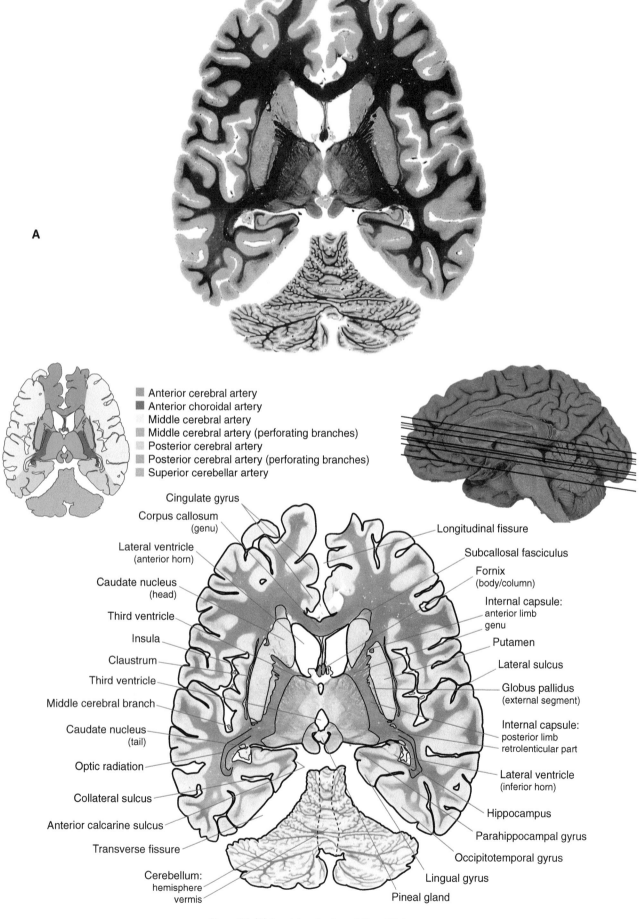

A

Anterior cerebral artery
Anterior choroidal artery
Middle cerebral artery
Middle cerebral artery (perforating branches)
Posterior cerebral artery
Posterior cerebral artery (perforating branches)
Superior cerebellar artery

Cingulate gyrus

Corpus callosum
(genu)

Lateral ventricle
(anterior horn)

Caudate nucleus
(head)

Third ventricle

Insula

Claustrum

Third ventricle

Middle cerebral branch

Caudate nucleus
(tail)

Optic radiation

Collateral sulcus

Anterior calcarine sulcus

Transverse fissure

Cerebellum:
hemisphere
vermis

Longitudinal fissure

Subcallosal fasciculus

Fornix
(body/column)

Internal capsule:
anterior limb
genu

Putamen

Lateral sulcus

Globus pallidus
(external segment)

Internal capsule:
posterior limb
retrolenticular part

Lateral ventricle
(inferior horn)

Hippocampus

Parahippocampal gyrus

Occipitotemporal gyrus

Lingual gyrus

Pineal gland

Figure 6.9 (A) An axial section through the midthalamus.

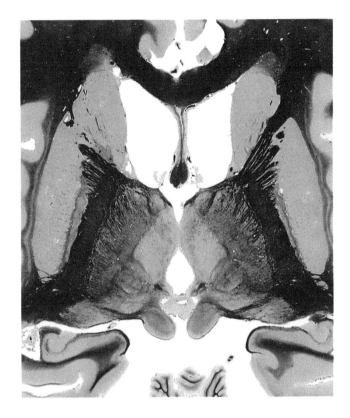

B

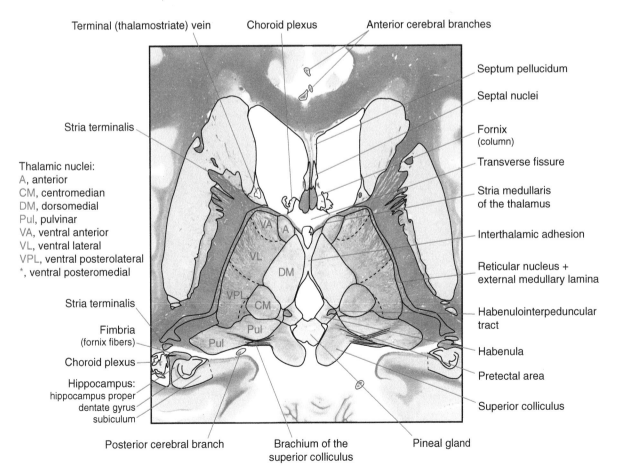

Terminal (thalamostriate) vein   Choroid plexus   Anterior cerebral branches

Septum pellucidum

Septal nuclei

Stria terminalis

Fornix
(column)

Transverse fissure

Thalamic nuclei:
A, anterior
CM, centromedian
DM, dorsomedial
Pul, pulvinar
VA, ventral anterior
VL, ventral lateral
VPL, ventral posterolateral
*, ventral posteromedial

Stria medullaris
of the thalamus

Interthalamic adhesion

Reticular nucleus +
external medullary lamina

Stria terminalis

Fimbria
(fornix fibers)

Choroid plexus

Hippocampus:
hippocampus proper
dentate gyrus
subiculum

Habenulointerpeduncular
tract

Habenula

Pretectal area

Superior colliculus

Posterior cerebral branch   Brachium of the
superior colliculus   Pineal gland

Figure 6.9 (Continued) **(B)** The central region of Fig. 6.9A, enlarged.

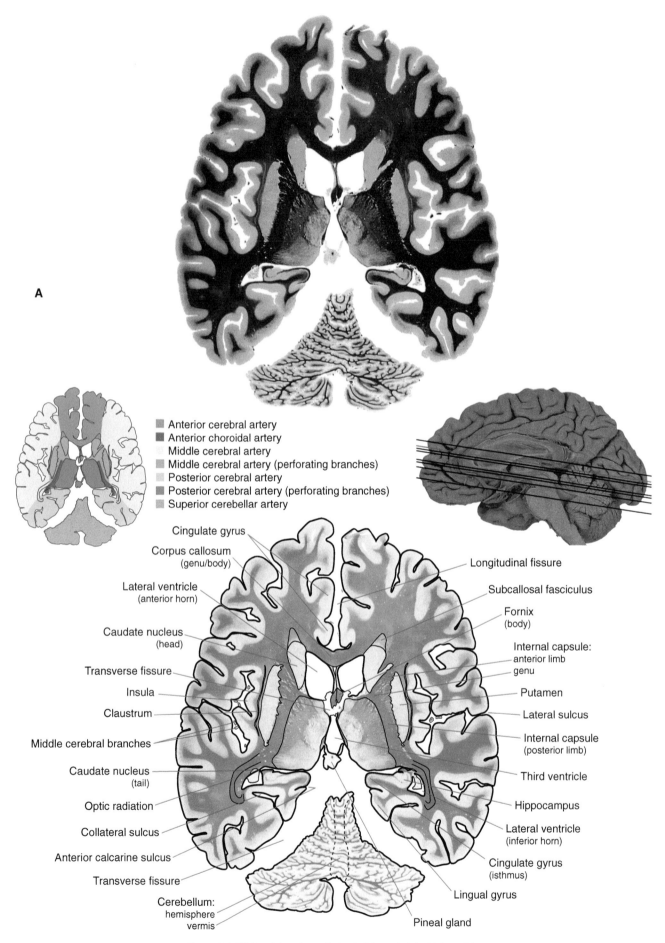

A

Anterior cerebral artery
Anterior choroidal artery
Middle cerebral artery
Middle cerebral artery (perforating branches)
Posterior cerebral artery
Posterior cerebral artery (perforating branches)
Superior cerebellar artery

Cingulate gyrus
Corpus callosum (genu/body)
Lateral ventricle (anterior horn)
Caudate nucleus (head)
Transverse fissure
Insula
Claustrum
Middle cerebral branches
Caudate nucleus (tail)
Optic radiation
Collateral sulcus
Anterior calcarine sulcus
Transverse fissure
Cerebellum: hemisphere vermis

Longitudinal fissure
Subcallosal fasciculus
Fornix (body)
Internal capsule: anterior limb genu
Putamen
Lateral sulcus
Internal capsule (posterior limb)
Third ventricle
Hippocampus
Lateral ventricle (inferior horn)
Cingulate gyrus (isthmus)
Lingual gyrus
Pineal gland

Figure 6.10 (A) An axial section at the level of the roof of the third ventricle.

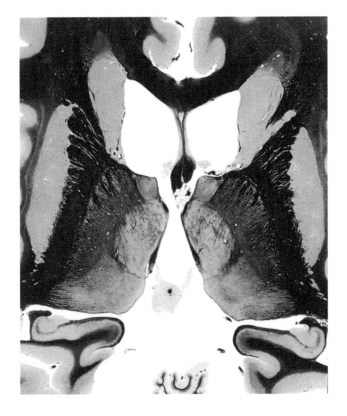

B

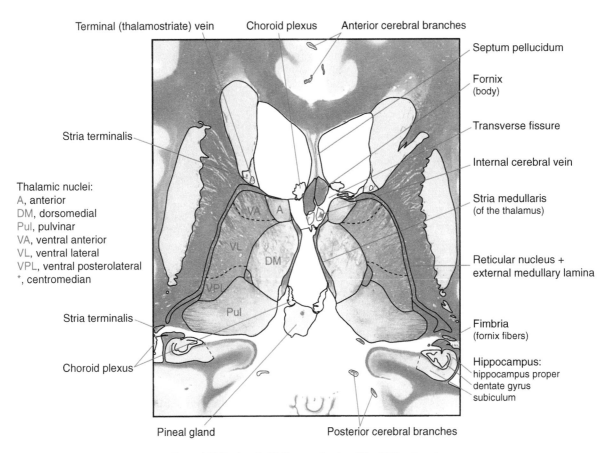

Terminal (thalamostriate) vein

Choroid plexus

Anterior cerebral branches

Septum pellucidum

Fornix
(body)

Stria terminalis

Transverse fissure

Internal cerebral vein

Thalamic nuclei:
A, anterior
DM, dorsomedial
Pul, pulvinar
VA, ventral anterior
VL, ventral lateral
VPL, ventral posterolateral
*, centromedian

Stria medullaris
(of the thalamus)

Reticular nucleus +
external medullary lamina

VA   A

VL

DM

VPL

Pul

Stria terminalis

Fimbria
(fornix fibers)

Choroid plexus

Hippocampus:
hippocampus proper
dentate gyrus
subiculum

Pineal gland

Posterior cerebral branches

Figure 6.10 (Continued) **(B)** The central region of Fig. 6.10A, enlarged.

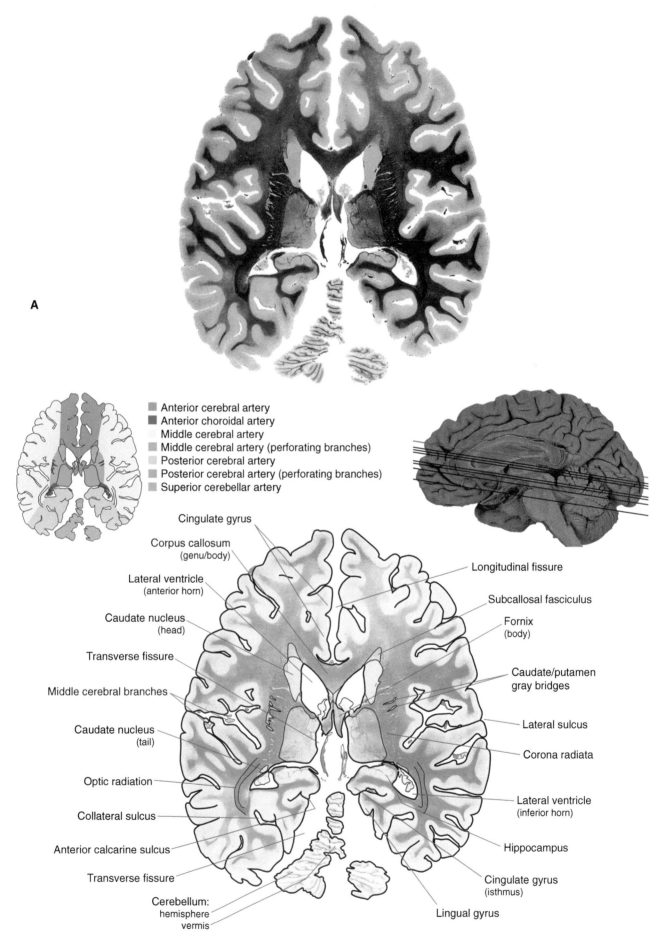

A

Anterior cerebral artery
Anterior choroidal artery
Middle cerebral artery
Middle cerebral artery (perforating branches)
Posterior cerebral artery
Posterior cerebral artery (perforating branches)
Superior cerebellar artery

Cingulate gyrus

Corpus callosum
(genu/body)

Lateral ventricle
(anterior horn)

Caudate nucleus
(head)

Transverse fissure

Middle cerebral branches

Caudate nucleus
(tail)

Optic radiation

Collateral sulcus

Anterior calcarine sulcus

Transverse fissure

Cerebellum:
hemisphere
vermis

Longitudinal fissure

Subcallosal fasciculus

Fornix
(body)

Caudate/putamen
gray bridges

Lateral sulcus

Corona radiata

Lateral ventricle
(inferior horn)

Hippocampus

Cingulate gyrus
(isthmus)

Lingual gyrus

Figure 6.11 (A) An axial section through the transverse fissure and internal cerebral veins.

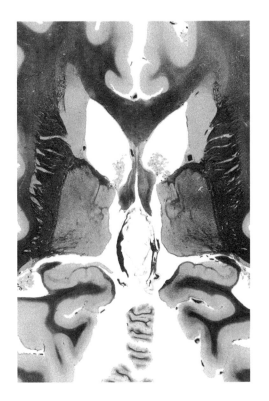

B

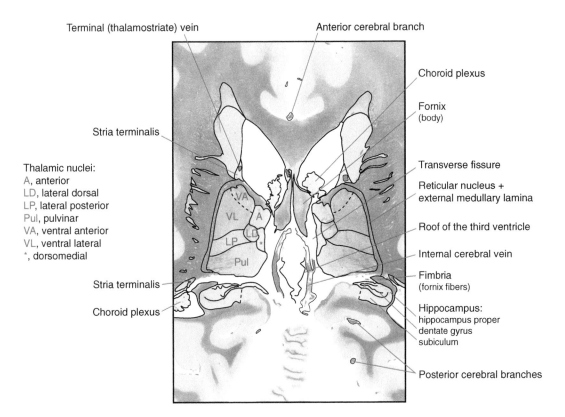

Terminal (thalamostriate) vein

Anterior cerebral branch

Choroid plexus

Fornix
(body)

Stria terminalis

Transverse fissure

Thalamic nuclei:
A, anterior
LD, lateral dorsal
LP, lateral posterior
Pul, pulvinar
VA, ventral anterior
VL, ventral lateral
*, dorsomedial

VA

VL   A

LD

LP   *

Pul

Reticular nucleus +
external medullary lamina

Roof of the third ventricle

Internal cerebral vein

Stria terminalis

Fimbria
(fornix fibers)

Choroid plexus

Hippocampus:
hippocampus proper
dentate gyrus
subiculum

Posterior cerebral branches

Figure 6.11 (Continued) **(B)** The central region of Fig. 6.11A, enlarged.

7

Sagittal Sections

This chapter, the last of three showing sections of entire human brains, illustrates para sagittal planes. Forebrain structures continue to be emphasized, but parts of the brainstem and cerebellum are indicated as well. The organization of various functional systems in the forebrain (e.g., thalamus, hippocampus) is presented in Chapter 8.

Colored diagrams showing typical areas of arterial supply in each section are provided in this and the preceding two chapters. We simplified these in two major ways. First, arterial territories are shown as sharply demarcated from each other when in reality there is significant interdigitation and overlap. Second, perforating arteries arise from all the vessels of the circle of Willis, but we lumped together those from the posterior communicating and posterior cerebral arteries and those from the anterior communicating and anterior cerebral arteries.

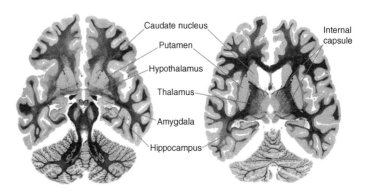

Figure 7.1 The axial sections from Figs. 6.3G and 6.3N, used in much of this chapter to indicate planes of section.

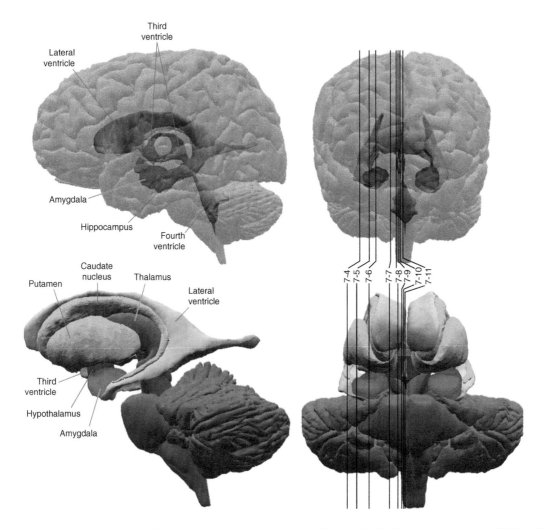

Figure 7.2 The planes of section shown in this chapter, indicated on three-dimensional reconstructions. (Courtesy Dr. John W. Sundsten, Department of Biological Structure, University of Washington School of Medicine.)

Figure 7.3 (A–P) Sixteen para sagittal sections of the right half of a brain. The sections are arranged in a lateral-to-medial sequence extending from the insula to the midline. Anterior is toward the left, so the view is as though you were backing through the brain, always looking from inside the brain out toward the lateral sulcus.

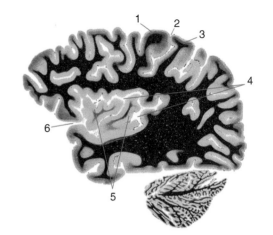

(A) The first section passes tangentially through the insula *(5)* and shows nicely how the lateral sulcus *(6)* leads to it and the circular sulcus *(4)* outlines it. The precentral *(1)* and postcentral *(3)* gyri can also be seen, separated from each other by the central sulcus *(2)*, which, cut obliquely, seems deeper than it really is.

(B) The circular sulcus *(1)* is still present, partially surrounding the insula *(2)*, but now the plane of section begins to reveal structures just deep to insular cortex—in this case the claustrum *(3, 6)*. The most lateral part of the lateral ventricle, the inferior horn *(5)*, also appears, with the tail of the caudate nucleus *(4)* cut tangentially in its wall.

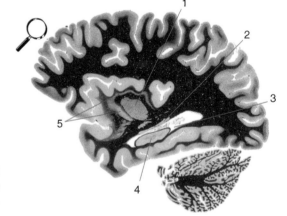

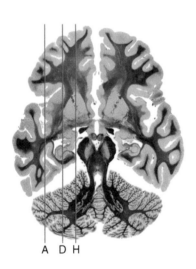

A D H

(C) Now the putamen *(1)* appears and the claustrum *(5)*, a sheet of gray matter that covers the curved lateral aspect of the putamen, appears to partially surround it in this two-dimensional view. The tail of the caudate nucleus *(2)* is cut tangentially in the wall of the inferior horn of the lateral ventricle *(3)*. Across the ventricle, the hippocampus *(4)* makes its appearance. Shown enlarged in Fig. 7.4.

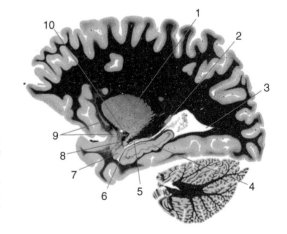

(D) The putamen *(1)* continues to increase in size, still partially surrounded by the claustrum *(9)*. The tail of the caudate nucleus *(2, 5)* is now cut in two places as it curves into the temporal lobe with the inferior horn of the lateral ventricle *(6)*. The posterior horn of the lateral ventricle *(3)* extends back toward the occipital lobe. The hippocampus *(4)* increases in size, and the amygdala *(7)* appears at its anterior end. A downward extension *(8)* of the putamen merges with the amygdala, much as the tail of the caudate nucleus merges with both in a nearby plane (see Fig. 7.3E). Fibers that have collected from the temporal lobe and will cross in the anterior commissure *(10)* mass underneath the putamen.

Figure 7.3 (Continued) Sagittal sections.

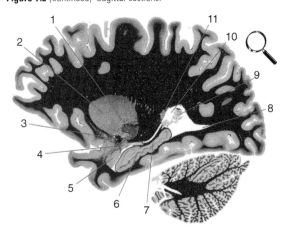

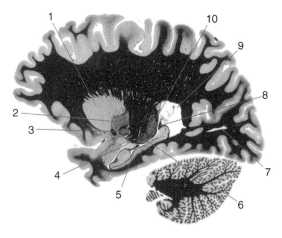

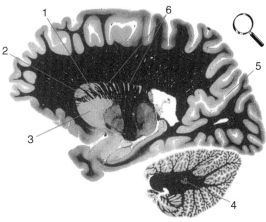

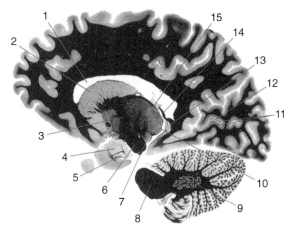

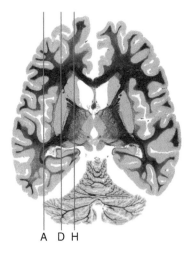

(E) The globus pallidus (*1*, part of its external segment) appears adjacent to the putamen *(2)*, with fibers of the anterior commissure *(3)* traveling beneath them. The caudate nucleus is again cut twice, once *(11)* as it curves around from the body to the inferior horn of the lateral ventricle and a second time *(4)* as it merges with the amygdala *(5)*. Fibers of the fimbria *(7)* are cut tangentially as they emerge from the hippocampus *(6)*. An enlarged mass of choroid plexus (*9*, the glomus) protrudes into the atrium of the lateral ventricle *(10)*, and the posterior horn of the ventricle *(8)* extends back into the occipital lobe. Shown enlarged in Fig. 7.5.

(F) Now both the internal *(3)* and external *(2)* segments of the globus pallidus can be seen adjacent to the putamen *(1)*. The plane of section has reached the thalamus; the pulvinar *(10)* appears, as well as the lateral geniculate nucleus *(6)* with the optic tract *(4)* ending in it. The fimbria, cut tangentially in Fig. 7.3E, is now cut in two places *(5, 8)*. The posterior horn of the lateral ventricle *(7)* appears in this plane to be a detached cavity in the occipital lobe but is in fact continuous with the atrium *(9)*.

(G) The head of the caudate nucleus *(2)* appears, with fibers of the anterior limb of the internal capsule *(1)* emerging from the cleft between it and the putamen *(3)*. Strands of gray matter *(6)* extend between the caudate nucleus and putamen, emphasizing the common embryological origin and similar pattern of connections of these two parts of the striatum. The most lateral of the deep cerebellar nuclei, the dentate nucleus *(4)*, can be seen, and the parietooccipital sulcus *(5)* is now distinct. Shown enlarged in Fig. 7.6.

(H) The head of the caudate nucleus *(2)* is cut tangentially in the wall of the anterior horn of the lateral ventricle *(1)*. The continuity between the internal capsule (*3*, here the genu) and cerebral peduncle *(6)* is apparent. In the temporal lobe, the amygdala *(4)* and the anterior end of the hippocampus *(5)* underlie the uncus, and the fimbria is in the process of separating from the most caudal bit of hippocampus *(13)* and continuing as the crus of the fornix *(14)*. The plane of section has moved deeper into the thalamus, and the medial geniculate nucleus *(7)*, pulvinar *(10)*, and nuclei of the lateral division (*15*, here the ventral posterolateral nucleus) can be seen. The dentate nucleus *(9)* is more fully formed, and visual cortex *(11)* occupies the banks of the calcarine sulcus *(12)*. The middle cerebellar peduncle *(8)* leaves the basal pons and enters the cerebellum.

Illustration continued on following page

Figure 7.3 (Continued) Sagittal sections.

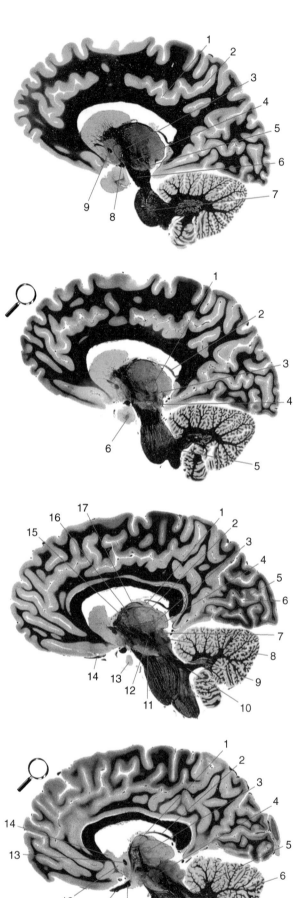

(I) As the plane of section moves medially, progressively more of the prominent sulci of the medial surface of the brain become apparent—in this case the cingulate sulcus *(1)* and its marginal branch *(2)*. The subthalamic nucleus *(4)* and substantia nigra *(5)* appear beneath the thalamus, and the continuous white-matter path from the internal capsule *(3)* through the cerebral peduncle *(6)* and into the basal pons *(7)* is shown nicely. The optic tract *(8)* proceeds posteriorly toward the lateral geniculate nucleus, and fibers of the anterior commissure *(9)* proceed toward (or away from) the midline.

(J) The subthalamic nucleus *(3)* and substantia nigra *(4)* are still apparent, and the centromedian nucleus *(1)* can now be seen in the thalamus. Fibers that formed the fimbria in previous sections of this series are now separated from the hippocampus and proceeding anteriorly as the crus of the fornix *(2)*. The inferior cerebellar peduncle *(5)* turns dorsally and enters the cerebellum. The uncus *(6)* dwindles in size. Shown enlarged in Fig. 7.7.

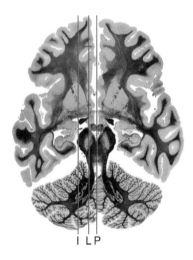

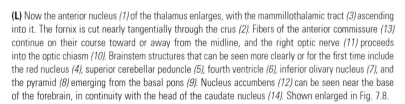

(K) Many thalamic nuclei are now distinct, including the lateral dorsal *(1)*, dorsomedial *(2)*, centromedian *(3)*, pulvinar *(4)*, ventral anterior *(15)*, ventral lateral *(16)*, and anterior *(17)* nuclei. The olfactory tract *(14)* moves posteriorly across the orbital surface of the frontal lobe. As the plane of section approaches the midline, more brainstem components begin to become apparent, including the superior *(7)* and inferior *(8)* colliculi and the red nucleus *(12)*, adjacent to the substantia nigra *(11)*. The superior cerebellar peduncle *(10)* emerges from the cerebellum, and the interposed nucleus *(9)* largely replaces the dentate nucleus. Visual cortex *(5)* lines the calcarine sulcus *(6)*. The last bit of the uncus *(13)*, the cortex covering its medial surface, is present.

(L) Now the anterior nucleus *(1)* of the thalamus enlarges, with the mammillothalamic tract *(3)* ascending into it. The fornix is cut nearly tangentially through the crus *(2)*. Fibers of the anterior commissure *(13)* continue on their course toward or away from the midline, and the right optic nerve *(11)* proceeds into the optic chiasm *(10)*. Brainstem structures that can be seen more clearly or for the first time include the red nucleus *(4)*, superior cerebellar peduncle *(5)*, fourth ventricle *(6)*, inferior olivary nucleus *(7)*, and the pyramid *(8)* emerging from the basal pons *(9)*. Nucleus accumbens *(12)* can be seen near the base of the forebrain, in continuity with the head of the caudate nucleus *(14)*. Shown enlarged in Fig. 7.8.

Figure 7.3 (Continued) Sagittal sections.

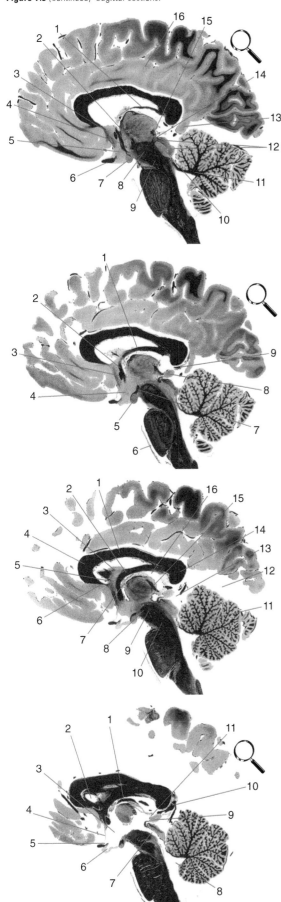

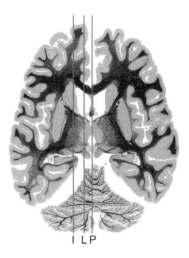

(M) The fornix is cut twice (although nearly tangentially in each instance): through the crus and body *(1)*, and as the column *(4)* ends in the mammillary body *(7)*, from which the mammillothalamic tract *(2)* emanates. The physical continuity between the septal nuclei *(3)* and the hypothalamus *(5)* is apparent. The cingulate gyrus *(16)* narrows into an isthmus *(13)* through which it is continuous with the parahippocampal gyrus. Half the fibers from each optic nerve cross the midline in the optic chiasm *(6)*, and the habenulointerpeduncular tract *(14)* descends from the habenula *(15)*. Brainstem and cerebellar structures include the superior and inferior colliculi *(12)*, periaqueductal gray *(10)*, fastigial nucleus *(11)*, and fibers of the superior cerebellar peduncle that emerge from their decussation *(9)* and pass through or around the red nucleus *(8)*. Shown enlarged in Fig. 7.9.

(N) The plane of section, now very near the midline, passes through the body *(1)* and column *(2)* of the fornix as the latter travels just behind the anterior commissure *(3)*. The hypothalamus *(4)*, including the mammillary body *(5)* and emerging mammillothalamic fibers *(7)*, forms the wall and floor of the third ventricle. Other near-midline structures include the basilar artery *(6)*, pineal gland *(8)*, and great cerebral vein of Galen *(9)*. Shown enlarged in Fig. 7.10.

(O) All the parts of the corpus callosum—the body *(1)*, genu *(4)*, rostrum *(6)*, and splenium *(14)*—are now apparent. The septum pellucidum *(3)* merges with the septal nuclei *(5)*, the fornix *(2)* is once again cut tangentially, and choroid plexus *(7)* passes through the interventricular foramen. The stria medullaris of the thalamus *(15)* proceeds posteriorly toward the habenula. Brainstem structures include the medial longitudinal fasciculus *(11)*, the decussating superior cerebellar peduncles *(10)*, and their continuation as cerebellothalamic fibers *(8)* surrounding the red nucleus *(9)*. A continuous cleft of subarachnoid space, here made up of the transverse fissure *(12, 16)* and superior cistern *(13)*, is interposed between the cerebral hemispheres and the rest of the brain.

(P) Almost exactly in the midline, an internal cerebral vein *(1)* travels posteriorly to join the great cerebral vein of Galen *(10)*. Much of the ventricular system can also be seen, including the cerebral aqueduct *(7)* and the fourth ventricle *(8)*. The section did not quite follow the entire septum pellucidum, and part of the anterior horn of the lateral ventricle *(2)* is visible through the resulting hole. The third ventricle *(3)* and its parts and boundaries are shown nicely: the lamina terminalis *(4)* at the rostral end of the ventricle, and the optic *(5)*, infundibular *(6)*, pineal *(9)*, and suprapineal *(11)* recesses. Shown enlarged in Fig. 7.11.

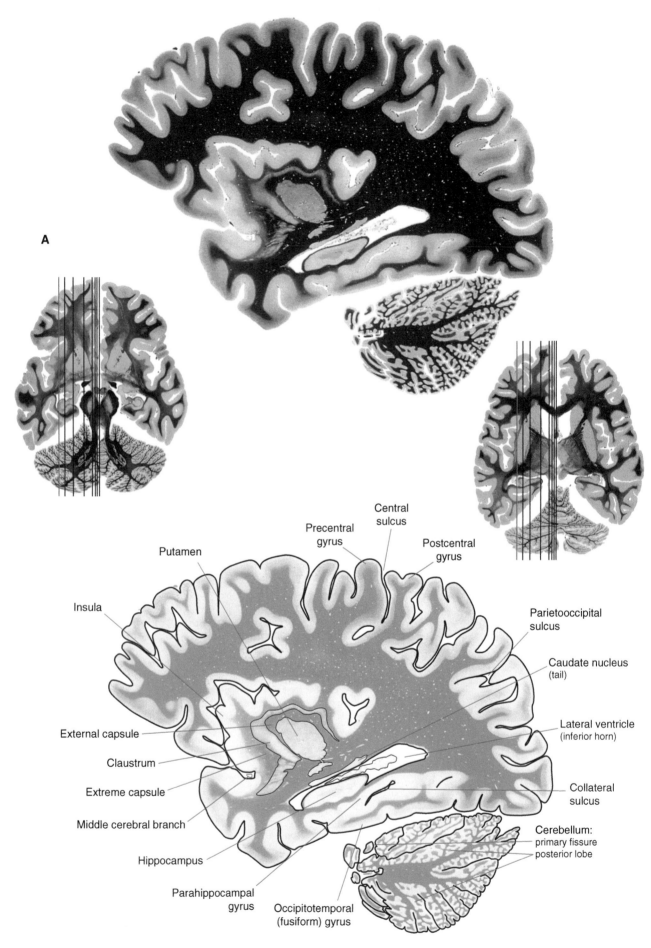

A

Central
sulcus
Precentral
gyrus
Postcentral
gyrus

Putamen

Insula

Parietooccipital
sulcus

Caudate nucleus
(tail)

External capsule

Claustrum

Lateral ventricle
(inferior horn)

Extreme capsule

Middle cerebral branch

Collateral
sulcus

Hippocampus

Cerebellum:
primary fissure
posterior lobe

Parahippocampal
gyrus

Occipitotemporal
(fusiform) gyrus

Figure 7.4 (A) A para sagittal section through lateral parts of the putamen and hippocampus.

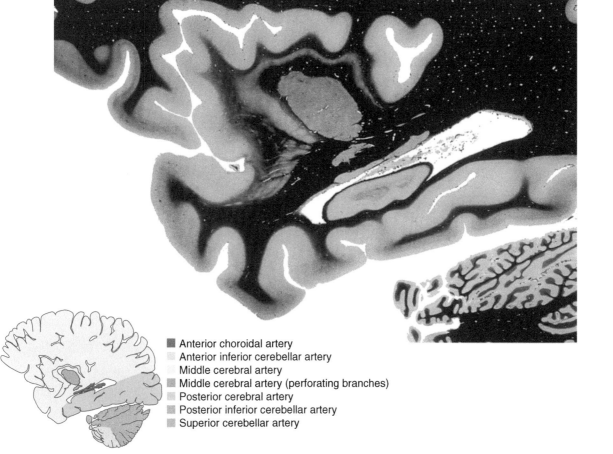

B

■ Anterior choroidal artery
▫ Anterior inferior cerebellar artery
▫ Middle cerebral artery
■ Middle cerebral artery (perforating branches)
▫ Posterior cerebral artery
▫ Posterior inferior cerebellar artery
▫ Superior cerebellar artery

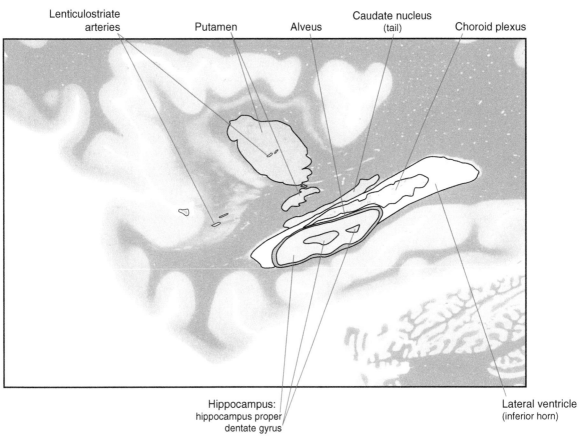

Lenticulostriate arteries

Putamen

Alveus

Caudate nucleus (tail)

Choroid plexus

Hippocampus:
hippocampus proper
dentate gyrus

Lateral ventricle (inferior horn)

Figure 7.4 (Continued) **(B)** The central region of Fig. 7.4A, enlarged.

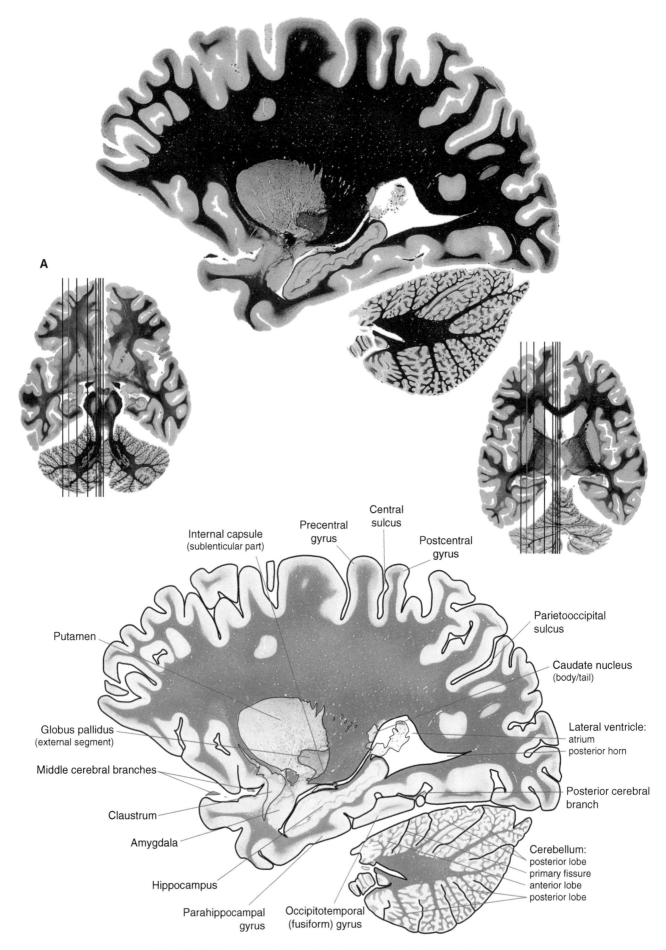

A

Internal capsule
(sublenticular part)

Precentral
gyrus

Central
sulcus

Postcentral
gyrus

Parietooccipital
sulcus

Putamen

Caudate nucleus
(body/tail)

Globus pallidus
(external segment)

Lateral ventricle:
atrium
posterior horn

Middle cerebral branches

Posterior cerebral
branch

Claustrum

Amygdala

Cerebellum:
posterior lobe
primary fissure
anterior lobe
posterior lobe

Hippocampus

Parahippocampal
gyrus

Occipitotemporal
(fusiform) gyrus

Figure 7.5 (A) A para sagittal section passing longitudinally through much of the hippocampus.

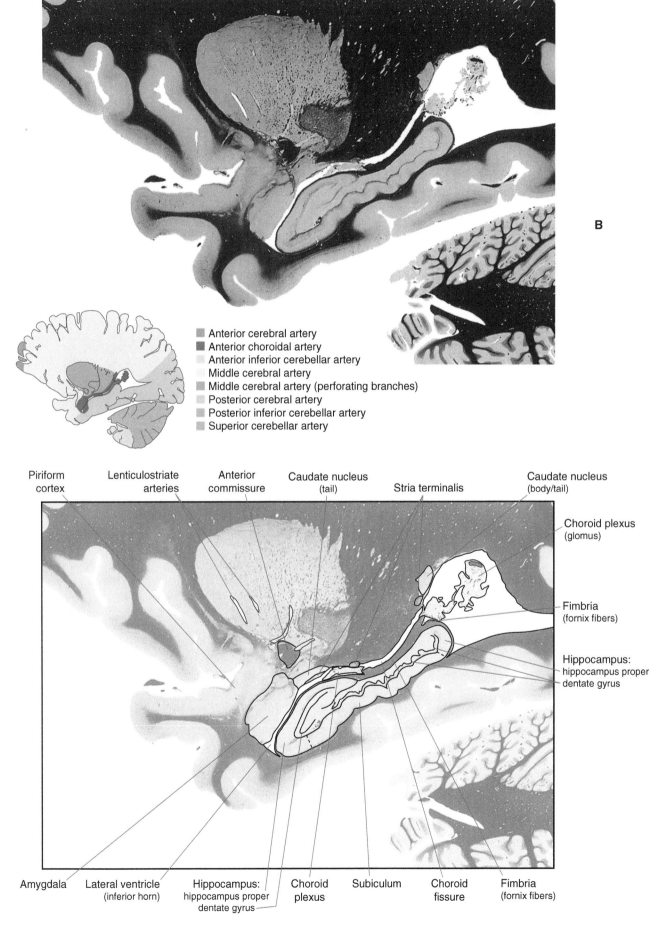

B

Anterior cerebral artery
Anterior choroidal artery
Anterior inferior cerebellar artery
Middle cerebral artery
Middle cerebral artery (perforating branches)
Posterior cerebral artery
Posterior inferior cerebellar artery
Superior cerebellar artery

Piriform cortex

Lenticulostriate arteries

Anterior commissure

Caudate nucleus (tail)

Stria terminalis

Caudate nucleus (body/tail)

Choroid plexus (glomus)

Fimbria (fornix fibers)

Hippocampus:
hippocampus proper
dentate gyrus

Amygdala

Lateral ventricle (inferior horn)

Hippocampus:
hippocampus proper
dentate gyrus

Choroid plexus

Subiculum

Choroid fissure

Fimbria (fornix fibers)

Figure 7.5 (Continued) **(B)** The central region of Fig. 7.5A, enlarged.

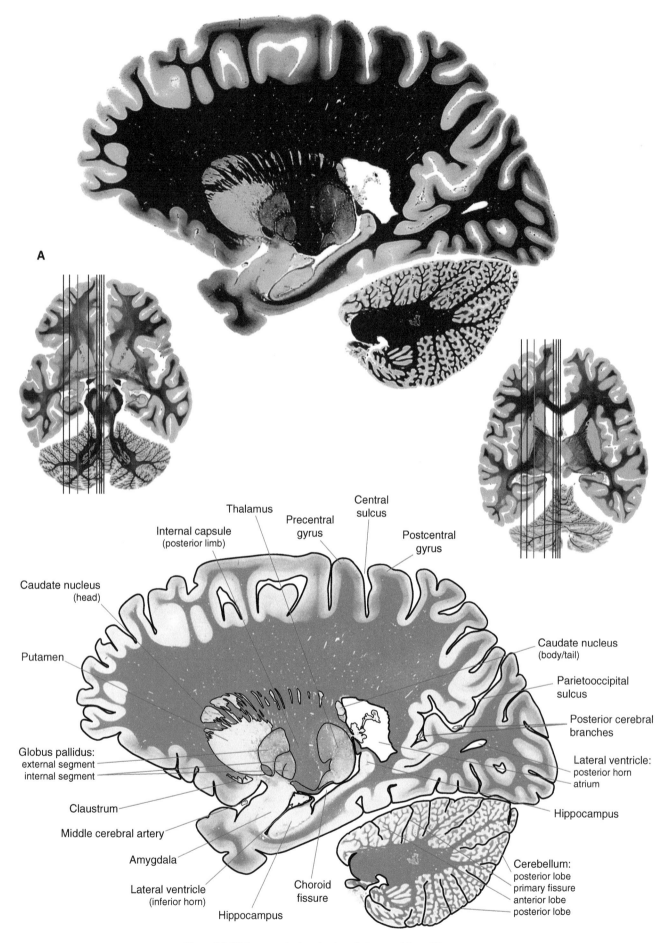

A

Caudate nucleus
(head)

Thalamus

Internal capsule
(posterior limb)

Precentral
gyrus

Central
sulcus

Postcentral
gyrus

Putamen

Caudate nucleus
(body/tail)

Parietooccipital
sulcus

Posterior cerebral
branches

Globus pallidus:
external segment
internal segment

Lateral ventricle:
posterior horn
atrium

Claustrum

Hippocampus

Middle cerebral artery

Amygdala

Cerebellum:
posterior lobe
primary fissure
anterior lobe
posterior lobe

Lateral ventricle
(inferior horn)

Choroid
fissure

Hippocampus

Figure 7.6 (A) A para sagittal section through the amygdala and hippocampus.

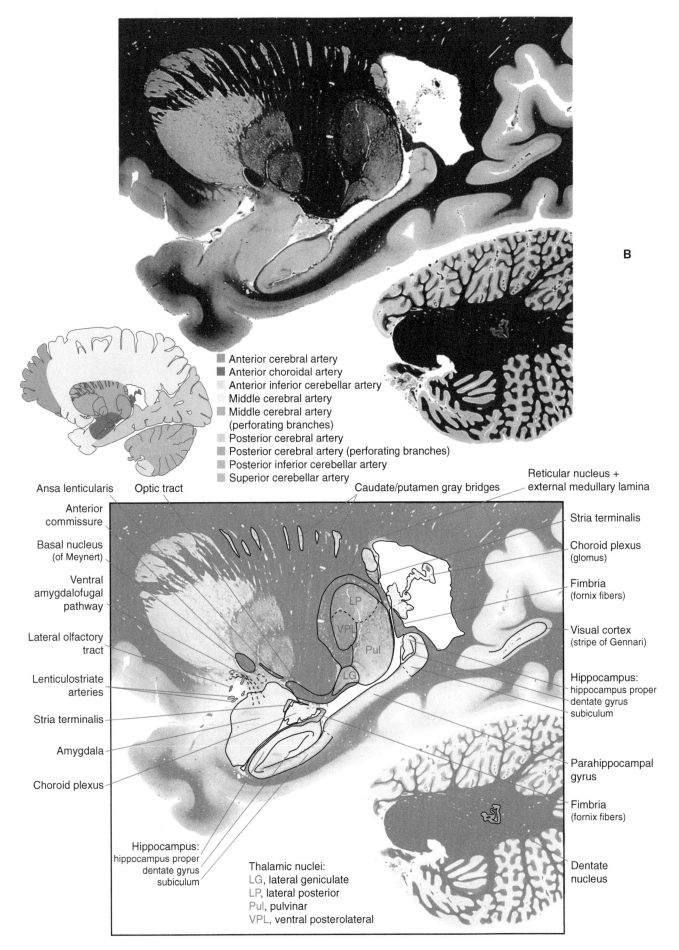

B

Anterior cerebral artery
Anterior choroidal artery
Anterior inferior cerebellar artery
Middle cerebral artery
Middle cerebral artery
(perforating branches)
Posterior cerebral artery
Posterior cerebral artery (perforating branches)
Posterior inferior cerebellar artery
Superior cerebellar artery

Ansa lenticularis
Anterior commissure
Basal nucleus (of Meynert)
Ventral amygdalofugal pathway
Lateral olfactory tract
Lenticulostriate arteries
Stria terminalis
Amygdala
Choroid plexus

Optic tract

Caudate/putamen gray bridges

Reticular nucleus + external medullary lamina
Stria terminalis
Choroid plexus (glomus)
Fimbria (fornix fibers)
Visual cortex (stripe of Gennari)
Hippocampus:
hippocampus proper
dentate gyrus
subiculum
Parahippocampal gyrus
Fimbria (fornix fibers)
Dentate nucleus

LP
VPL
Pul
LG

Hippocampus:
hippocampus proper
dentate gyrus
subiculum

Thalamic nuclei:
LG, lateral geniculate
LP, lateral posterior
Pul, pulvinar
VPL, ventral posterolateral

Figure 7.6 (Continued) **(B)** The central region of Fig. 7.6A, enlarged.

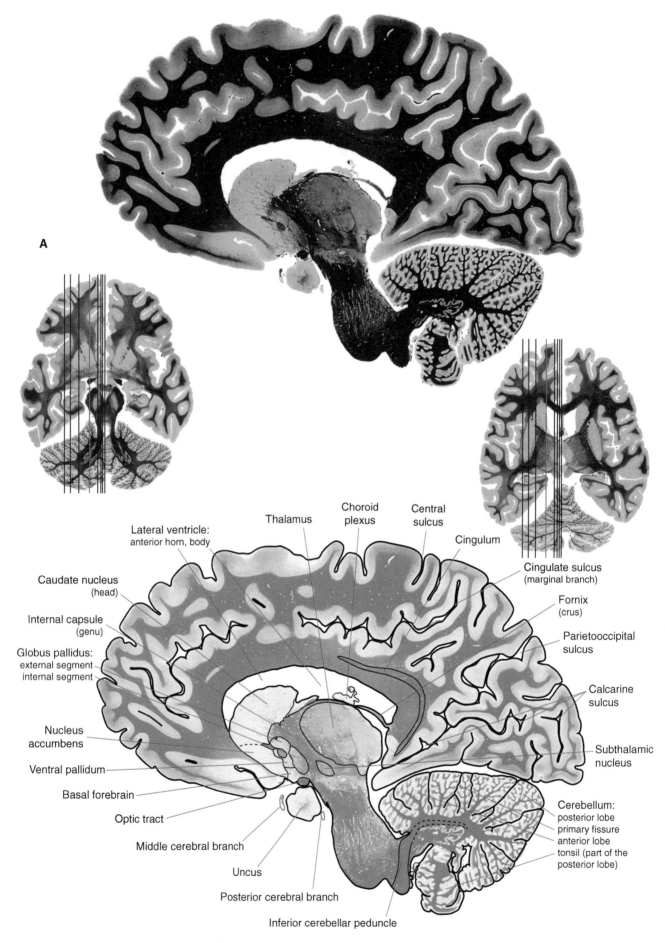

A

Lateral ventricle:
anterior horn, body

Caudate nucleus
(head)

Internal capsule
(genu)

Globus pallidus:
external segment
internal segment

Nucleus
accumbens

Ventral pallidum

Basal forebrain

Optic tract

Middle cerebral branch

Uncus

Posterior cerebral branch

Inferior cerebellar peduncle

Thalamus

Choroid
plexus

Central
sulcus

Cingulum

Cingulate sulcus
(marginal branch)

Fornix
(crus)

Parietooccipital
sulcus

Calcarine
sulcus

Subthalamic
nucleus

Cerebellum:
posterior lobe
primary fissure
anterior lobe
tonsil (part of the
posterior lobe)

Figure 7.7 (A) A para sagittal section through the uncus and the middle of the thalamus.

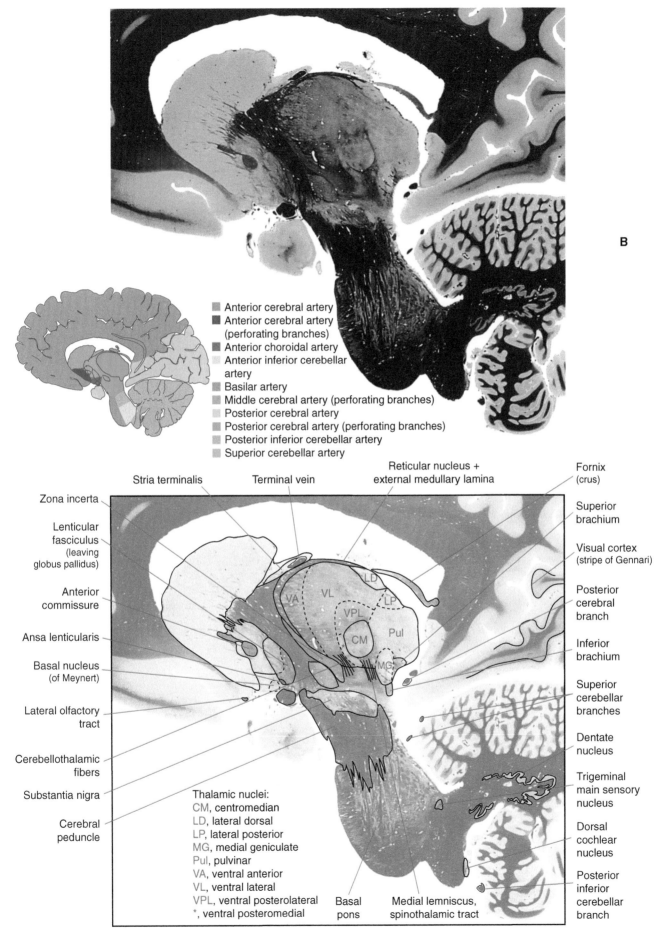

B

Anterior cerebral artery
Anterior cerebral artery
(perforating branches)
Anterior choroidal artery
Anterior inferior cerebellar
artery
Basilar artery
Middle cerebral artery (perforating branches)
Posterior cerebral artery
Posterior cerebral artery (perforating branches)
Posterior inferior cerebellar artery
Superior cerebellar artery

Stria terminalis
Terminal vein
Reticular nucleus +
external medullary lamina
Fornix
(crus)

Zona incerta
Superior
brachium

Lenticular
fasciculus
(leaving
globus pallidus)
Visual cortex
(stripe of Gennari)

LD
VL
LP
Posterior
cerebral
branch

Anterior
commissure
VA
VPL

Ansa lenticularis
CM
Pul
Inferior
brachium

Basal nucleus
(of Meynert)
MG
Superior
cerebellar
branches

Lateral olfactory
tract
Dentate
nucleus

Cerebellothalamic
fibers
Trigeminal
main sensory
nucleus

Substantia nigra
Thalamic nuclei:
CM, centromedian
LD, lateral dorsal
LP, lateral posterior
MG, medial geniculate
Pul, pulvinar
VA, ventral anterior
VL, ventral lateral
VPL, ventral posterolateral
*, ventral posteromedial
Dorsal
cochlear
nucleus

Cerebral
peduncle

Basal
pons
Medial lemniscus,
spinothalamic tract
Posterior
inferior
cerebellar
branch

Figure 7.7 (Continued) **(B)** The central region of Fig. 7.7A, enlarged.

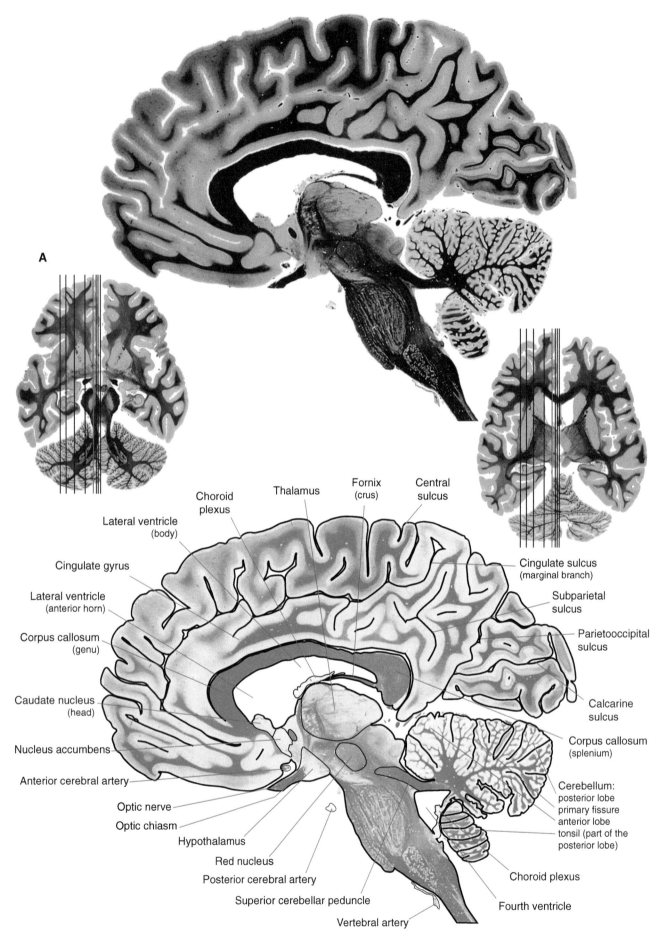

A

Choroid plexus

Lateral ventricle (body)

Thalamus

Fornix (crus)

Central sulcus

Cingulate gyrus

Cingulate sulcus (marginal branch)

Lateral ventricle (anterior horn)

Subparietal sulcus

Corpus callosum (genu)

Parietooccipital sulcus

Caudate nucleus (head)

Calcarine sulcus

Nucleus accumbens

Corpus callosum (splenium)

Anterior cerebral artery

Cerebellum: posterior lobe primary fissure anterior lobe tonsil (part of the posterior lobe)

Optic nerve

Optic chiasm

Hypothalamus

Red nucleus

Choroid plexus

Posterior cerebral artery

Superior cerebellar peduncle

Fourth ventricle

Vertebral artery

Figure 7.8 (A) A para sagittal section through the mammillothalamic tract.

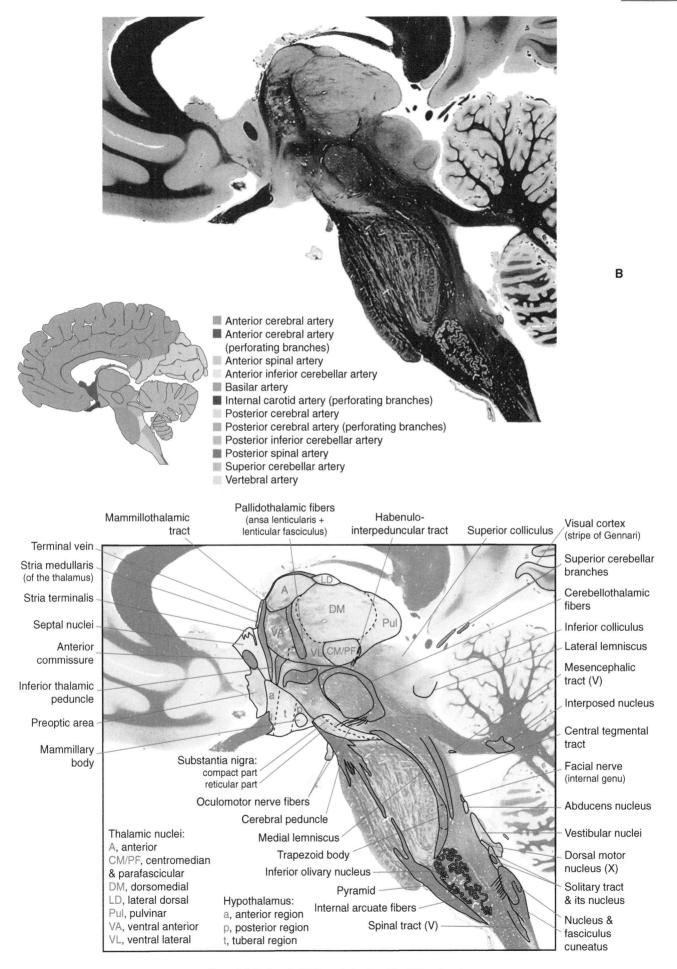

B

Anterior cerebral artery
Anterior cerebral artery (perforating branches)
Anterior spinal artery
Anterior inferior cerebellar artery
Basilar artery
Internal carotid artery (perforating branches)
Posterior cerebral artery
Posterior cerebral artery (perforating branches)
Posterior inferior cerebellar artery
Posterior spinal artery
Superior cerebellar artery
Vertebral artery

Mammillothalamic tract
Pallidothalamic fibers (ansa lenticularis + lenticular fasciculus)
Habenulo-interpeduncular tract
Superior colliculus
Visual cortex (stripe of Gennari)

Terminal vein
Stria medullaris (of the thalamus)
Stria terminalis
Septal nuclei
Anterior commissure
Inferior thalamic peduncle
Preoptic area
Mammillary body

Superior cerebellar branches
Cerebellothalamic fibers
Inferior colliculus
Lateral lemniscus
Mesencephalic tract (V)
Interposed nucleus
Central tegmental tract
Facial nerve (internal genu)
Abducens nucleus
Vestibular nuclei
Dorsal motor nucleus (X)
Solitary tract & its nucleus
Nucleus & fasciculus cuneatus

Substantia nigra:
compact part
reticular part
Oculomotor nerve fibers
Cerebral peduncle
Medial lemniscus
Trapezoid body
Inferior olivary nucleus
Pyramid
Internal arcuate fibers
Spinal tract (V)

Thalamic nuclei:
A, anterior
CM/PF, centromedian & parafascicular
DM, dorsomedial
LD, lateral dorsal
Pul, pulvinar
VA, ventral anterior
VL, ventral lateral

Hypothalamus:
a, anterior region
p, posterior region
t, tuberal region

Figure 7.8 (Continued) **(B)** The central region of Fig. 7.8A, enlarged.

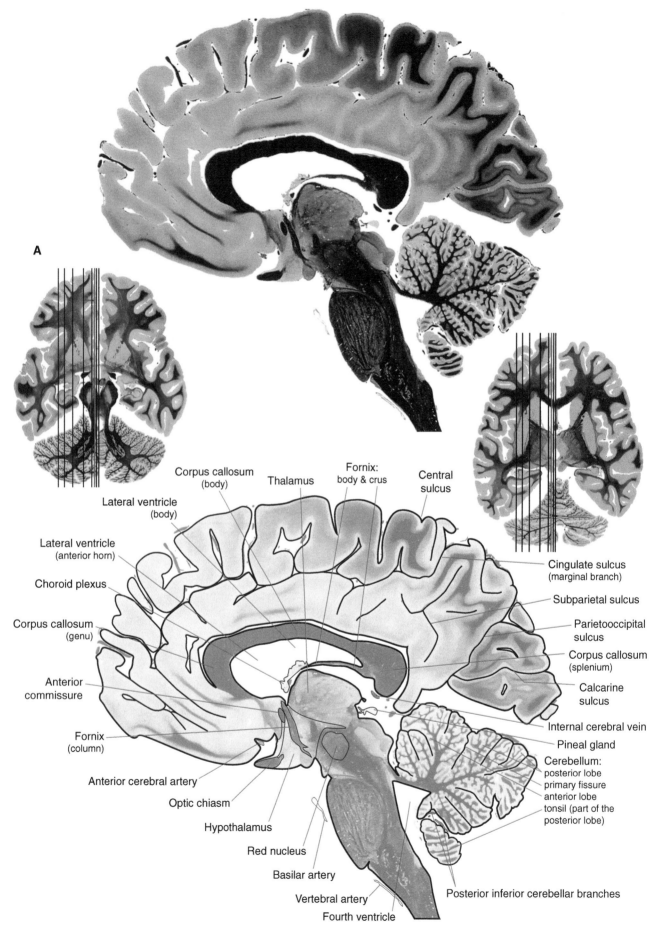

A

Corpus callosum (body)
Thalamus
Fornix: body & crus
Central sulcus

Lateral ventricle (body)

Lateral ventricle (anterior horn)

Choroid plexus

Corpus callosum (genu)

Anterior commissure

Fornix (column)

Anterior cerebral artery

Optic chiasm

Hypothalamus

Red nucleus

Basilar artery

Vertebral artery

Fourth ventricle

Cingulate sulcus (marginal branch)

Subparietal sulcus

Parietooccipital sulcus

Corpus callosum (splenium)

Calcarine sulcus

Internal cerebral vein

Pineal gland

Cerebellum: posterior lobe primary fissure anterior lobe tonsil (part of the posterior lobe)

Posterior inferior cerebellar branches

Figure 7.9 (A) A sagittal section through the column of the fornix as it enters the mammillary body.

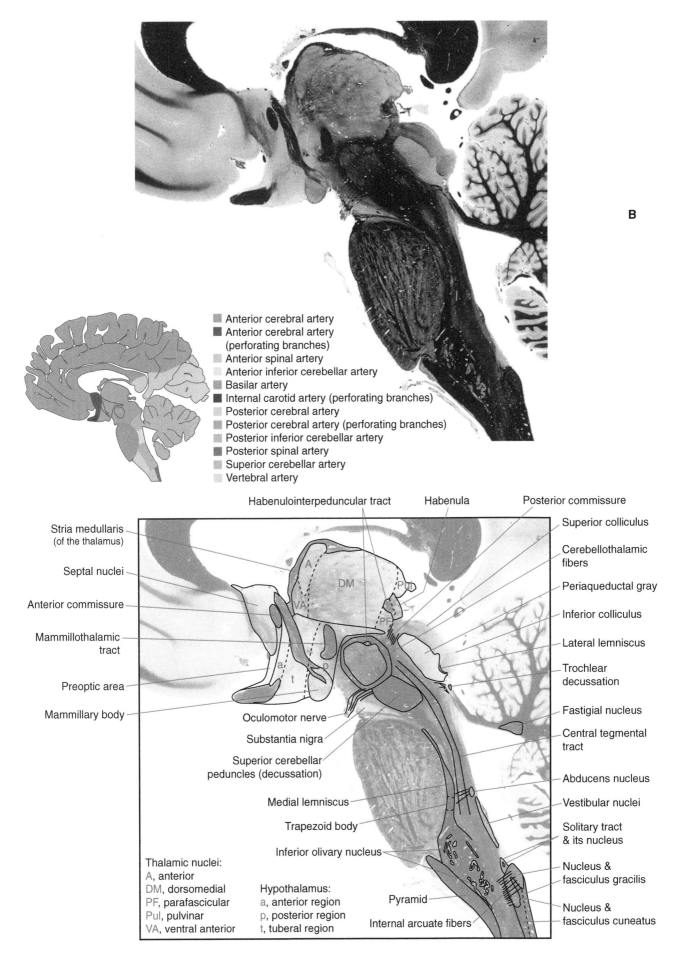

B

Anterior cerebral artery
Anterior cerebral artery (perforating branches)
Anterior spinal artery
Anterior inferior cerebellar artery
Basilar artery
Internal carotid artery (perforating branches)
Posterior cerebral artery
Posterior cerebral artery (perforating branches)
Posterior inferior cerebellar artery
Posterior spinal artery
Superior cerebellar artery
Vertebral artery

Habenulointerpeduncular tract   Habenula   Posterior commissure
Stria medullaris (of the thalamus)
Septal nuclei
Anterior commissure
Mammillothalamic tract
Preoptic area
Mammillary body
Oculomotor nerve
Substantia nigra
Superior cerebellar peduncles (decussation)
Medial lemniscus
Trapezoid body
Inferior olivary nucleus
Superior colliculus
Cerebellothalamic fibers
Periaqueductal gray
Inferior colliculus
Lateral lemniscus
Trochlear decussation
Fastigial nucleus
Central tegmental tract
Abducens nucleus
Vestibular nuclei
Solitary tract & its nucleus
Nucleus & fasciculus gracilis
Pyramid
Internal arcuate fibers
Nucleus & fasciculus cuneatus

Thalamic nuclei:
A, anterior
DM, dorsomedial
PF, parafascicular
Pul, pulvinar
VA, ventral anterior

Hypothalamus:
a, anterior region
p, posterior region
t, tuberal region

Figure 7.9 (Continued) **(B)** The central region of Fig. 7.9A, enlarged.

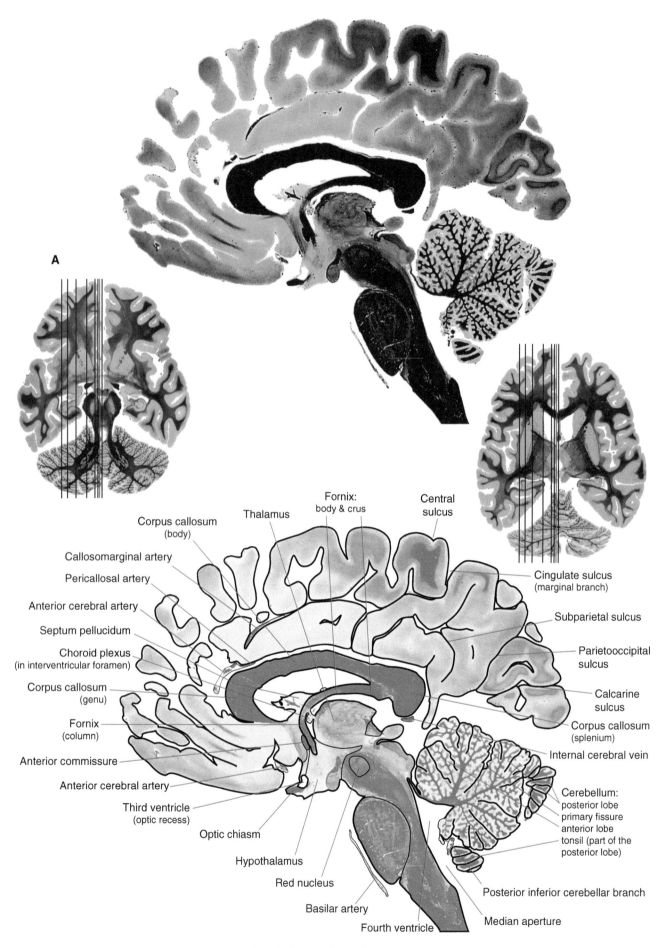

A

Corpus callosum
(body)

Callosomarginal artery

Pericallosal artery

Anterior cerebral artery

Septum pellucidum

Choroid plexus
(in interventricular foramen)

Corpus callosum
(genu)

Fornix
(column)

Anterior commissure

Anterior cerebral artery

Third ventricle
(optic recess)

Optic chiasm

Hypothalamus

Red nucleus

Basilar artery

Fourth ventricle

Thalamus

Fornix:
body & crus

Central
sulcus

Cingulate sulcus
(marginal branch)

Subparietal sulcus

Parietooccipital
sulcus

Calcarine
sulcus

Corpus callosum
(splenium)

Internal cerebral vein

Cerebellum:
posterior lobe
primary fissure
anterior lobe
tonsil (part of the
posterior lobe)

Posterior inferior cerebellar branch

Median aperture

Figure 7.10 (A) A para sagittal section near the midline.

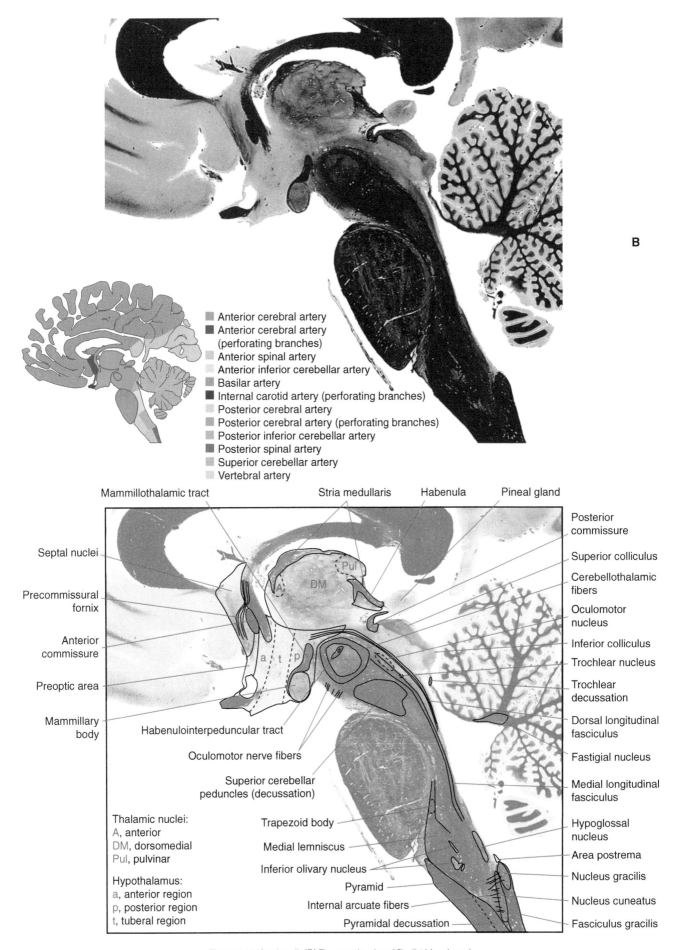

B

Anterior cerebral artery
Anterior cerebral artery
(perforating branches)
Anterior spinal artery
Anterior inferior cerebellar artery
Basilar artery
Internal carotid artery (perforating branches)
Posterior cerebral artery
Posterior cerebral artery (perforating branches)
Posterior inferior cerebellar artery
Posterior spinal artery
Superior cerebellar artery
Vertebral artery

Mammillothalamic tract
Stria medullaris
Habenula
Pineal gland

Septal nuclei
Precommissural fornix
Anterior commissure
Preoptic area
Mammillary body

Posterior commissure
Superior colliculus
Cerebellothalamic fibers
Oculomotor nucleus
Inferior colliculus
Trochlear nucleus
Trochlear decussation
Dorsal longitudinal fasciculus
Fastigial nucleus
Medial longitudinal fasciculus
Hypoglossal nucleus
Area postrema
Nucleus gracilis
Nucleus cuneatus
Fasciculus gracilis

Pul
A
DM

a t p

Habenulointerpeduncular tract
Oculomotor nerve fibers
Superior cerebellar peduncles (decussation)

Thalamic nuclei:
A, anterior
DM, dorsomedial
Pul, pulvinar

Hypothalamus:
a, anterior region
p, posterior region
t, tuberal region

Trapezoid body
Medial lemniscus
Inferior olivary nucleus
Pyramid
Internal arcuate fibers
Pyramidal decussation

Figure 7.10 (Continued) **(B)** The central region of Fig. 7.10A, enlarged.

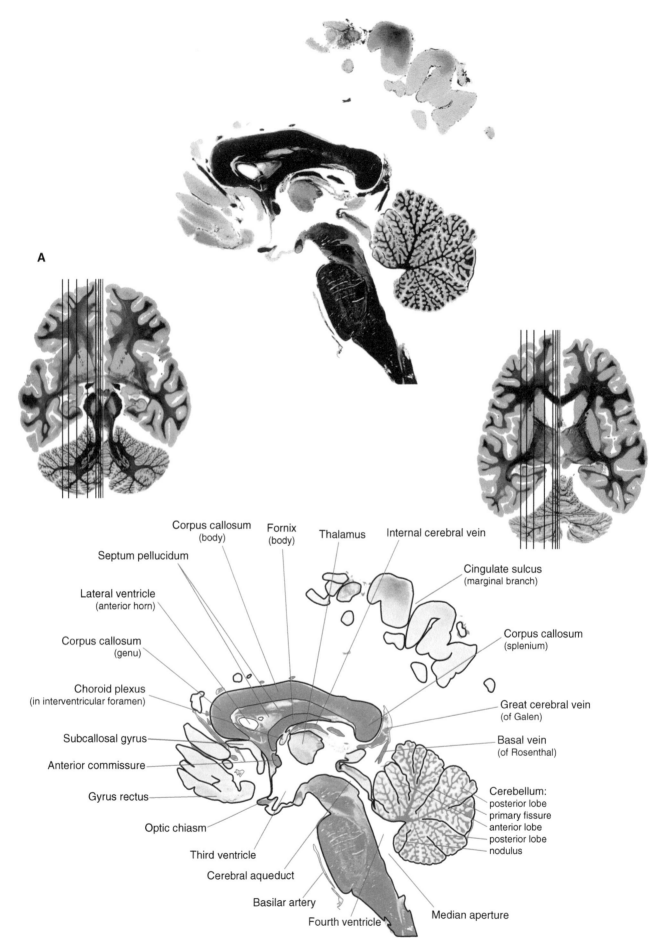

A

Corpus callosum
(body)
Fornix
(body)
Thalamus
Internal cerebral vein
Septum pellucidum
Cingulate sulcus
(marginal branch)
Lateral ventricle
(anterior horn)
Corpus callosum
(genu)
Corpus callosum
(splenium)
Choroid plexus
(in interventricular foramen)
Great cerebral vein
(of Galen)
Subcallosal gyrus
Basal vein
(of Rosenthal)
Anterior commissure
Gyrus rectus
Cerebellum:
posterior lobe
primary fissure
anterior lobe
posterior lobe
nodulus
Optic chiasm
Third ventricle
Cerebral aqueduct
Basilar artery
Fourth ventricle
Median aperture

Figure 7.11 (A) A sagittal section almost exactly in the midline.

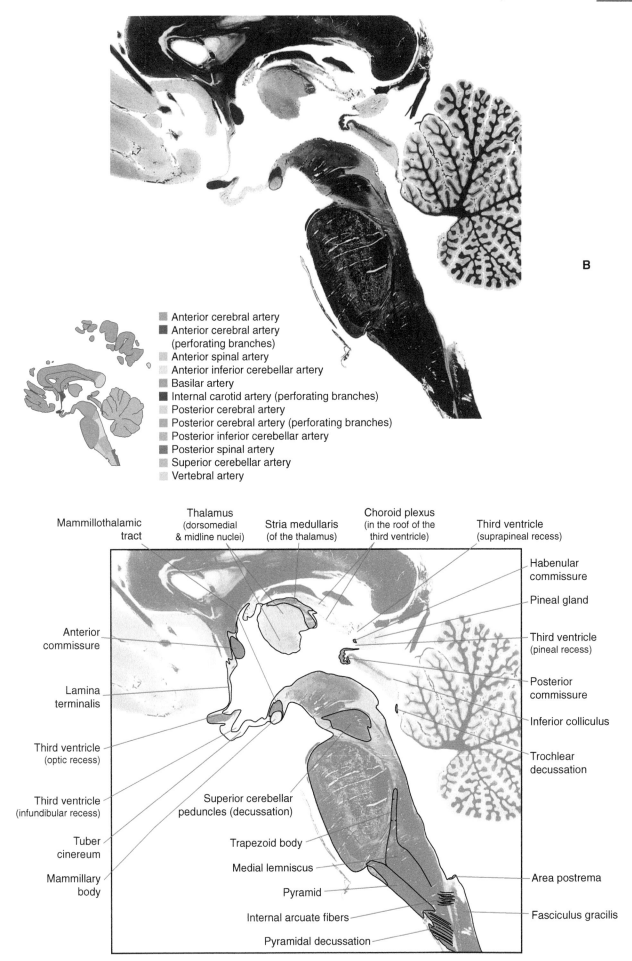

B

Anterior cerebral artery
Anterior cerebral artery
(perforating branches)
Anterior spinal artery
Anterior inferior cerebellar artery
Basilar artery
Internal carotid artery (perforating branches)
Posterior cerebral artery
Posterior cerebral artery (perforating branches)
Posterior inferior cerebellar artery
Posterior spinal artery
Superior cerebellar artery
Vertebral artery

Mammillothalamic tract

Thalamus
(dorsomedial
& midline nuclei)

Stria medullaris
(of the thalamus)

Choroid plexus
(in the roof of the
third ventricle)

Third ventricle
(suprapineal recess)

Habenular commissure

Pineal gland

Anterior commissure

Third ventricle
(pineal recess)

Lamina terminalis

Posterior commissure

Inferior colliculus

Third ventricle
(optic recess)

Trochlear decussation

Third ventricle
(infundibular recess)

Superior cerebellar peduncles (decussation)

Tuber cinereum

Trapezoid body

Medial lemniscus

Mammillary body

Area postrema

Pyramid

Internal arcuate fibers

Fasciculus gracilis

Pyramidal decussation

Figure 7.11 (Continued) **(B)** The central region of Fig. 7.11A, enlarged.

8

Functional Systems

The preceding chapters presented the major structures seen at individual levels of the central nervous system (CNS) or in particular views of the brain. This chapter is complementary, using many of the same sections and views to indicate the structures and connections involved in particular neurological functions.

We have taken a "bare-bones" approach to this task and indicated only major pathways and connections. Much of the circuitry discussed in standard textbooks has been omitted in the interest of simplicity. The locations of neuronal cell bodies, the trajectories of their axons in tracts, and the locations of their synaptic endings are usually indicated by cartoon neurons like this one:

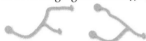

Neuronal cell body   Axon   Synaptic ending

In addition, some anatomical liberties were taken to keep the diagrams relatively simple. The number of lines was minimized by indicating axons as diverging or converging:

(Axons frequently branch to innervate multiple targets, but this is not what we mean to indicate in any of these figures; moreover, axons from multiple neurons never converge to form a single axon.)

Finally, colors were used to make it easier to follow particular pathways in each figure. Their use is consistent within a given figure but not across figures: We were unable to devise a meaningful color scheme that would accommodate all the different functional systems. Hence a given color seldom has a functional implication.

LONG TRACTS OF THE SPINAL CORD AND BRAINSTEM

- Fig. 8.1. Touch sensation and proprioception: the posterior column–medial lemniscus system
- Fig. 8.2. Pain and temperature sensation: the anterolateral system
- Fig. 8.3. Voluntary movement: the corticospinal tract

SENSORY SYSTEMS OF THE BRAINSTEM AND CEREBRUM

- Fig. 8.4. Connections of the trigeminal nerve
- Fig. 8.5. Chemical senses: gustatory system
- Fig. 8.6. Chemical senses: olfactory system
- Fig. 8.7. Connections of the eighth nerve: auditory system
- Fig. 8.8. Connections of the eighth nerve: vestibular system
- Fig. 8.9. Visual system and visual fields

CRANIAL NERVE MOTOR NUCLEI

- Fig. 8.10. Cranial nerve nuclei that innervate ordinary skeletal muscle (via cranial nerves III, IV, VI, and XII)
- Fig. 8.11. Cranial nerve nuclei that innervate muscles of branchial arch origin (via cranial nerves V, VII, IX, X, and XI)

- Fig. 8.12. Voluntary movement of muscles of the head and neck: the corticobulbar tract

VISCERAL AFFERENTS AND EFFERENTS

- Fig. 8.13. Visceral and gustatory afferents, preganglionic sympathetic and parasympathetic neurons

BASAL GANGLIA

- Fig. 8.14. The major circuit of the basal ganglia
- Fig. 8.15. Connections of the striatum (caudate nucleus, putamen, nucleus accumbens)
- Fig. 8.16. Connections of the globus pallidus
- Fig. 8.17. Connections of the substantia nigra
- Fig. 8.18. Connections of the subthalamic nucleus

CEREBELLUM

- Fig. 8.19. Gross anatomy
- Fig. 8.20. Cerebellar circuitry: afferent and efferent routes through the cerebellar peduncles
- Fig. 8.21. Cerebellar circuitry: structure of cerebellar cortex
- Fig. 8.22. Inputs to the cerebellum
- Fig. 8.23. Outputs from the cerebellum to the forebrain
- Fig. 8.24. Outputs from the cerebellum to the brainstem

THALAMUS AND CEREBRAL CORTEX

- Fig. 8.25. Projections of thalamic relay nuclei to the cerebral cortex
- Fig. 8.26. Projections of thalamic association nuclei to the cerebral cortex
- Fig. 8.27. Internal capsule

HYPOTHALAMUS AND LIMBIC SYSTEM

- Figs. 8.28 and 8.29. Connections of the hypothalamus
- Fig. 8.30. An overview of the limbic system
- Figs. 8.31 and 8.32. Major input/output pathways of the limbic system
- Fig. 8.33. Inputs to the amygdala
- Fig. 8.34. Outputs from the amygdala
- Fig. 8.35. Inputs to the hippocampus
- Fig. 8.36. Outputs from the hippocampus

CHEMICALLY CODED NEURONAL SYSTEMS

- Fig. 8.37. Cholinergic neurons and pathways
- Fig. 8.38. Noradrenergic neurons and pathways
- Fig. 8.39. Dopaminergic neurons and pathways
- Fig. 8.40. Serotonergic neurons and pathways
- Fig. 8.41. Modulatory outputs from the hypothalamus

Figure 8.1 (A) The posterior column–medial lemniscus system.

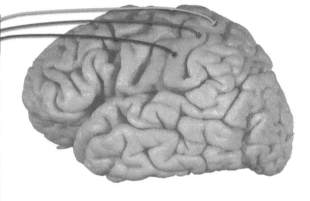

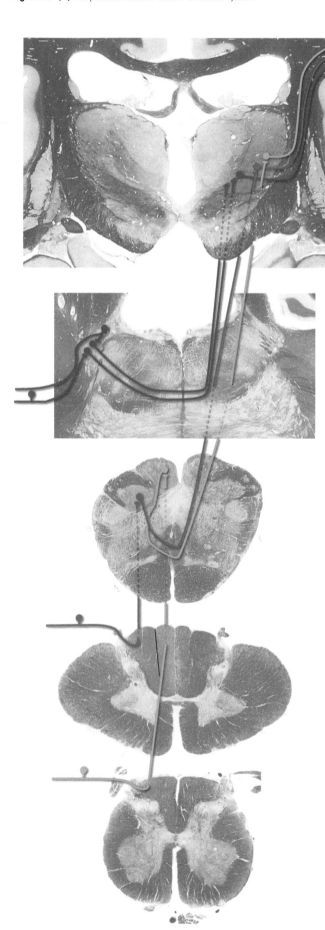

Large-diameter primary afferent fibers, conveying information about limb position and movement and the details of tactile stimuli, enter the spinal cord in the **medial division** of each dorsal rootlet (Fig. 8.1B [*inset 1*]). The principal route through which this information reaches consciousness is the **posterior column–medial lemniscus pathway**. Branches of the primary afferents ascend through the ipsilateral **posterior funiculus** (**posterior column**). Entering fibers add onto the lateral aspect of fibers already present in the posterior funiculus (Fig. 8.1B [*inset 2*]), so by the time they reach the medulla, fibers conveying information from the leg are located in the more medial **fasciculus gracilis** and those conveying information from the arm in the more lateral **fasciculus cuneatus**. This is the beginning of a **somatotopic** arrangement that is maintained (with some twists and turns) throughout the remainder of this pathway.

Each posterior column terminates in the ipsilateral **posterior column nuclei** (**nuclei gracilis** and **cuneatus**), whose axons cross the midline and ascend to the **ventral posterolateral nucleus** (**VPL**) of the thalamus. VPL in turn projects to **primary somatosensory cortex** in the **postcentral gyrus**.

An analogous pathway conveying similar information from the face involves primary afferents with cell bodies in the **trigeminal ganglion** and the **mesencephalic nucleus** of the trigeminal nerve (see Fig. 8.4). Central processes of these afferents terminate in the **main sensory nucleus** of the trigeminal nerve. Their axons cross the midline, join the somatotopically appropriate region of the medial lemniscus, and ascend to the **ventral posteromedial nucleus** (**VPM**) of the thalamus. VPM in turn projects to the face area of the postcentral gyrus.

Tactile and proprioceptive information can also reach consciousness by way of postsynaptic fibers arising from spinal cord neurons. Some of these projections travel in the posterior columns, but others travel in pathways outside the posterior funiculus (e.g., tactile information in the anterolateral system described in Fig. 8.2), so posterior column damage does not cause total loss of touch and position sensation.

Figure 8.1 (Continued) **(B)** The posterior column–medial lemniscus system, continued. (Inset 2 redrawn from Mettler FA. *Neuroanatomy*. 2nd ed. St Louis: Mosby; 1948.)

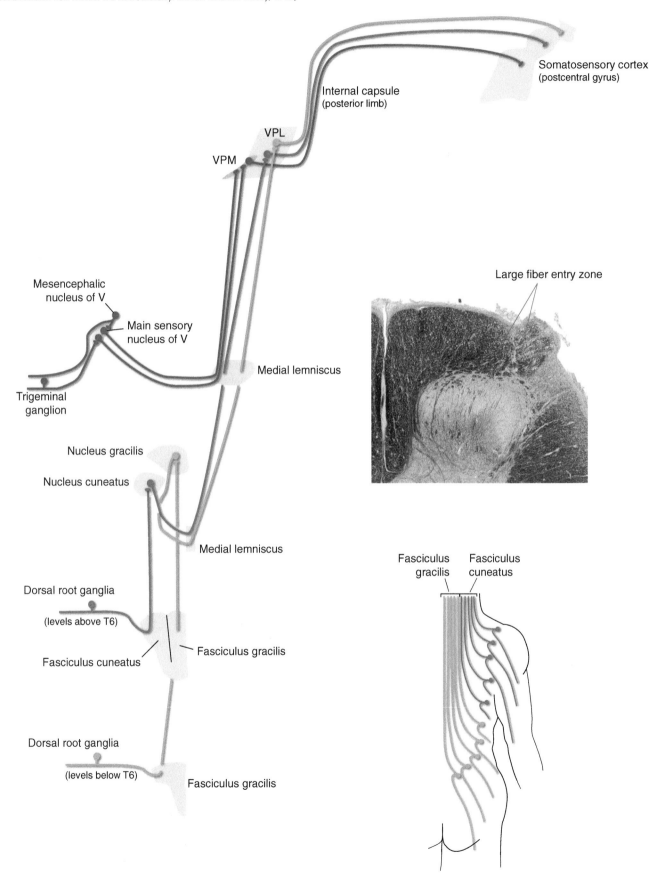

Somatosensory cortex
(postcentral gyrus)

Internal capsule
(posterior limb)

VPL

VPM

Large fiber entry zone

Mesencephalic
nucleus of V

Main sensory
nucleus of V

Medial lemniscus

Trigeminal
ganglion

Nucleus gracilis

Nucleus cuneatus

Medial lemniscus

Dorsal root ganglia

(levels above T6)

Fasciculus gracilis

Fasciculus
gracilis

Fasciculus
cuneatus

Fasciculus cuneatus

Fasciculus gracilis

Dorsal root ganglia

(levels below T6)

Fasciculus gracilis

Figure 8.2 (A) The anterolateral system.

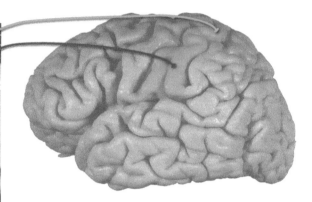

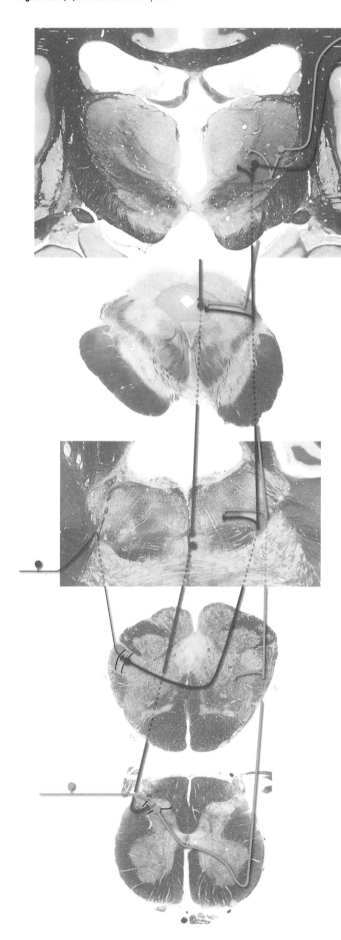

Small-diameter afferent fibers conveying pain and temperature (and a limited amount of tactile) information enter the spinal cord in the **lateral division** of each dorsal rootlet. The principal route through which this information reaches consciousness is the **spinothalamic tract**. Primary afferents terminate on tract cells in the **posterior horn**, whose axons cross and join the spinothalamic tract, adding onto the ventromedial aspect of fibers already present. This is the beginning of a **somatotopic** arrangement that is maintained (relatively unchanged) throughout the pathway. Spinothalamic fibers then ascend to **VPL** of the thalamus, which projects to **primary somatosensory cortex** in the **postcentral gyrus**.

The analogous pathway dealing with the face involves **trigeminal ganglion cells** whose central processes descend through the **spinal trigeminal tract** to caudal parts of the **spinal trigeminal nucleus** (see Fig. 8.4). Axons of these second-order neurons cross the midline, join the somatotopically appropriate region of the spinothalamic tract, and ascend to **VPM** of the thalamus. VPM in turn projects to the face area of the postcentral gyrus.

Pain and temperature information is in fact more widely distributed than this simplified account would indicate and reaches the reticular formation, additional thalamic nuclei, and multiple cortical areas. Several additional pain pathways travel with or near the spinothalamic tract, and all are commonly referred to collectively as the **anterolateral system**.

Access to the spinothalamic tract is modulated by small neurons of the **substantia gelatinosa** (and at several other sites). One important pain-control pathway originates in the **periaqueductal gray matter** of the midbrain and involves a relay in the **raphe nuclei** (see Fig. 8.40) and nearby **reticular formation** of the medulla and caudal pons. The periaqueductal gray sums up anterolateral and limbic inputs to help determine when to turn this pathway on.

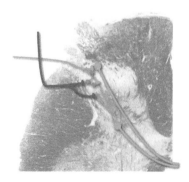

Figure 8.2 (Continued) **(B)** The anterolateral system, continued.

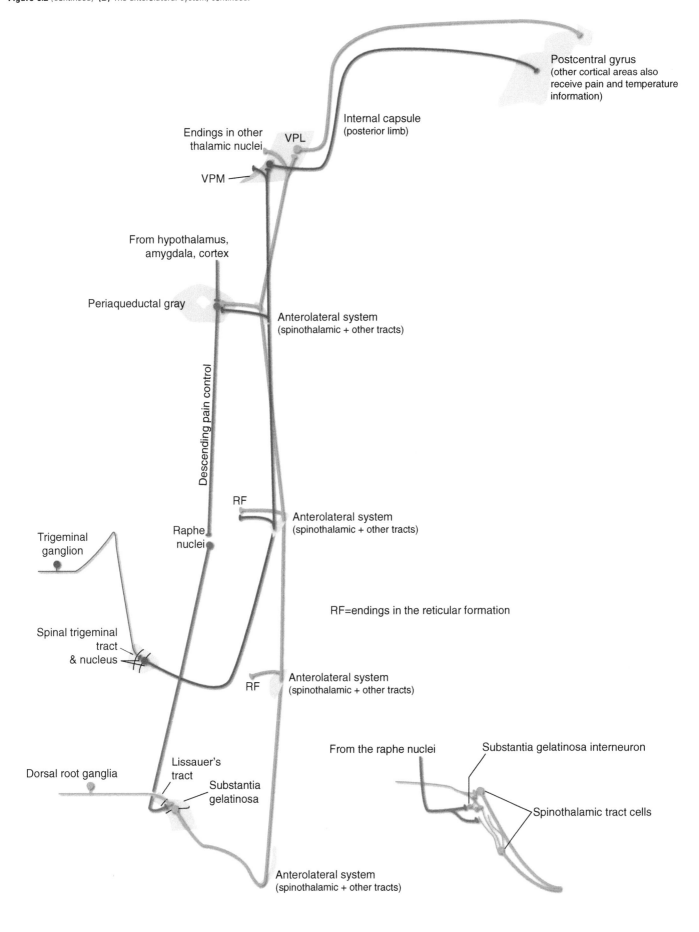

Figure 8.3 (A) The corticospinal tract.

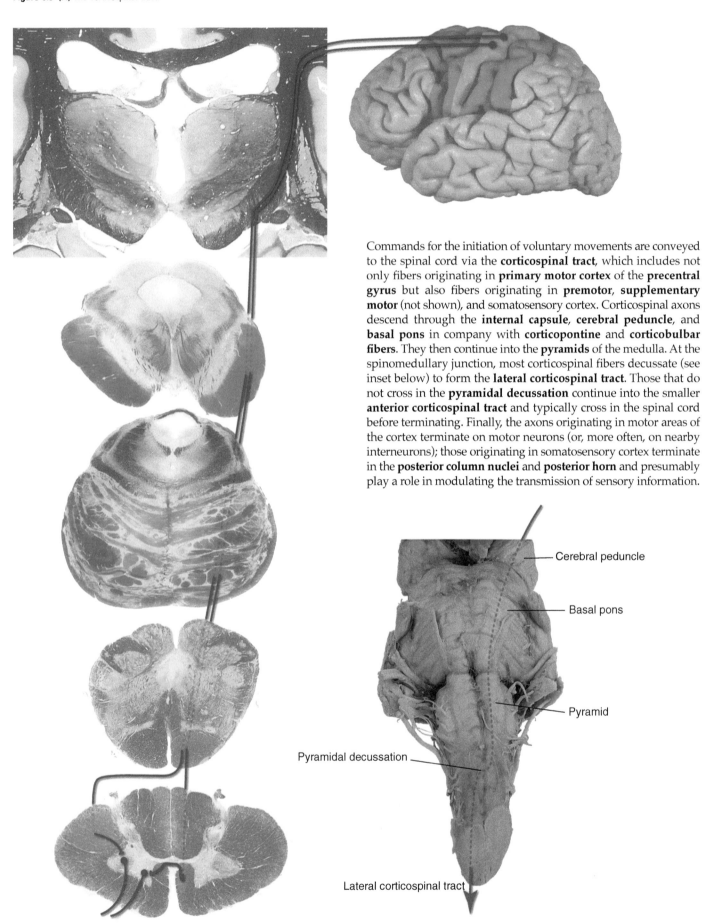

Commands for the initiation of voluntary movements are conveyed to the spinal cord via the **corticospinal tract**, which includes not only fibers originating in **primary motor cortex** of the **precentral gyrus** but also fibers originating in **premotor**, **supplementary motor** (not shown), and somatosensory cortex. Corticospinal axons descend through the **internal capsule**, **cerebral peduncle**, and **basal pons** in company with **corticopontine** and **corticobulbar fibers**. They then continue into the **pyramids** of the medulla. At the spinomedullary junction, most corticospinal fibers decussate (see inset below) to form the **lateral corticospinal tract**. Those that do not cross in the **pyramidal decussation** continue into the smaller **anterior corticospinal tract** and typically cross in the spinal cord before terminating. Finally, the axons originating in motor areas of the cortex terminate on motor neurons (or, more often, on nearby interneurons); those originating in somatosensory cortex terminate in the **posterior column nuclei** and **posterior horn** and presumably play a role in modulating the transmission of sensory information.

Cerebral peduncle

Basal pons

Pyramid

Pyramidal decussation

Lateral corticospinal tract

Figure 8.3 (Continued) **(B)** The corticospinal tract, continued.

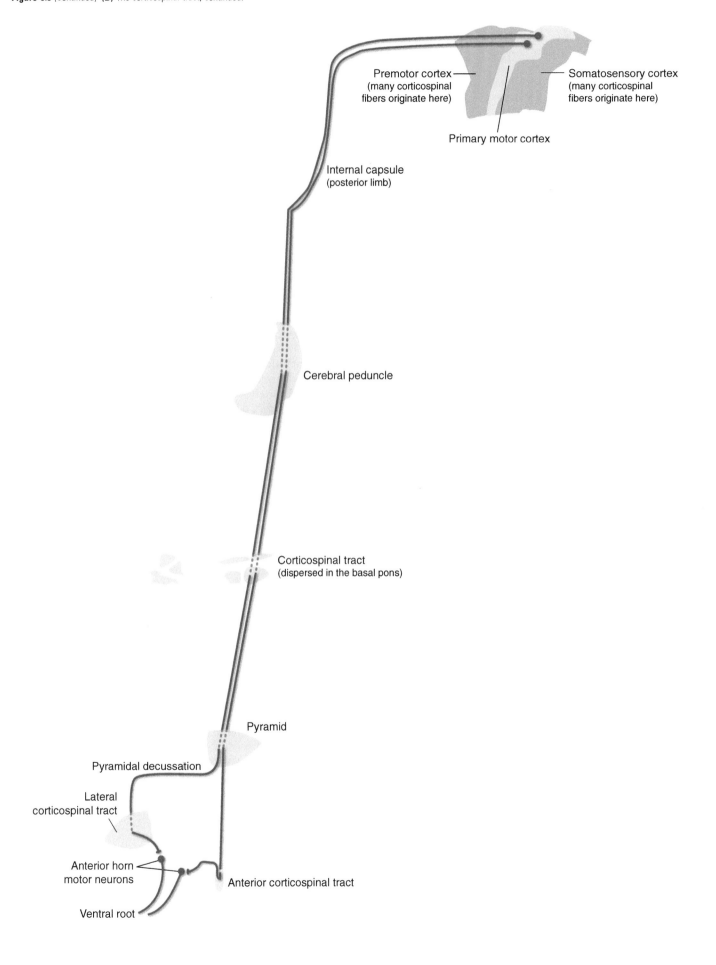

Figure 8.4 (A) Central connections of the trigeminal nerve.

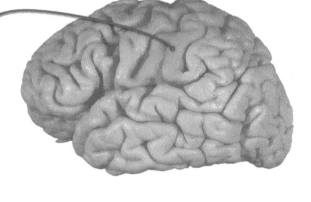

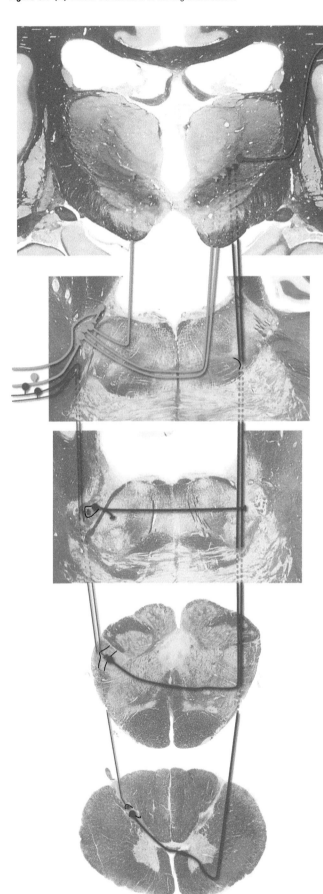

The **trigeminal nerve** conveys somatic sensory information from most of the head, and it is also the motor nerve for most muscles of mastication. Connections of the **trigeminal motor nucleus** are noted in Fig. 8.11, and sensory connections are reviewed here. The connections of somatosensory components bear many similarities to those of spinal nerves (see Figs. 8.1 and 8.2), but there are important differences as well.

Large-diameter trigeminal afferents have cell bodies in the **trigeminal ganglion** or in the **mesencephalic nucleus** of the trigeminal (in effect, a bit of the trigeminal ganglion located within the CNS instead of in the periphery). Many central processes terminate in the **main sensory nucleus** of the trigeminal, which in turn projects through the contralateral **medial lemniscus** to VPM of the thalamus. (Part of the main sensory nucleus, where the mouth is represented, sends an uncrossed projection, the dorsal trigeminal tract, to the ipsilateral VPM; the functional significance of this uncrossed projection is unclear.) Other central processes project to the trigeminal motor nucleus as part of the masseter stretch reflex arc, or to **trigeminocerebellar** neurons in rostral parts of the **spinal trigeminal nucleus**.

Small-diameter trigeminal afferents, all with cell bodies in the trigeminal ganglion, travel through the **spinal trigeminal tract** to termination sites at various levels of the spinal trigeminal nucleus. The most caudal levels of the spinal trigeminal tract and nucleus are essentially rostral extensions of **Lissauer's tract** and the **posterior horn**, respectively, of the upper cervical spinal cord and have an analogous function. That is, they convey information about facial pain and temperature to VPM. This seemingly odd location of the second-order neurons for facial pain and temperature ensures that, moving from the spinal cord into the brainstem, there is a smooth continuation of the somatotopic pain/temperature map. More rostral levels participate in trigeminocerebellar projections and in other reflexes, notably the bilateral **blink reflex** in response to an object touching either cornea.

Figure 8.4 (Continued) **(B)** Central connections of the trigeminal nerve, continued.

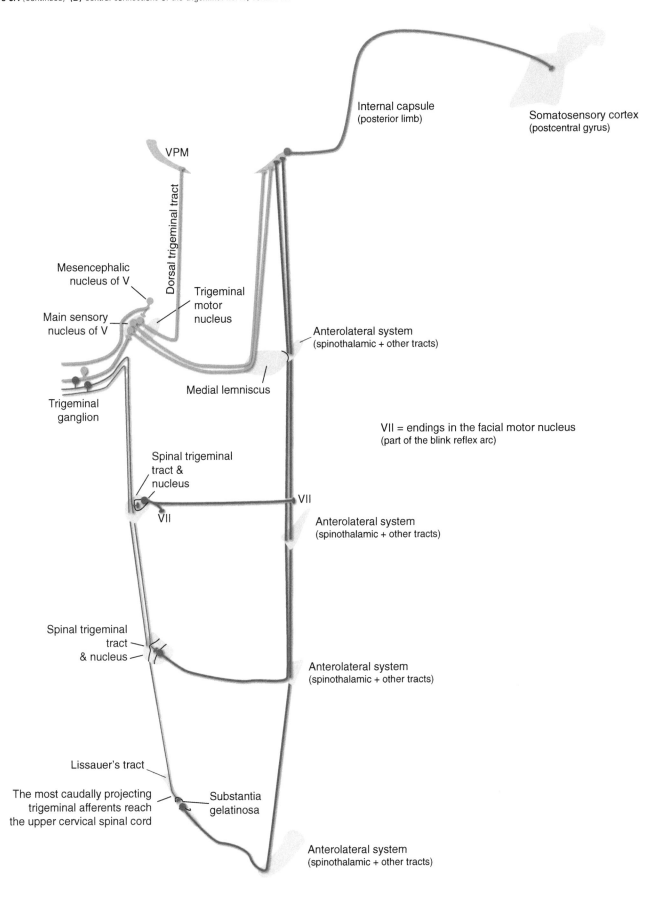

Figure 8.5 (A) Central gustatory connections.

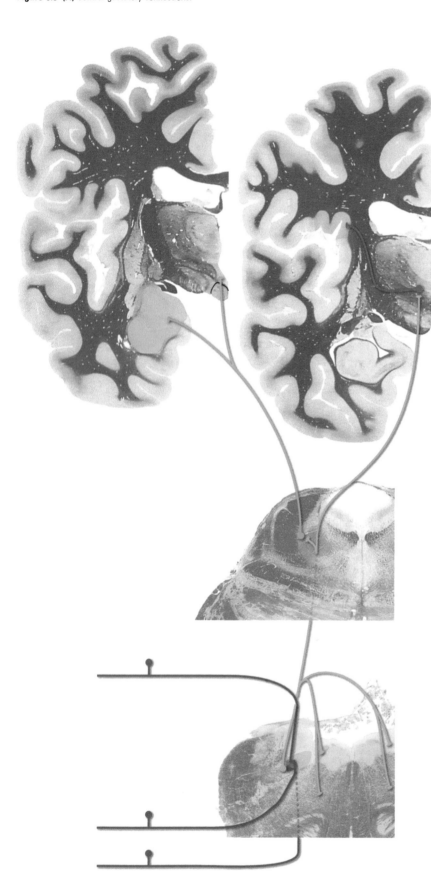

What we commonly refer to as "taste" is actually a complex sensation. Sensory information from **taste buds** is an important contributor, but this is combined with information from **olfactory receptors** (aroma) and **trigeminal endings** (texture, spiciness, temperature). To avoid ambiguity the sensations initiated in taste buds are referred to as **gustatory** sensations.

Receptor cells in taste buds synapse on peripheral processes of fibers in the **facial (VII)**, **glossopharyngeal (IX)**, and **vagus (X)** nerves. Facial endings innervate taste buds on the anterior two thirds of the tongue, glossopharyngeal endings innervate those on the posterior third, and vagal endings innervate scattered taste buds of the epiglottis and esophagus. Central processes of these gustatory primary afferents travel through the **solitary tract** to reach second-order neurons in rostral parts of the **nucleus of the solitary tract**.

Second-order gustatory neurons influence feeding-related behavior and autonomic functions by projecting to the **dorsal motor nucleus of the vagus**, to the nearby **reticular formation**, and even to **preganglionic sympathetic neurons** in the spinal cord (not indicated in the accompanying figures). Conscious perception of taste is mediated by a largely uncrossed projection from the nucleus of the solitary tract to the thalamus (**VPM**), and from there to the **gustatory cortex** in the **insula** and the adjacent **frontal operculum**.

Gustatory information also reaches the **hypothalamus** and **amygdala**, where it influences metabolic regulation and feelings of hunger, satiety, and pleasantness or unpleasantness accompanying various tastes. The route utilized involves, at least partially, a projection from gustatory cortex to the amygdala. In many animals, gustatory information is also transmitted to the hypothalamus and amygdala more directly, through a projection from the **parabrachial nuclei** of the pontine reticular formation. Whether this pathway exists in humans is doubtful, as implied by question marks in Fig. 8.5B.

Figure 8.5 (Continued) **(B)** Central gustatory connections, continued.

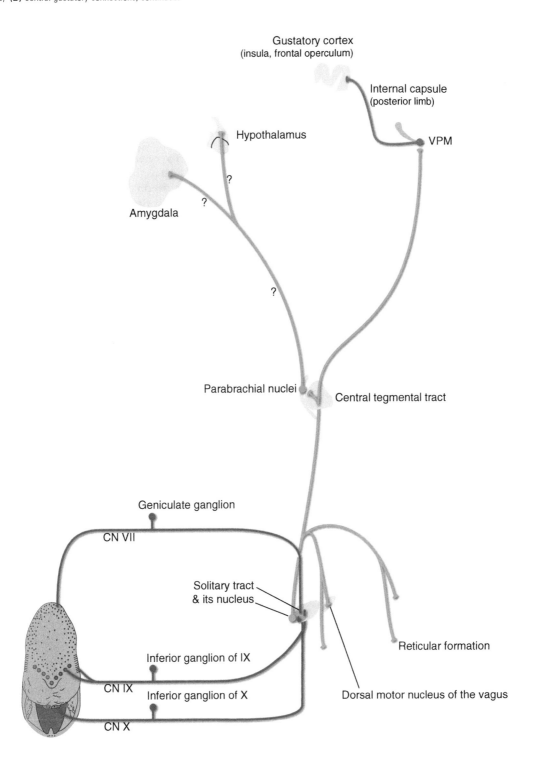

Figure 8.6 (A) Central olfactory connections.

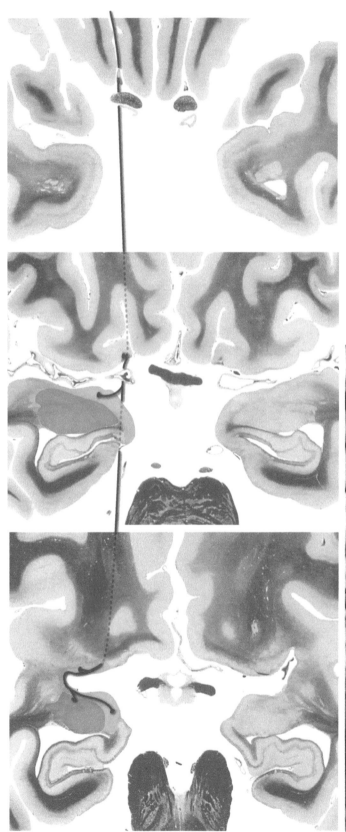

The **olfactory bulb** develops as an outgrowth of the **cerebral hemisphere**, leading to a unique arrangement of connections in the olfactory system. The axons of **olfactory receptor neurons**, collectively making up **cranial nerve I**, pass through the **cribriform plate** of the **ethmoid bone** and terminate in the olfactory bulb. Second-order olfactory neurons then project through the **olfactory tract** to a variety of nearby sites, all part of the ipsilateral cerebral hemisphere. Some olfactory tract fibers terminate in the **anterior olfactory nucleus** (which in turn projects through the **anterior commissure** to the contralateral olfactory bulb) or the **olfactory tubercle** (an inconspicuous part of the **anterior perforated substance** at the base of the cerebrum). The remaining fibers curve toward the temporal lobe as the **lateral olfactory tract** to reach olfactory cortical areas (**piriform cortex** adjacent to the lateral olfactory tract, **periamygdaloid cortex** overlying part of the **amygdala**, and **entorhinal cortex** at the anterior end of the **parahippocampal gyrus**) and a restricted part of the amygdala. This is the only known example of sensory information reaching the cerebral cortex directly, without a stop in the thalamus.

Olfactory information is subsequently distributed more widely, both by projections from these primary olfactory receiving areas and by relays in the thalamus. Some of these olfactory projections converge with **gustatory** and **somatosensory** information in an area of **orbital cortex** important for integrated judgments of flavor.

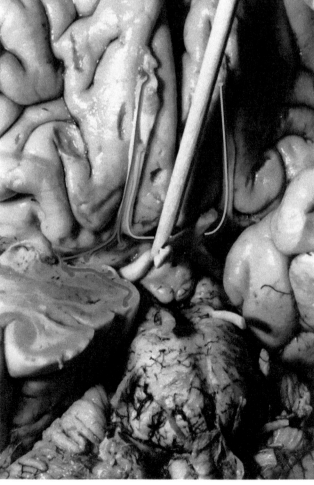

Figure 8.6 (Continued) **(B)** Central olfactory connections, continued.

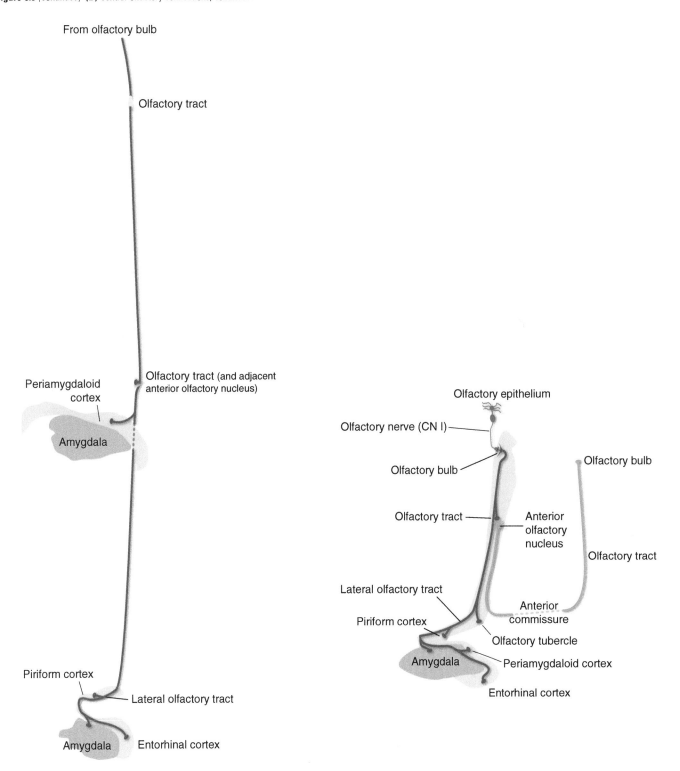

Figure 8.7 (A) The auditory system.

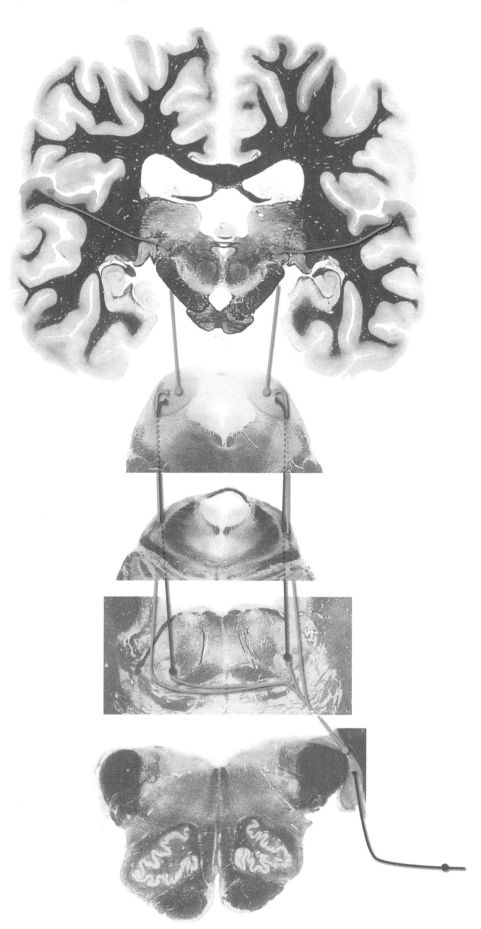

Auditory information reaches the brainstem via the **cochlear division** of **cranial nerve VIII**, a collection of primary afferent fibers with cell bodies in the **spiral ganglion** (embedded in the cochlea), peripheral processes that innervate cochlear **hair cells**, and central processes that terminate in the **dorsal** and **ventral cochlear nuclei** at the pontomedullary junction.

In contrast to the somatosensory system, the second-order neurons of the cochlear nuclei project bilaterally (crossing fibers in the **trapezoid body**) to higher levels of the auditory system, allowing for sound localization by comparing inputs from the two ears. The first site where such binaural comparisons occur is the **superior olivary nucleus**. Efferents from each superior olivary nucleus, together with crossed and uncrossed projections from the cochlear nuclei, ascend to the **inferior colliculus** through the **lateral lemniscus**. The inferior colliculus then projects through the **brachium of the inferior colliculus** to the **medial geniculate nucleus** of the thalamus, which in turn projects to **auditory cortex** in the temporal lobe. Primary auditory cortex is located in the aptly named **transverse temporal gyri** (of **Heschl**) on the superior surface of the **superior temporal gyrus**.

One consequence of this bilateral representation of each ear at all levels beyond the cochlear nuclei is that serious hearing loss restricted to one ear implies damage at the level of the cochlear nuclei or (more likely) the middle or inner ear or the eighth nerve.

Figure 8.7 (Continued) **(B)** The auditory system, continued.

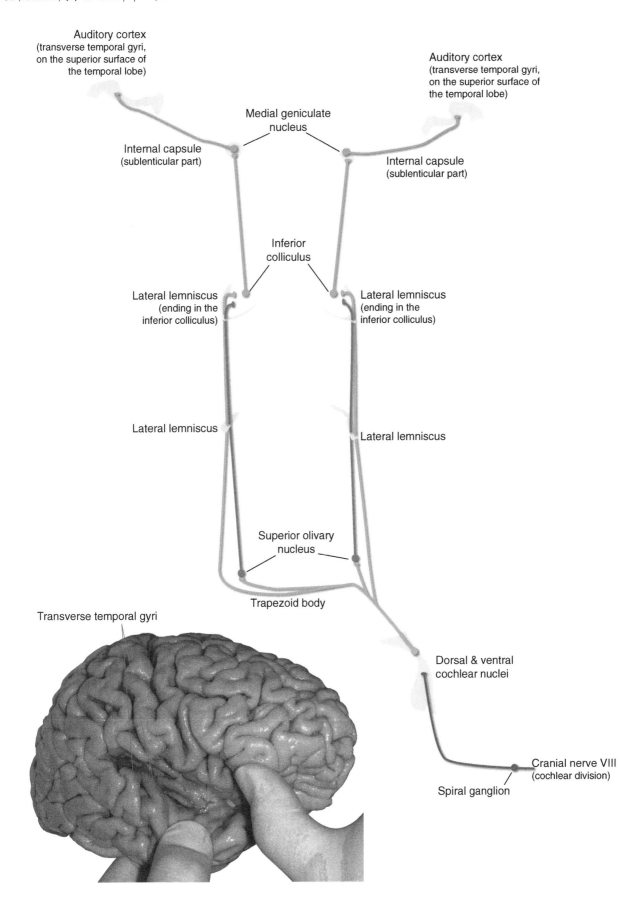

Auditory cortex
(transverse temporal gyri,
on the superior surface of
the temporal lobe)

Auditory cortex
(transverse temporal gyri,
on the superior surface of
the temporal lobe)

Medial geniculate
nucleus

Internal capsule
(sublenticular part)

Internal capsule
(sublenticular part)

Inferior
colliculus

Lateral lemniscus
(ending in the
inferior colliculus)

Lateral lemniscus
(ending in the
inferior colliculus)

Lateral lemniscus

Lateral lemniscus

Superior olivary
nucleus

Trapezoid body

Transverse temporal gyri

Dorsal & ventral
cochlear nuclei

Cranial nerve VIII
(cochlear division)

Spiral ganglion

Figure 8.8 **(A)** The vestibular system.

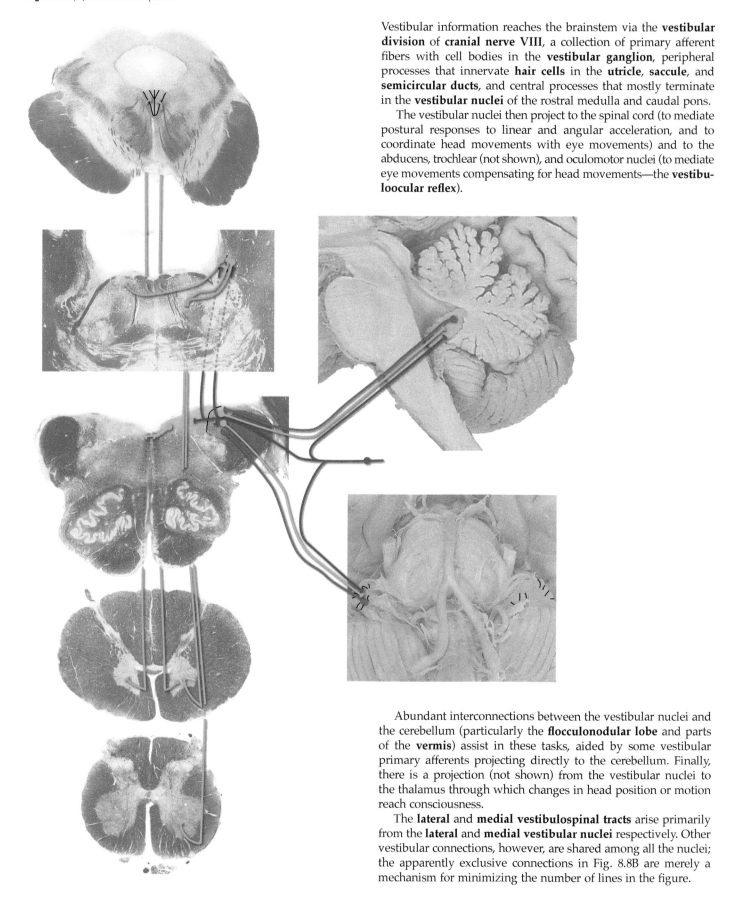

Vestibular information reaches the brainstem via the **vestibular division** of **cranial nerve VIII**, a collection of primary afferent fibers with cell bodies in the **vestibular ganglion**, peripheral processes that innervate **hair cells** in the **utricle**, **saccule**, and **semicircular ducts**, and central processes that mostly terminate in the **vestibular nuclei** of the rostral medulla and caudal pons.

The vestibular nuclei then project to the spinal cord (to mediate postural responses to linear and angular acceleration, and to coordinate head movements with eye movements) and to the abducens, trochlear (not shown), and oculomotor nuclei (to mediate eye movements compensating for head movements—the **vestibuloocular reflex**).

Abundant interconnections between the vestibular nuclei and the cerebellum (particularly the **flocculonodular lobe** and parts of the **vermis**) assist in these tasks, aided by some vestibular primary afferents projecting directly to the cerebellum. Finally, there is a projection (not shown) from the vestibular nuclei to the thalamus through which changes in head position or motion reach consciousness.

The **lateral** and **medial vestibulospinal tracts** arise primarily from the **lateral** and **medial vestibular nuclei** respectively. Other vestibular connections, however, are shared among all the nuclei; the apparently exclusive connections in Fig. 8.8B are merely a mechanism for minimizing the number of lines in the figure.

Figure 8.8 (Continued) **(B)** The vestibular system, continued.

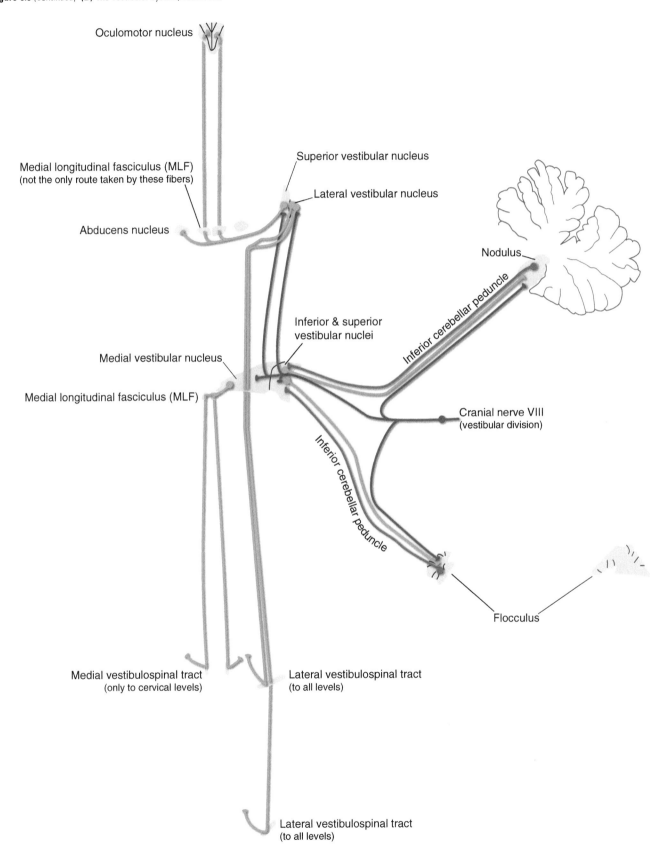

Oculomotor nucleus

Medial longitudinal fasciculus (MLF)
(not the only route taken by these fibers)

Superior vestibular nucleus

Lateral vestibular nucleus

Abducens nucleus

Nodulus

Inferior & superior
vestibular nuclei

Inferior cerebellar peduncle

Medial vestibular nucleus

Cranial nerve VIII
(vestibular division)

Medial longitudinal fasciculus (MLF)

Inferior cerebellar peduncle

Flocculus

Medial vestibulospinal tract
(only to cervical levels)

Lateral vestibulospinal tract
(to all levels)

Lateral vestibulospinal tract
(to all levels)

Figure 8.9 (A) The visual system.

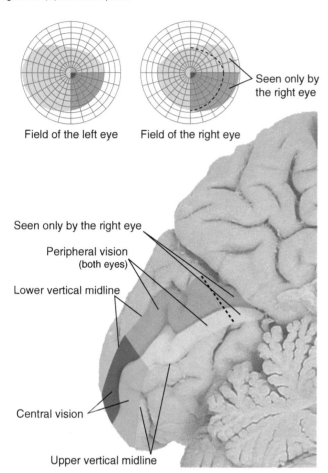

Field of the left eye   Field of the right eye

Seen only by
the right eye

Seen only by the right eye

Peripheral vision
(both eyes)

Lower vertical midline

Central vision

Upper vertical midline

1. The map of the right visual field (of both eyes) in primary visual cortex of the left occipital lobe. The foveal representation is most posterior and extends over the occipital pole. (Most visual cortex is actually in the walls of the calcarine sulcus.)

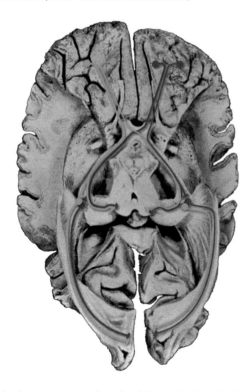

2. The visual pathway, shown over a dissection of the ventral surface of the brain. (Modified from Ludwig E, Klingler J: *Atlas cerebri humani*. Boston: Little, Brown & Co.; 1956.)

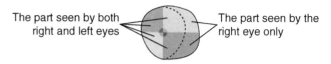

The part seen by both
right and left eyes

The part seen by the
right eye only

3. The visual field of the right eye.

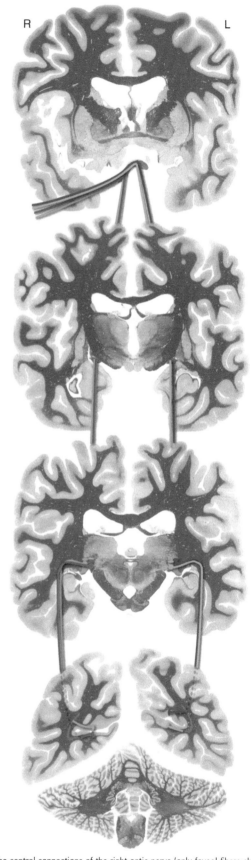

R   L

4. The central connections of the right optic nerve (only foveal fibers shown).

Figure 8.9 (Continued) **(B)** The visual system.

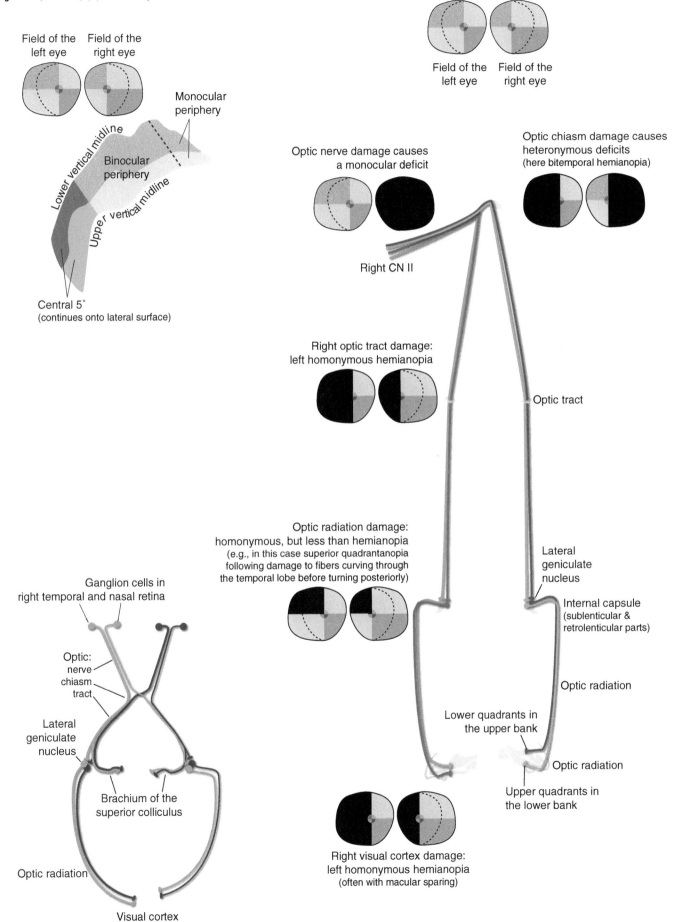

Figure 8.10 Cranial nerve nuclei that innervate ordinary skeletal muscle.

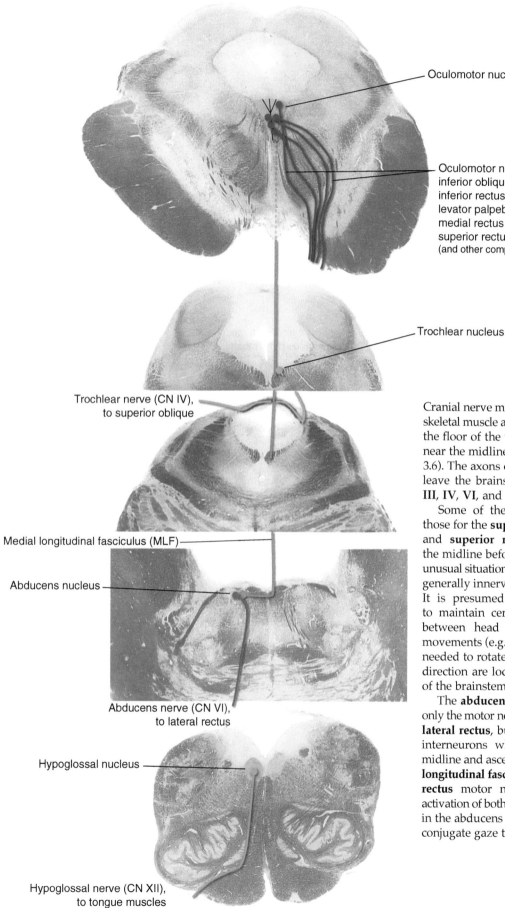

Oculomotor nucleus

Oculomotor nerve (CN III), to:
inferior oblique
inferior rectus
levator palpebrae superioris
medial rectus
superior rectus
(and other components shown in Fig. 8.13)

Trochlear nucleus

Trochlear nerve (CN IV),
to superior oblique

Medial longitudinal fasciculus (MLF)

Abducens nucleus

Abducens nerve (CN VI),
to lateral rectus

Hypoglossal nucleus

Hypoglossal nerve (CN XII),
to tongue muscles

Cranial nerve motor nuclei for ordinary skeletal muscle are typically located near the floor of the ventricular system and near the midline (see Figs. 3.3, 3.4, and 3.6). The axons of these motor neurons leave the brainstem in **cranial nerves III, IV, VI, and XII**.

Some of these axons—specifically, those for the **superior oblique** (CN IV) and **superior rectus** (CN III)—cross the midline before they exit. This is an unusual situation because motor neurons generally innervate ipsilateral muscles. It is presumed to be an adaptation to maintain certain interrelationships between head movements and eye movements (e.g., all the motor neurons needed to rotate both eyes in the same direction are located on the same side of the brainstem).

The **abducens nucleus** contains not only the motor neurons for the ipsilateral **lateral rectus**, but also a population of interneurons whose axons cross the midline and ascend through the **medial longitudinal fasciculus (MLF)** to **medial rectus** motor neurons. Simultaneous activation of both populations of neurons in the abducens nucleus thus results in conjugate gaze to the ipsilateral side.

Figure 8.11 Cranial nerve nuclei that innervate skeletal muscle of branchial arch origin.

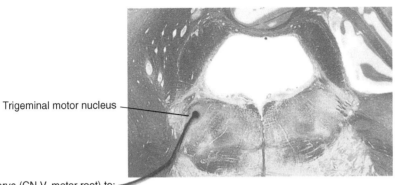

Trigeminal motor nucleus

Trigeminal nerve (CN V, motor root) to:
muscles of mastication (masseter,
temporalis, pterygoids, others);
tensor tympani

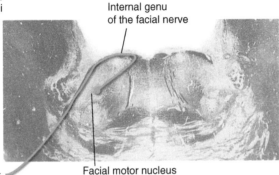

Internal genu
of the facial nerve

Facial motor nucleus

Facial nerve (CN VII) to:
buccinator, orbicularis oris,
orbicularis oculi, other facial muscles;
stapedius
(see Fig. 8.13 for other components)

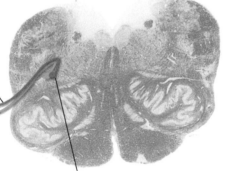

Glossopharyngeal nerve (CN IX),
to stylopharyngeus
(see Fig. 8.13 for other components)

Vagus nerve (CN X),
to laryngeal and pharyngeal muscles
(see Fig. 8.13 for other components)

Nucleus ambiguus (extends longitudinally
through the rostral medulla)

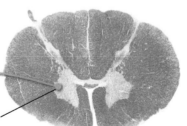
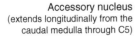

Accessory nerve (CN XI), to:
sternocleidomastoid
trapezius

Accessory nucleus
(extends longitudinally from the
caudal medulla through C5)

Cranial nerve motor nuclei for skeletal muscle derived embryologically from **branchial arches** are typically located farther from both the midline and the floor of the ventricular system than are their counterparts for ordinary skeletal muscle (see Figs. 3.3, 3.4, and 3.6).

The axons of these motor neurons leave the brainstem in **cranial nerves V, VII, IX, X,** and **XI.** Many of them make an odd, hairpin turn before their exit. Axons leaving the **facial motor nucleus** provide the most striking example, hooking around the **abducens nucleus** in an **internal genu** (accounting for the **facial colliculus** in the floor of the **fourth ventricle**—see Fig. 1.11A).

Figure 8.12 (A) The corticobulbar tract.

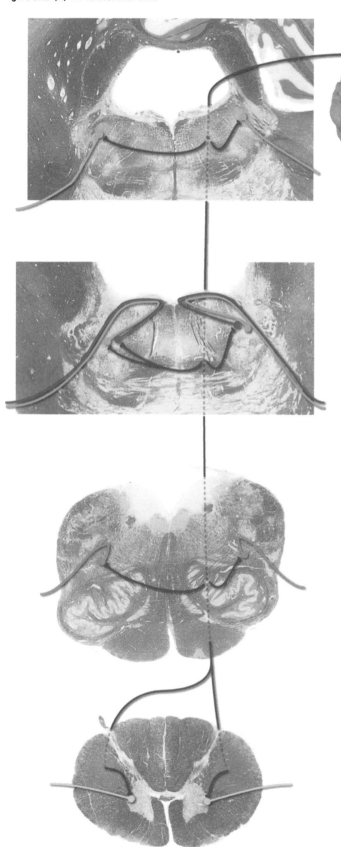

Commands for the initiation of voluntary movements mediated by cranial nerves are conveyed to the brainstem via the **corticobulbar tract**, which includes not only fibers originating in **primary motor cortex** of the **precentral gyrus** but also fibers originating in **premotor, supplementary motor** (not shown), and somatosensory cortex. Corticobulbar axons descend through the **internal capsule, cerebral peduncle, basal pons**, and **medullary pyramids** in company with **corticopontine** and **corticospinal fibers**. At the levels of the motor nuclei of **cranial nerves V, VII, IX, X, XI,** and **XII**, contingents of these fibers peel off and terminate on motor neurons there (or, more often, on nearby interneurons). In contrast to the **corticospinal tract**, which mostly crosses in the **pyramidal decussation**, the corticobulbar fibers from each hemisphere are distributed bilaterally. This corresponds to the way in which muscles on both sides of the face and head are typically used simultaneously (e.g., chewing, swallowing, speaking). As a result of this bilateral distribution, unilateral damage to the internal capsule or corticobulbar tract typically does not cause substantial, lasting weakness of these muscles. The major exception is the muscles of the lower face, whose motor neurons receive a predominantly crossed corticobulbar input (corresponding to the way in which we can make asymmetrical lower facial expressions). Hence, weakness of one lower quadrant of the face is an important clinical sign of contralateral corticobulbar damage. (The nuclei of cranial nerves III, IV, and VI receive no direct corticobulbar inputs, because cortical projections instead reach brainstem pattern generators that in turn drive coordinated movements of the two eyes.)

Figure 8.12 (Continued) **(B)** The corticobulbar tract, continued.

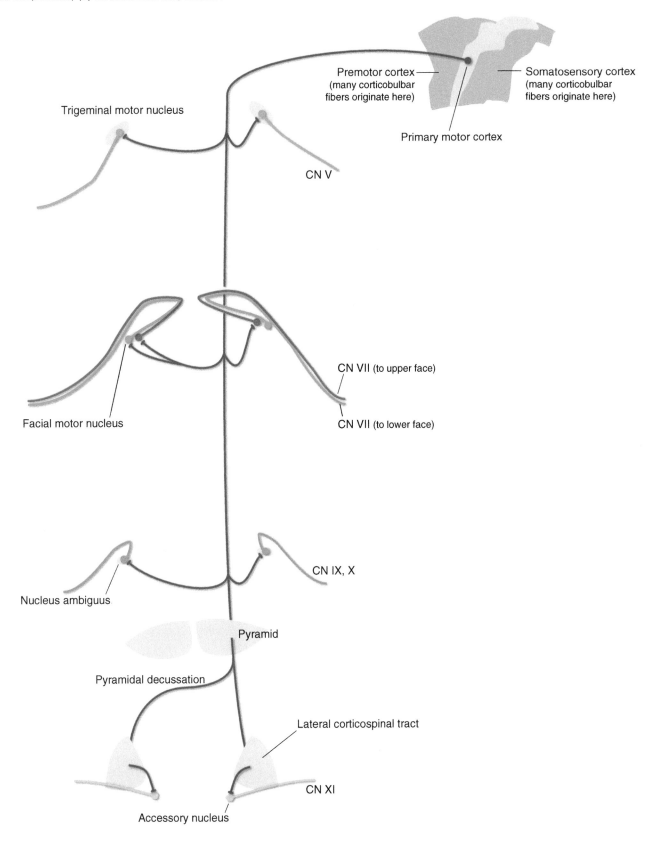

Figure 8.13 (A) Visceral and gustatory afferents (right side of the figure); preganglionic sympathetic and parasympathetic neurons (left side of the figure). Relatively minor elements (e.g., visceral afferents in the facial nerve) and some elements lacking a distinct CNS nucleus (e.g., preganglionic parasympathetics mediating lacrimation and salivation via the facial and glossopharyngeal nerves) have been omitted.

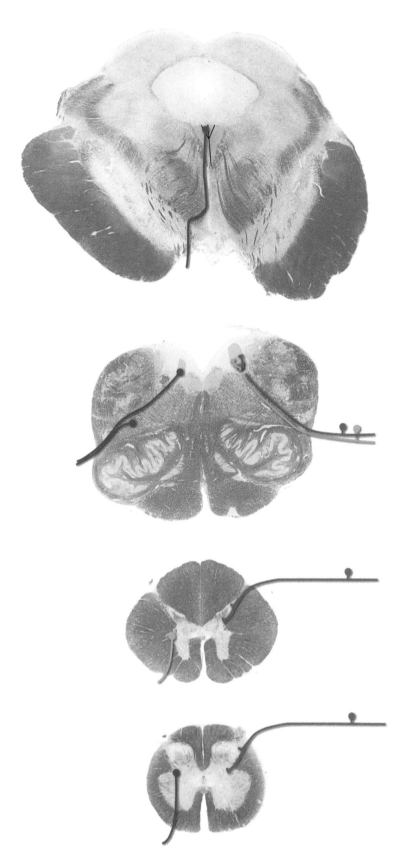

Figure 8.13 (Continued) **(B)** Visceral afferents and efferents, continued.

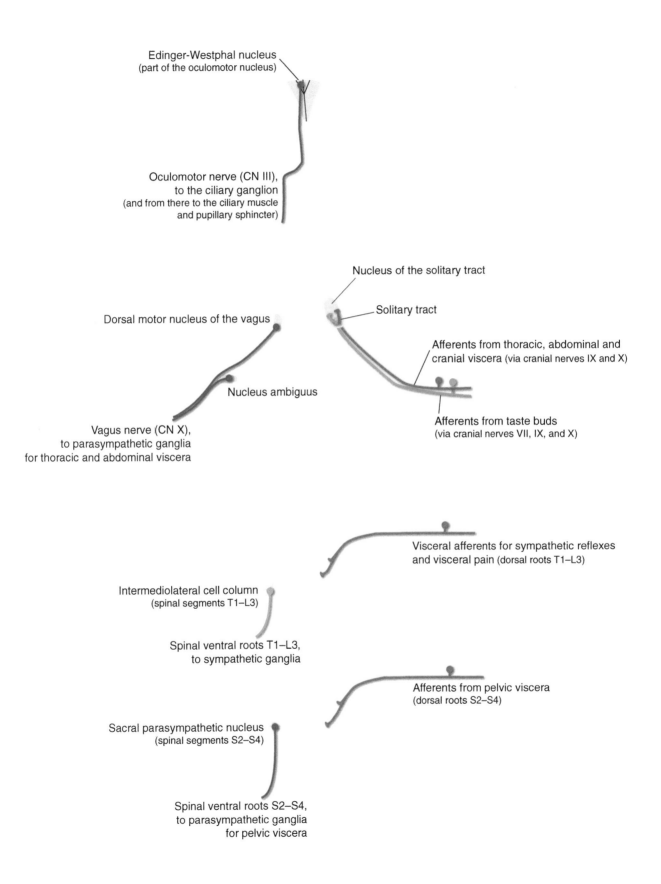

Edinger-Westphal nucleus
(part of the oculomotor nucleus)

Oculomotor nerve (CN III),
to the ciliary ganglion
(and from there to the ciliary muscle
and pupillary sphincter)

Nucleus of the solitary tract

Solitary tract

Dorsal motor nucleus of the vagus

Afferents from thoracic, abdominal and
cranial viscera (via cranial nerves IX and X)

Nucleus ambiguus

Vagus nerve (CN X),
to parasympathetic ganglia
for thoracic and abdominal viscera

Afferents from taste buds
(via cranial nerves VII, IX, and X)

Visceral afferents for sympathetic reflexes
and visceral pain (dorsal roots T1–L3)

Intermediolateral cell column
(spinal segments T1–L3)

Spinal ventral roots T1–L3,
to sympathetic ganglia

Afferents from pelvic viscera
(dorsal roots S2–S4)

Sacral parasympathetic nucleus
(spinal segments S2–S4)

Spinal ventral roots S2–S4,
to parasympathetic ganglia
for pelvic viscera

Figure 8.14 The principal circuit of the basal ganglia, shown for the putamen (left side of the figure) and caudate nucleus (right side of the figure). Excitatory connections are shown in *green*, inhibitory connections in *red*.

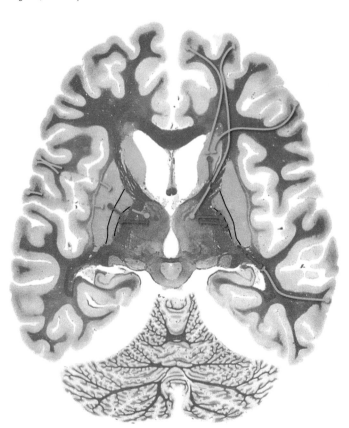

The **basal ganglia**, which include the **striatum**,[a] **globus pallidus**, **subthalamic nucleus**, and **substantia nigra**, are prominently involved in motor control (and in cognitive functions as well, through parallel connections with other CNS areas). They affect movement not by projecting to motor neurons in the spinal cord or brainstem, but rather by influencing the output of the cerebral cortex. The principal anatomical circuit underlying this influence is a series of parallel loops of the type indicated in the inset below: A relatively widespread area of cerebral cortex projects to a particular region of the striatum, which by way of the globus pallidus and thalamus feeds back to the cerebral cortex (typically to a frontal or limbic area).

Most parts of the cerebral cortex, and the **hippocampus** and **amygdala** as well, participate in such loops. **Association areas** of cortex are related most prominently to the **caudate nucleus**, **somatosensory** and **motor cortex** to the **putamen**, and **limbic areas** to the **ventral striatum**.

The substantia nigra and subthalamic nucleus form parts of additional basal ganglia circuitry, as indicated in Figs. 8.17 and 8.18.

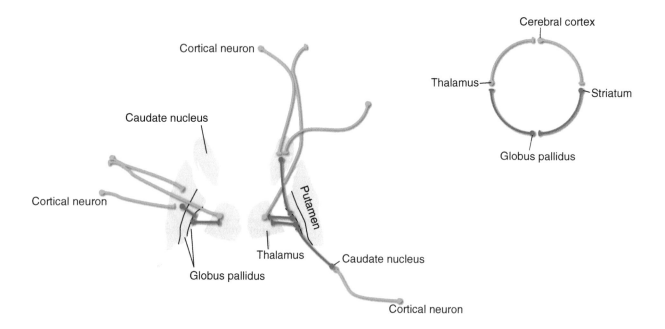

---

[a]*Striatum* refers to the combination of caudate nucleus, putamen, and nucleus accumbens. (Nucleus accumbens and adjacent parts of the caudate, putamen, and basal forebrain are often referred to as the *ventral striatum.*)

Figure 8.15 Major connections of the striatum; afferents on the left, efferents on the right. Excitatory connections are shown in *green*, inhibitory connections in *red*. (Inputs from the compact part of the substantia nigra are shown in a third color because they excite some striatal neurons and inhibit others.)

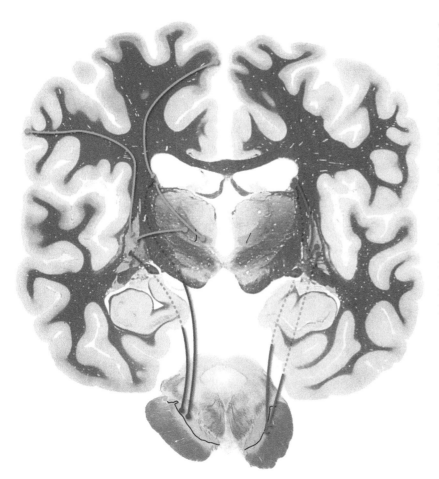

The most prominent afferents to the **striatum** arise in the cerebral cortex, **substantia nigra (compact part)**, and **intralaminar nuclei** of the thalamus (especially the **centromedian** and **parafascicular nuclei**). Although not portrayed in this figure, cortical inputs are topographically organized: **Association areas** project mainly to the **caudate nucleus**, **somatosensory** and **motor areas** to the **putamen**, and **limbic areas** (including the **hippocampus** and **amygdala**) to the **ventral striatum**. The implication of these differing inputs, borne out by other aspects of basal ganglia connections and by behavioral studies, is that the different parts of the striatum have distinct functions.

Striatal efferents form the next stage in the path back to cerebral cortex by projecting to both segments of the **globus pallidus** and to the **reticular part** of the **substantia nigra**, which in most respects may be considered an extension of the globus pallidus (**internal segment**).

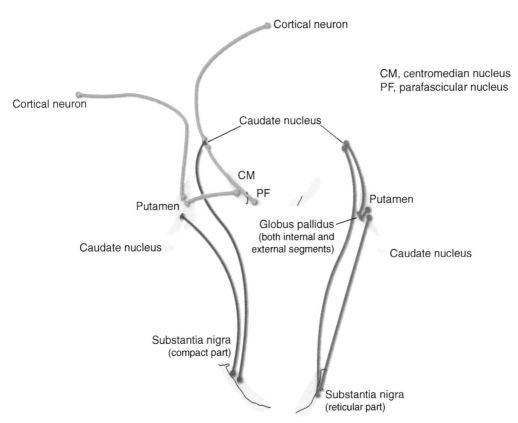

Figure 8.16 Major connections of the globus pallidus; afferents on the left, efferents on the right. Excitatory connections are shown in *green*, inhibitory connections in *red*.

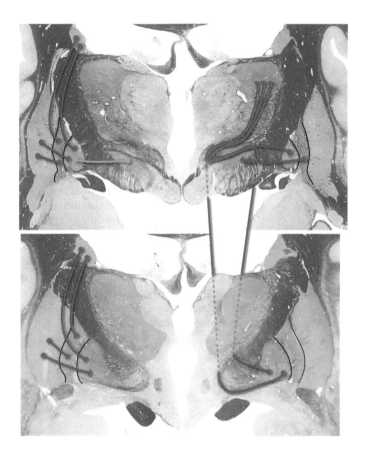

The globus pallidus is prominently subdivided over most of its extent into an **external segment** (adjacent to the **putamen**) and an **internal segment** (adjacent to the **internal capsule**). Both segments (as well as the **reticular part** of the **substantia nigra, SNr**) receive inputs from the **striatum**. The **subthalamic nucleus** provides a prominent excitatory input to the internal segment through fibers that penetrate the internal capsule as a series of small bundles collectively called the **subthalamic fasciculus**.

The external (**GPe**) and internal (**GPi**) segments of the globus pallidus have distinct efferent projections. GPe projects to the subthalamic nucleus through the subthalamic fasciculus. (GPe also has widespread inhibitory outputs to other parts of the basal ganglia, omitted from this figure to keep it from getting too complicated.) GPi and SNr, in contrast, form the next stage in the path back to cerebral cortex, by projecting to the thalamus. Some efferents from GPi penetrate the internal capsule as a series of small fiber bundles collectively called the **lenticular fasciculus**; others emerge from the inferior surface of GPi and hook around the internal capsule in the **ansa lenticularis**. The ansa lenticularis and lenticular fasciculus join **cerebellar efferents** underneath the thalamus to form the **thalamic fasciculus**.

Although pallidal efferents in this figure are portrayed as ending in the **ventral lateral nucleus**, many actually end in the **ventral anterior nucleus**. Others reach more widespread thalamic sites (as might be expected in view of the striatal inputs from diverse cortical areas), such as the **dorsomedial nucleus**.

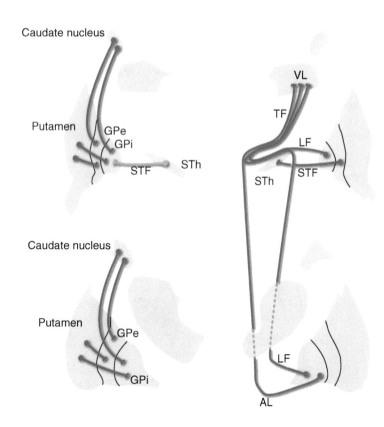

Abbreviations:
AL, ansa lenticularis
GPe, globus pallidus (external segment)
GPi, globus pallidus (internal segment)
LF, lenticular fasciculus
STF, subthalamic fasciculus
STh, subthalamic nucleus
TF, thalamic fasciculus
VL, ventral lateral nucleus of the thalamus

Figure 8.17 Connections of the substantia nigra. Excitatory connections are shown in *green*, inhibitory connections in *red*. (Projections from the compact part of the substantia nigra are shown in a third color because they excite some striatal neurons and inhibit others.)

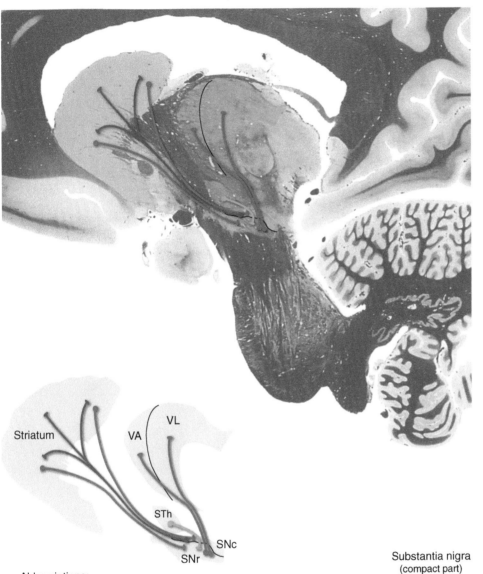

Abbreviations:
SNc, substantia nigra (compact part)
SNr, substantia nigra (reticular part)
STh, subthalamic nucleus
VA, ventral anterior nucleus of the thalamus
VL, ventral lateral nucleus of the thalamus

The **substantia nigra** is almost like two separate and distinct neural structures laminated together. The **reticular part (SNr)**, adjacent to the corticospinal and corticopontine fibers of the **cerebral peduncle**, is functionally a displaced part of the **globus pallidus (internal segment)**; it receives inputs from the **striatum** and **subthalamic nucleus** and projects to the thalamus. (As in the case of the globus pallidus, its thalamic projections extend beyond the **ventral anterior** and **ventral lateral nuclei**, although this is not indicated in this figure.)

The **compact part (SNc)** is a collection of darkly pigmented neurons (from which the substantia nigra derives its name) that receive inputs from the striatum and other sites, then project to the **putamen** and **caudate nucleus** and release **dopamine** there; their degeneration leads to Parkinson's disease. A comparable set of dopaminergic neurons in the nearby **ventral tegmental area** projects to the **ventral striatum, frontal cortex**, and **amygdala**.

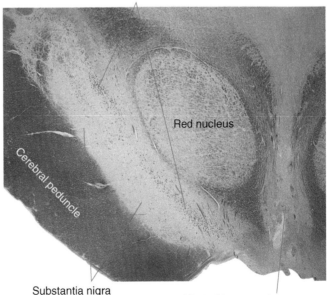

Figure 8.18 Connections of the subthalamic nucleus. Excitatory connections are shown in *green*, inhibitory connections in *red*.

Despite its relatively small size, the **subthalamic nucleus** has surprisingly widespread connections, with inputs from the cerebral cortex (especially **motor cortex**) and interconnections with the thalamus and **reticular formation** and with several other nuclei of the basal ganglia.

The most important of these connections from a functional standpoint may be inputs from the **external segment** of the **globus pallidus** and outputs to the **internal segment** of the **globus pallidus** (and to the **reticular part** of the **substantia nigra**). These form part

of an **indirect route** through the basal ganglia (see inset below). One general strategy used by the basal ganglia may be to facilitate some cortical activities by means of signals conveyed in the **direct route** (described in Fig. 8.14), while simultaneously suppressing competing cortical activities by means of signals in this indirect route. However, there is undoubtedly more to the story than this; it does not take into account, for example, the widespread inhibitory projections of GPe to sites other than the subthalamic nucleus.

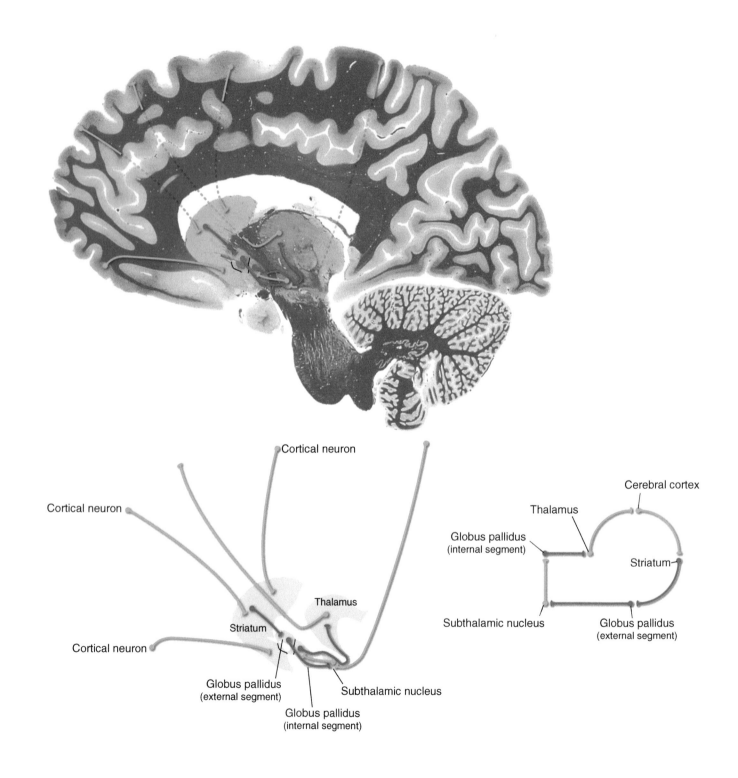

Figure 8.19 Gross anatomy of the cerebellum; shown here is the medial surface of a hemisected cerebellum **(A)**, and the same cerebellum before hemisection seen from superior **(B)**, posterior **(C)**, and anterior **(D)** viewpoints. (See Fig. 1.9 for additional views of the same cerebellum).

The **cerebellum** is even more highly convoluted than the cerebral hemispheres; this makes room for a large expanse of uniformly organized **cerebellar cortex** (see Fig. 8.21). Its **fissures** are mostly oriented transversely, and prominent ones are used as landmarks to divide the cerebellum into lobes and lobules. Thus the very deep **primary fissure** separates the **anterior** and **posterior lobes**, and the **posterolateral fissure** separates the posterior and **flocculonodular** lobes.

Along lines roughly at right angles to the fissures, the entire cerebellum is divided into a narrow **vermis** that straddles the midline and a much larger **hemisphere** on each side.

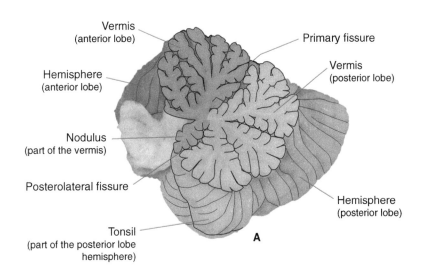

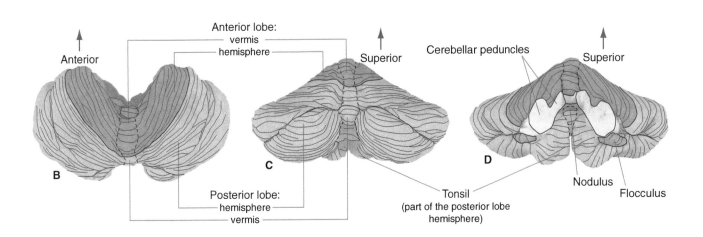

Figure 8.20 Routes into and out of the cerebellum: the cerebellar peduncles.

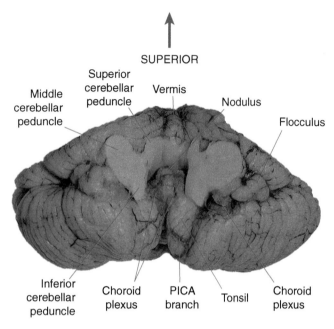

SUPERIOR

Middle
cerebellar
peduncle

Superior
cerebellar
peduncle

Vermis

Nodulus

Flocculus

Inferior
cerebellar
peduncle

Choroid
plexus

PICA
branch

Tonsil

Choroid
plexus

(A) Ventral surface of a cerebellum that had been removed from the brainstem by severing the cerebellar peduncles. The view is as if one were looking dorsally from the floor of the fourth ventricle toward its roof. *PICA*, Posterior inferior cerebellar artery.

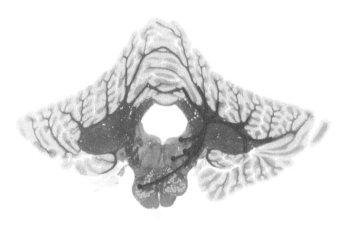

(B) The inferior cerebellar peduncle is the major input route for fibers from the inferior olivary nucleus, vestibular nuclei, trigeminal nuclei, reticular formation, and spinal cord. (The inferior peduncle also contains some cerebellar efferents, particularly those bound for vestibular nuclei.)

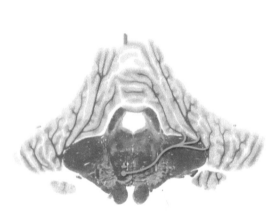

(C) The middle cerebellar peduncle is the input route for information from cerebral cortex. Corticopontine fibers traverse the internal capsule and cerebral peduncle and terminate in pontine nuclei. Pontocerebellar fibers then project through the contralateral middle cerebellar peduncle to nearly all areas of the cerebellar cortex.

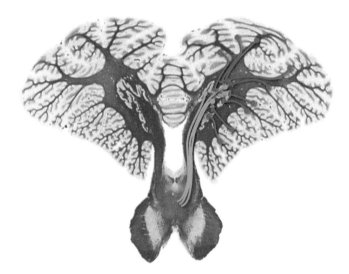

(D) The superior cerebellar peduncle is the major output route from the cerebellum. Cerebellar cortex projects to a series of deep cerebellar nuclei, most of whose axons leave the cerebellum through this peduncle. (A few spinocerebellar afferents also travel through the superior peduncle.)

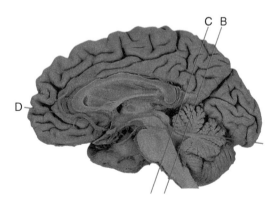

C B

D

(E) The planes of section shown in this figure. (The odd-looking section in *D* is part of Fig. 6.5A turned upside down so that its orientation more closely resembles that of *B* and *C*.)

Figure 8.21 The structure of cerebellar cortex. **(A)** Cross section of a single folium (as indicated in the *inset*). **(B)** Oblique longitudinal section of a folium. **(C)** Longitudinal section of a folium. **(D)** Cross section of a single folium from a human cerebellum, stained with hematoxylin and eosin. ([**A–C**] Modified from Ramón y Cajal S. Histologie du système nerveux de l'homme et des vertébres, Paris, 1909–1911, Norbert Maloine. [**D**] Provided by Dr. Nathaniel T. McMullen, Department of Cellular and Molecular Medicine, The University of Arizona College of Medicine.)

The lobes and lobules of the cerebellum are further subdivided by smaller sulci into a large number of **folia**. Each **folium** is covered by a remarkably uniform and precisely ordered **cortex**. Most of the various cell types contained in this cortex are indicated in *A*, but the basic organization is one in which two types of afferent fibers (**mossy fibers** and **climbing fibers**) enter the cortex and one type of axon (**Purkinje cell** axons) leaves to convey information to the **deep cerebellar nuclei**.

The climbing fibers all come from one place—the contralateral **inferior olivary nucleus**—and wrap around the proximal dendrites of Purkinje cells, forming powerful excitatory synapses.

All other cerebellar afferents (other than a complement of the diffuse modulatory inputs indicated in Figs. 8.38 to 8.41) enter the cerebellum as mossy fibers and terminate on the vast numbers of tiny **granule cells** in the **granular layer**. (Granule cells account for half of the neurons in the CNS.) Granule cell axons ascend toward the cerebellar surface and bifurcate in the **molecular layer** to form **parallel fibers**, which run parallel to the long axis of a given folium. In so doing, each parallel fiber intersects the flattened, transversely oriented dendritic trees of hundreds of Purkinje cells, where they make excitatory synapses.

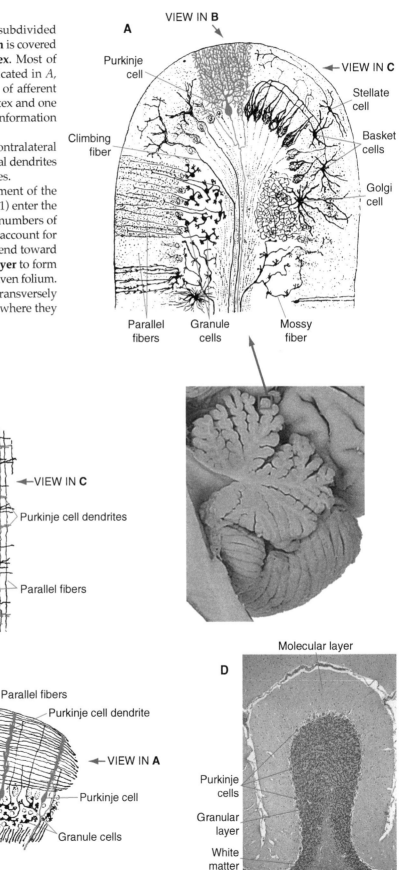

Figure 8.22 **(A)** Afferents to the cerebellum.

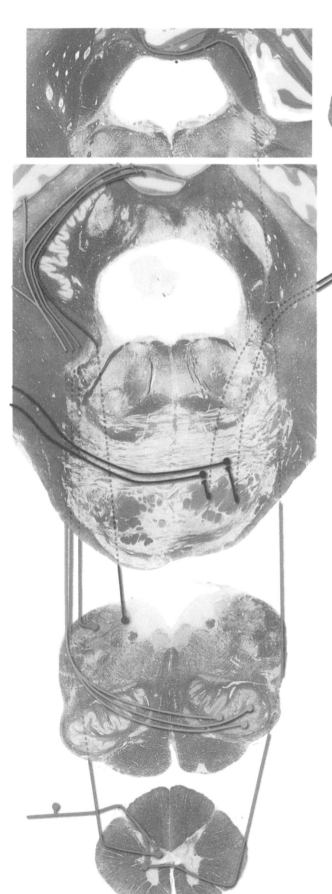

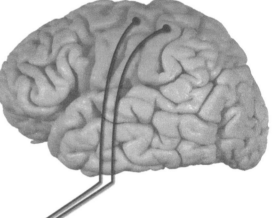

The cerebellum receives afferent inputs of three broad categories: afferents conveying information from the cerebral cortex, afferents conveying sensory information from a variety of subcortical sites, and **climbing fibers** from the contralateral **inferior olivary nucleus**.

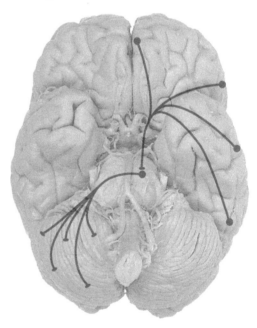

Cerebral cortical input (mostly, but not entirely, from **motor** and **somatosensory areas**) reaches the cerebellum through the **middle cerebellar peduncle** after a relay in the **pontine nuclei**. Most sensory information, arising most prominently in the **spinal cord** and **vestibular nuclei**, arrives via the **inferior cerebellar peduncle** (although a small amount traverses the **superior peduncle**). Axons leaving each inferior olivary nucleus travel through the contralateral inferior cerebellar peduncle before ending in the cerebellum as climbing fibers.

(The connections of the cerebellum are actually more widespread than this simple account would indicate, and it seems to have correspondingly broader functions. For example, interconnections between the cerebellum and the hypothalamus have been described, and the cerebellum plays a role in coordinating autonomic functions. Cortical inputs from association areas such as prefrontal cortex indicate that the cerebellum, like the basal ganglia, is also involved in higher cognitive functions.)

Figure 8.22 (Continued) **(B)** Afferents to the cerebellum, continued.

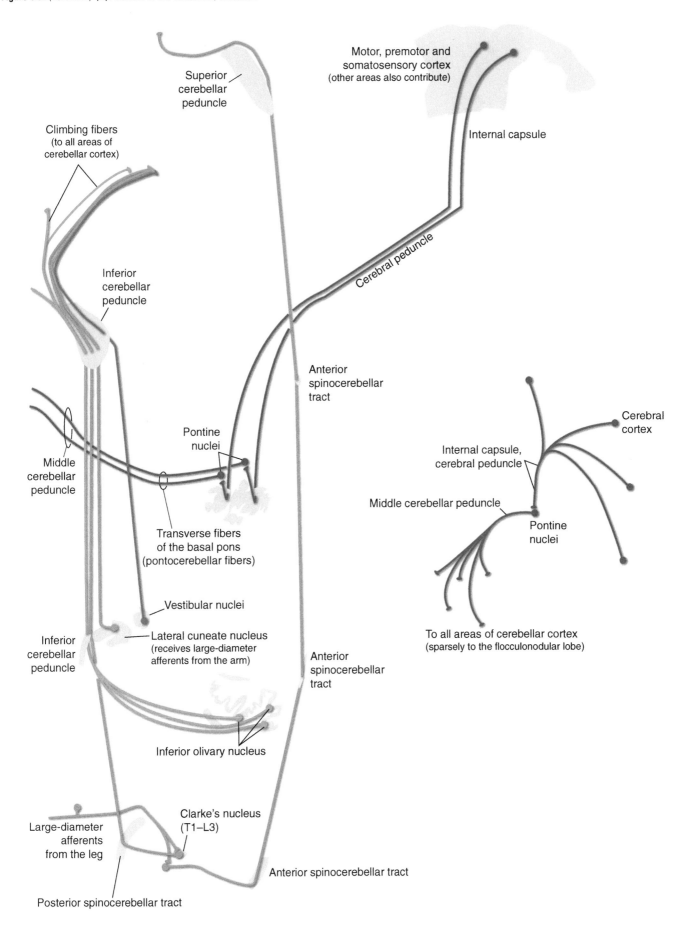

Figure 8.23 (A) Efferents from the cerebellum to the forebrain.

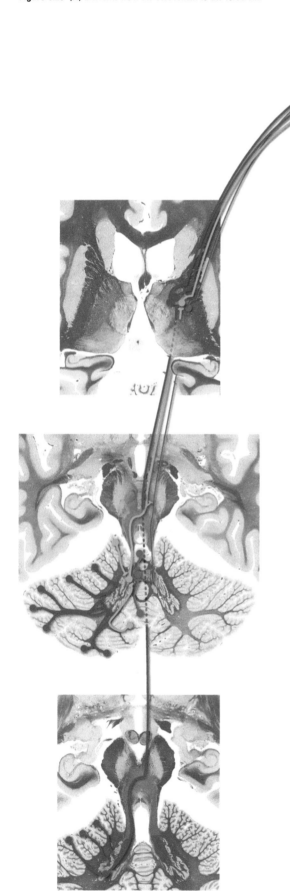

Purkinje cell axons are the sole output from **cerebellar cortex**. Some leave the cerebellum entirely, through the **inferior cerebellar peduncle**, to reach the **vestibular nuclei**. Most, however, project to a series of **deep cerebellar nuclei** in the roof of the fourth ventricle, which in turn provide most of the output from the cerebellum.

There are three deep cerebellar nuclei on each side, arranged in a lateral-to-medial sequence: the **dentate, interposed,**[b] and **fastigial nuclei**. This arrangement of the nuclei corresponds to three longitudinal zones of cerebellar cortex: the large, **lateral part** of the **hemisphere**; a smaller, **medial part** of the hemisphere (also called the **intermediate zone**); and the **vermis** most medially. The pairing of deep nuclei and longitudinal zones of cortex is a reflection of functional subdivisions within the cerebellum that are also reflected in cerebellar inputs and outputs.

The lateral part of each cerebellar hemisphere receives its major inputs from the cerebral cortex (motor, somatosensory, and other, more widespread areas) via **pontine nuclei**. Its outputs then influence the activity of **motor** and **premotor cortex** through a pathway involving the dentate nucleus and contralateral thalamus (primarily the **ventral lateral nucleus**). It is thought to play a role in planning skilled movements.

The medial part of each cerebellar hemisphere receives information about the limbs from two major sources—motor cortex (via pontine nuclei) and the **spinal cord** (via **spinocerebellar tracts**). It is thus strategically positioned to compare intended and actual movements and to assist with moment-to-moment correction of movement by way of connections with the interposed nucleus and motor cortex (via the thalamus).

The vermis receives information about axial muscles and body position from the vestibular nuclei and spinal cord and, through the fastigial nucleus, is involved in the maintenance and adjustment of posture. Most of this is accomplished at the level of the brainstem (see Fig. 8.24), and the connections of the fastigial nucleus with the thalamus are relatively minor.

Finally, the **flocculonodular lobe** (which does not fit comfortably into this longitudinal zonation scheme) is critically involved in eye movements by way of its connections with the **vestibular nuclei**.

[b]The interposed nucleus is itself a combination of the more lateral emboliform nucleus and more medial globose nucleus.

Figure 8.23 (Continued) **(B)** Efferents from the cerebellum to the forebrain, continued.

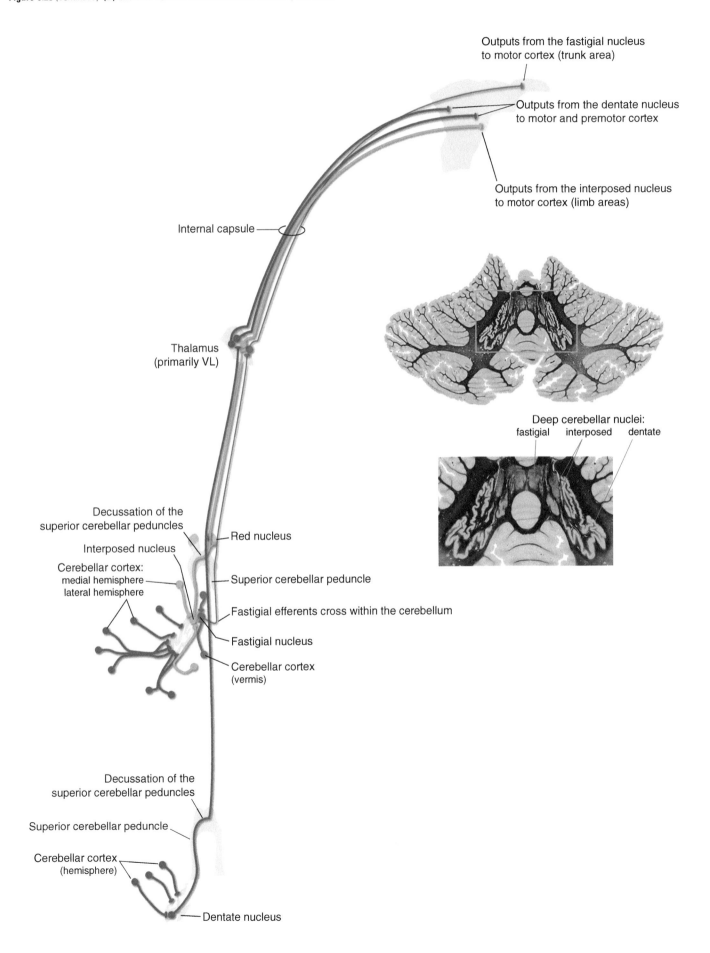

Outputs from the fastigial nucleus
to motor cortex (trunk area)

Outputs from the dentate nucleus
to motor and premotor cortex

Outputs from the interposed nucleus
to motor cortex (limb areas)

Internal capsule

Thalamus
(primarily VL)

Deep cerebellar nuclei:
fastigial   interposed   dentate

Decussation of the
superior cerebellar peduncles

Interposed nucleus

Red nucleus

Cerebellar cortex:
medial hemisphere
lateral hemisphere

Superior cerebellar peduncle

Fastigial efferents cross within the cerebellum

Fastigial nucleus

Cerebellar cortex
(vermis)

Decussation of the
superior cerebellar peduncles

Superior cerebellar peduncle

Cerebellar cortex
(hemisphere)

Dentate nucleus

Figure 8.24 (A) Efferents from the cerebellum to the brainstem.

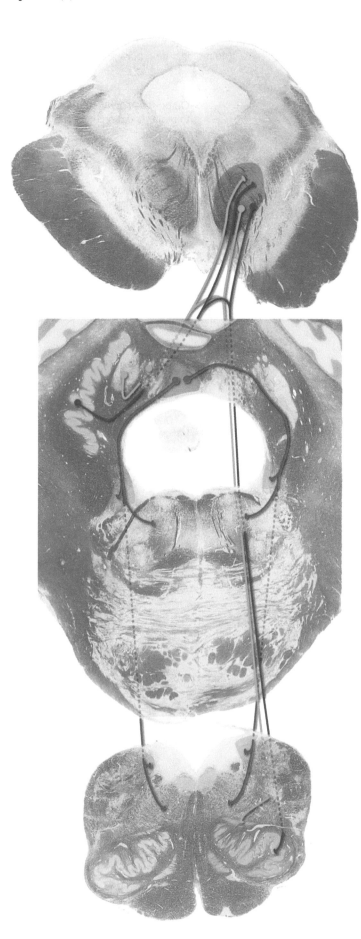

Each of the **deep cerebellar nuclei** also has outputs to sites in the brainstem; in the case of the **fastigial nucleus**, these represent its major connections.

As the **superior cerebellar peduncle** passes through or around the **red nucleus**, some of its fibers synapse on rubral neurons (*nucleus ruber* is Latin for "red nucleus"). A relatively small part of the red nucleus gives rise to the **rubrospinal tract**, which decussates and proceeds to the spinal cord. This is one route through which the cerebellum helps make corrections to ongoing movements, but it is relatively unimportant in humans. Most neurons of the red nucleus project instead to the ipsilateral **inferior olivary nucleus** via the **central tegmental tract**. In addition, some fibers leave the superior cerebellar peduncle as it traverses the brainstem, turn caudally, cross as the **descending limb** of the superior cerebellar peduncle, and reach the inferior olivary nucleus directly. The functional significance of these cerebellum–(red nucleus)–inferior olivary nucleus connections is not known with certainty, but they may play a role in motor learning.

The fastigial nucleus, consistent with its role in postural adjustments, projects bilaterally to the **vestibular nuclei** and **reticular formation**. Some of its efferents leave the cerebellum uncrossed through the **inferior cerebellar peduncle**. Others cross the midline within the cerebellum, hook over the top of the superior cerebellar peduncle (as the **uncinate fasciculus**), and join the contralateral inferior cerebellar peduncle.

Figure 8.24 (Continued) **(B)** Efferents from the cerebellum to the brainstem, continued.

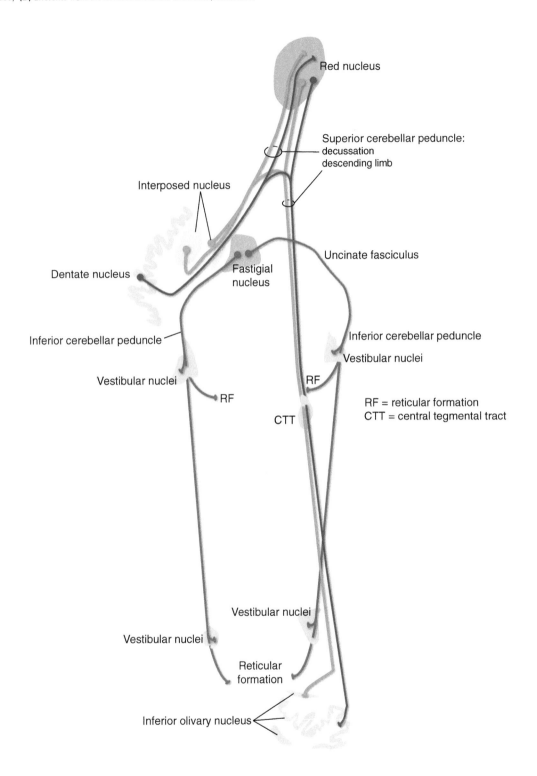

Figure 8.25 (A) Projections of thalamic relay nuclei to the cerebral cortex (not shown: gustatory projections from VPM to the insula).

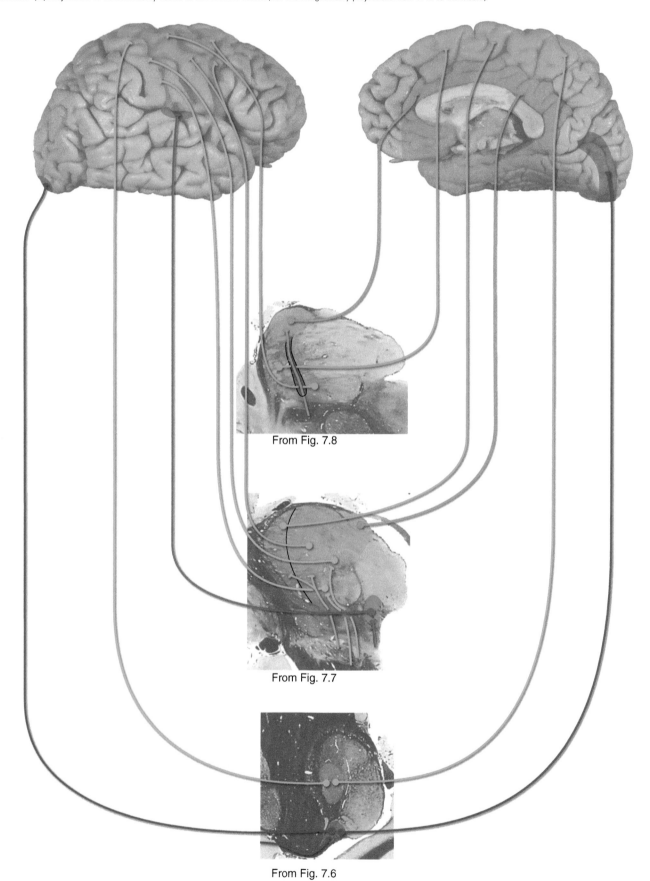

From Fig. 7.8

From Fig. 7.7

From Fig. 7.6

Figure 8.25 (Continued) **(B)** Projections of thalamic relay nuclei to the cerebral cortex, continued (numbers = Brodmann's areas).

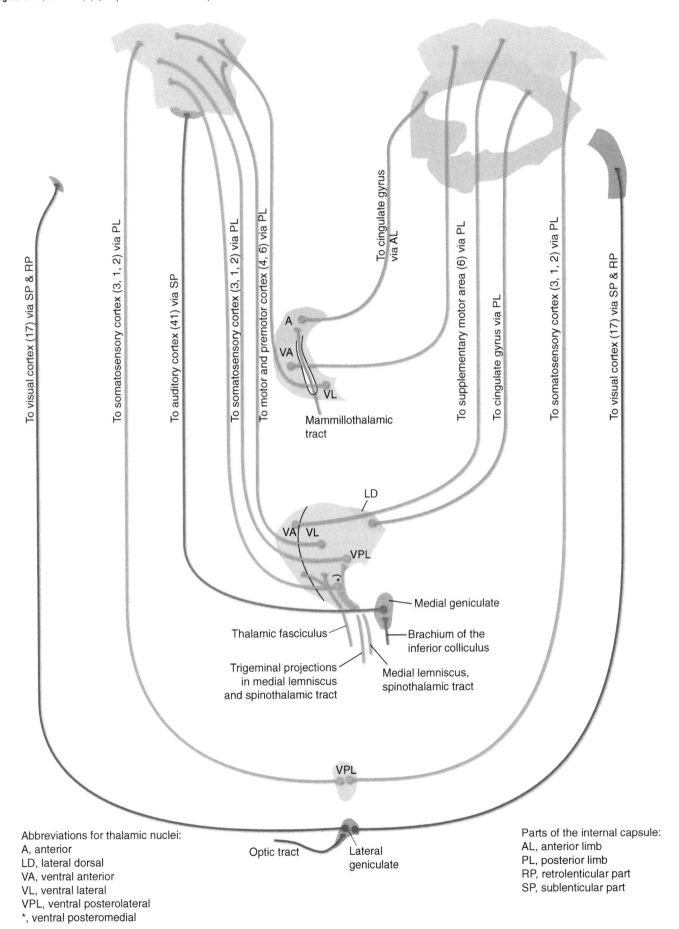

To visual cortex (17) via SP & RP

To somatosensory cortex (3, 1, 2) via PL

To auditory cortex (41) via SP

To somatosensory cortex (3, 1, 2) via PL

To motor and premotor cortex (4, 6) via PL

To cingulate gyrus via AL

To supplementary motor area (6) via PL

To cingulate gyrus via PL

To somatosensory cortex (3, 1, 2) via PL

To visual cortex (17) via SP & RP

A

VA

VL

Mammillothalamic tract

LD

VA VL

VPL

*

Medial geniculate

Thalamic fasciculus

Brachium of the inferior colliculus

Trigeminal projections in medial lemniscus and spinothalamic tract

Medial lemniscus, spinothalamic tract

VPL

Optic tract Lateral geniculate

Abbreviations for thalamic nuclei:
A, anterior
LD, lateral dorsal
VA, ventral anterior
VL, ventral lateral
VPL, ventral posterolateral
*, ventral posteromedial

Parts of the internal capsule:
AL, anterior limb
PL, posterior limb
RP, retrolenticular part
SP, sublenticular part

Figure 8.26 (A) Projections of thalamic association nuclei to the cerebral cortex.

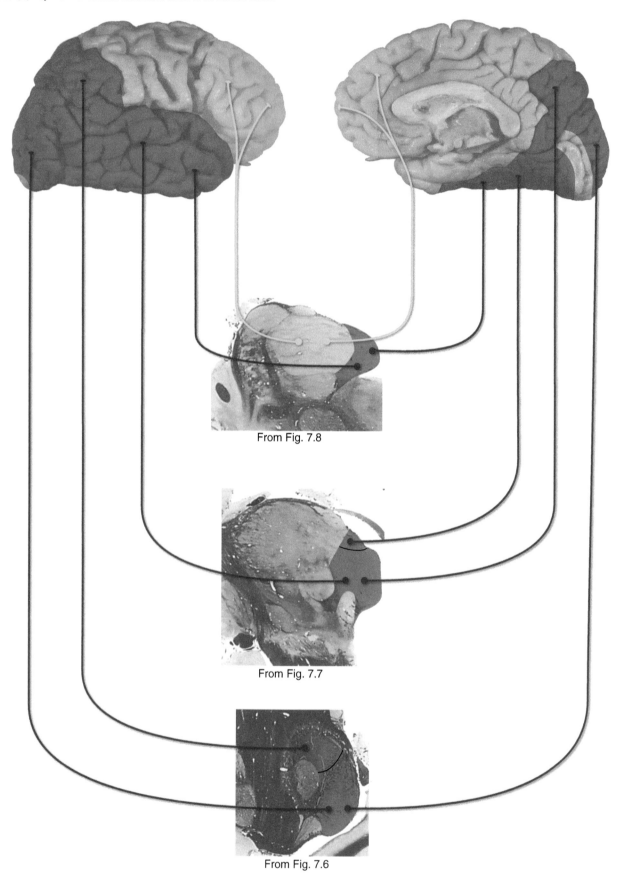

From Fig. 7.8

From Fig. 7.7

From Fig. 7.6

Figure 8.26 (Continued) **(B)** Projections of thalamic association nuclei to the cerebral cortex, continued (numbers = Brodmann's areas).

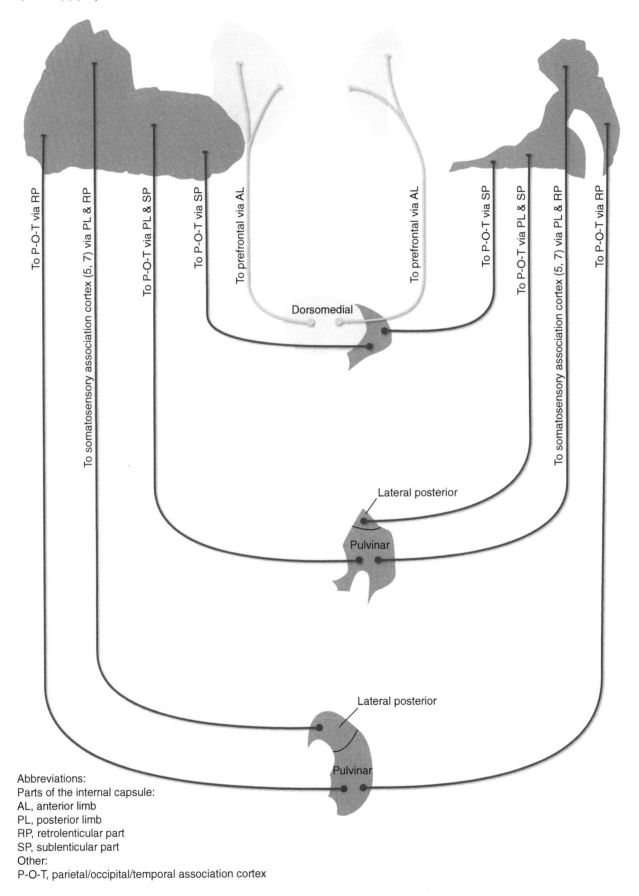

Abbreviations:
Parts of the internal capsule:
AL, anterior limb
PL, posterior limb
RP, retrolenticular part
SP, sublenticular part
Other:
P-O-T, parietal/occipital/temporal association cortex

Figure 8.27 (A) The internal capsule.

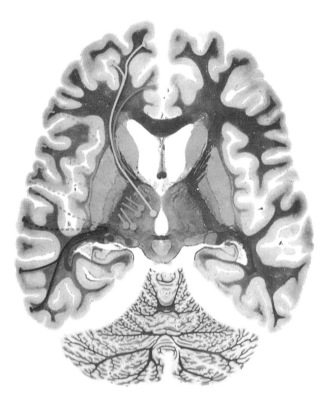

1. An axial section, demonstrating four of the five parts of the internal capsule.

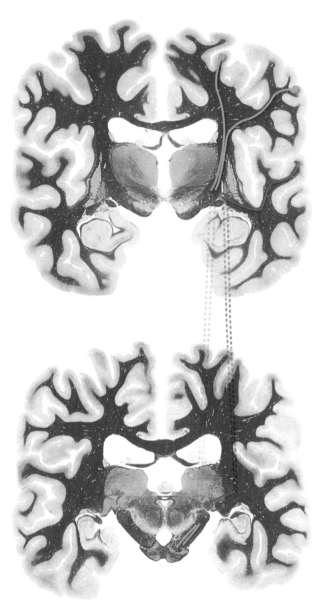

2. The posterior limb and the retrolenticular and sublenticular parts of the internal capsule in coronal sections.

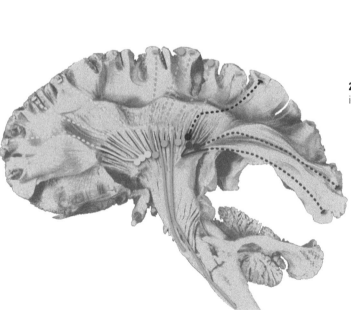

3. The entire internal capsule, shown in a dissection of the lateral surface of the brain. Because the temporal lobe was removed in this dissection, fibers traveling through the sublenticular part from the medial geniculate nucleus to auditory cortex are no longer present. (Modified from Ludwig E, Klingler J. *Atlas cerebri humani.* Boston: Little, Brown & Co.; 1956.)

The **internal capsule** is a compact bundle of fibers traveling to or from the cerebral cortex. Above the internal capsule, the same fibers fan out within the hemisphere as the **corona radiata**; below it, many of them continue on into the **cerebral peduncle**.

The internal capsule is shaped somewhat like an incomplete cone that partly surrounds the **lenticular nucleus**. Relationships between parts of the cone and the lenticular nucleus are used to define five regions: the **anterior limb**, between the lenticular nucleus and the **head** of the **caudate nucleus**; the **posterior limb**, between the lenticular nucleus and the **thalamus**; the **genu**, at the junction of the anterior and posterior limbs; the **retrolenticular part**, behind the lenticular nucleus; and the **sublenticular part**, dipping under the posterior end of the lenticular nucleus.

Figure 8.27 (Continued) **(B)** The internal capsule, continued.

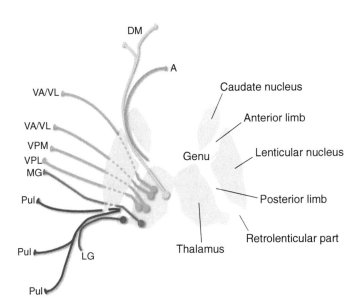

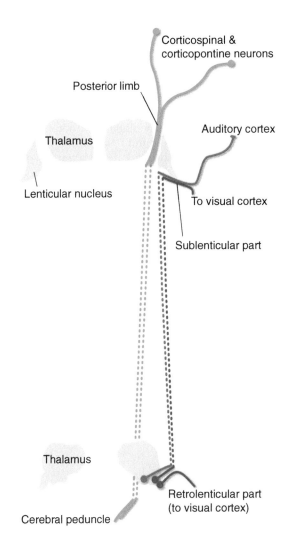

Sources of thalamocortical fibers:
A, anterior nucleus
DM, dorsomedial nucleus
LG, lateral geniculate nucleus
MG, medial geniculate nucleus
Pul, pulvinar
VA/VL, ventral anterior and ventral lateral nuclei
VPL, ventral posterolateral nucleus
VPM, ventral posteromedial nucleus

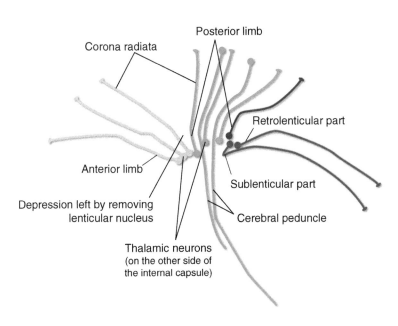

Figure 8.28 Afferents to the hypothalamus. Various kinds of afferents are mapped out systematically in different parts of the hypothalamus, but this is not indicated in the figure. With the exception of inputs from the retina and endings in the mammillary body (MB), the exact location of endings in this figure has no significance.

The **hypothalamus** is tiny, accounting for much less than 1% of the weight of the CNS, but is centrally involved in essentially all homeostatic and drive-related functions. As such, it has a multitude of connections, most of them predictable from these functions.

Many hypothalamic afferents are sensory, dealing with metabolic variables and the general condition of the body. Some of these are **visceral afferents**, arriving from places such as the **spinal cord**, the **nucleus of the solitary tract**, the **parabrachial nuclei**, and the **periaqueductal gray**. Some are collaterals of fibers in pathways to the thalamus, most prominently the **spinothalamic tract**. Most of these inputs arrive through the **medial forebrain bundle**, which travels through the reticular formation, or through the **dorsal longitudinal fasciculus**, which travels through the periventricular and periaqueductal gray matter; both of these bundles also convey hypothalamic efferents. Other relevant inputs arrive via the

bloodstream (not indicated in the figure): Certain hypothalamic neurons are directly sensitive to the temperature of blood passing through the hypothalamus, to its osmolality, or to its concentration of glucose, other metabolites, or various hormones. Finally, there is a direct input from a subset of **retinal ganglion cells** to the **suprachiasmatic nucleus** of the hypothalamus. The suprachiasmatic nucleus contains the master clock for circadian rhythms, and the retinal inputs help to synchronize this clock with actual day length.

The hypothalamus also receives numerous inputs from **prefrontal** and **limbic cortex**, the **hippocampus**, the **amygdala**, and other subcortical limbic nuclei. Afferents from the hippocampus arrive through the **fornix** and largely terminate in the ipsilateral **mammillary body**; those from the amygdala travel through the **stria terminalis** or the **ventral amygdalofugal pathway**.

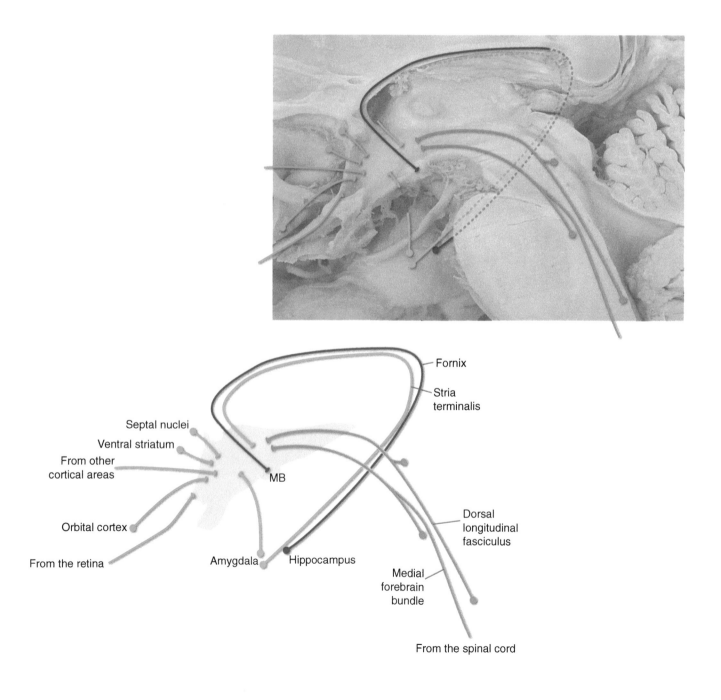

Figure 8.29 Efferents from the hypothalamus. Various kinds of efferents leave systematically from different parts of the hypothalamus, but this is not indicated in the figure: With the exception of neurons in the mammillary body *(MB)*, the exact location of neurons in this figure has no significance. Other abbreviations: *A*, Anterior nucleus of the thalamus; *Am*, amygdala; *DM*, dorsomedial nucleus of the thalamus (as well as some other thalamic nuclei); *MTT*, mammillothalamic tract.

The hypothalamus projects back to some of the same sites from which it receives inputs, often via the same bundles. For example, it projects through the **medial forebrain bundle** to **preganglionic autonomic neurons** and other autonomic centers in the **brainstem** and **spinal cord**. It also projects back to **prefrontal** and **limbic cortex** and to the **hippocampus**, but in these cases, a thalamic relay is involved. The hippocampal projection involves the anatomically prominent **mammillothalamic tract**, extending from the **mammillary body** to the **anterior nucleus** of the thalamus. There are also outputs that reach the cerebral cortex directly, but these are diffuse modulatory projections that reach widespread cortical regions (see Fig. 8.41).

A final set of hypothalamic outputs contributes to homeostasis by controlling the release of hormones from the **pituitary gland**.

The pituitary is a two-part gland, with an **anterior lobe** derived from the roof of the mouth and a **posterior lobe** that develops as an outgrowth from the hypothalamus. Hypothalamic control is exercised through a corresponding two-part system. Neurons in the walls of the third ventricle near the **infundibulum** produce factors (mostly peptides) that promote or inhibit the secretion of anterior lobe hormones. These factors are released near capillaries in the **median eminence** (which lacks a blood–brain barrier), travel down **portal veins** in the infundibulum, and are rereleased in the anterior pituitary. Posterior pituitary hormones are actually produced in the hypothalamus itself. Neurons in the **supraoptic** and **paraventricular nuclei** of the anterior hypothalamus produce **oxytocin** or **vasopressin**, which travels down the axons of these neurons and is released into the circulation in the posterior pituitary.

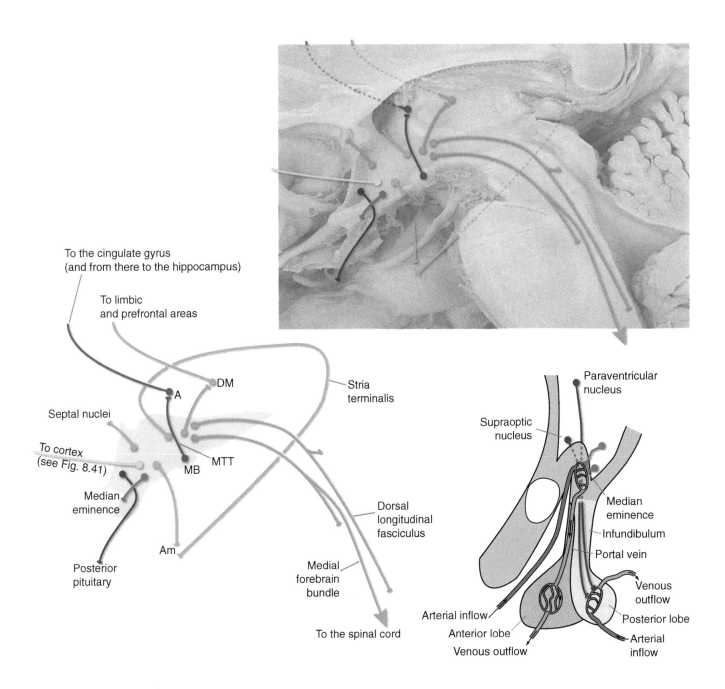

Figure 8.30 An overview of the limbic system.

The **limbic system** is a set of intricately interconnected structures that form a functional bridge between large areas of cerebral cortex and the input/output structures of the nervous system. It forms the basis of autonomic, endocrine, and behavioral responses to homeostatic challenges and events with implications for survival and reproduction, and it helps to ensure that such events are remembered.

The principal structures of the limbic system are the **hippocampus** and **amygdala** in the **medial temporal lobe**, a collection of nuclei in and near the **hypothalamus**, a ring of **limbic cortex** that provides a link with the rest of the cerebral cortex, and the interconnections of all these areas. They are shown here in three-dimensional reconstructions of the limbic system of the same brain shown in sagittal sections in Chapter 7. Limbic structures were outlined on serial sections by Jay B. Angevine Jr.; outlines were assembled into 3D reconstructions by Cheryl Cotman.

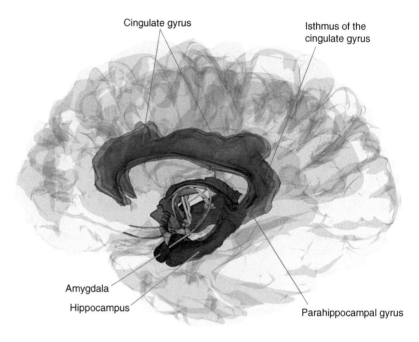

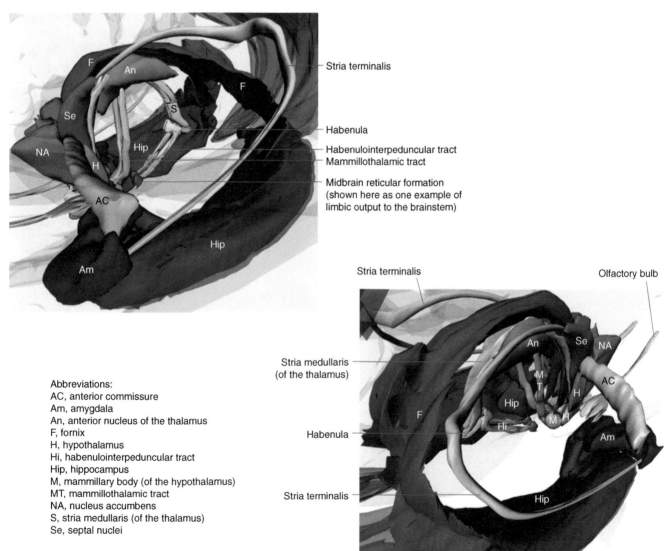

Abbreviations:
AC, anterior commissure
Am, amygdala
An, anterior nucleus of the thalamus
F, fornix
H, hypothalamus
Hi, habenulointerpeduncular tract
Hip, hippocampus
M, mammillary body (of the hypothalamus)
MT, mammillothalamic tract
NA, nucleus accumbens
S, stria medullaris (of the thalamus)
Se, septal nuclei

Figure 8.31 The amygdala and its input/output pathways. (3D reconstruction provided by Cheryl Cotman.)

The **amygdala** and **hippocampus** in humans are prominent examples of structures that wind up in the temporal lobe as a consequence of the **C-shaped growth** of the cerebral hemispheres (see Fig. 4.1). As a result, some of the pathways associated with them trace the same C shape as other parts of the hemisphere.

Most connections between the amygdala and the **hypothalamus** and nearby areas travel through one of two routes: (1) the **stria terminalis**, a small but long, curved bundle of fibers that travels in the wall of the **lateral ventricle** adjacent to the **caudate nucleus**, and (2) the **ventral amygdalofugal pathway** (a misleading name because it contains both afferents and efferents), a loosely organized group of fibers that pass underneath the **lenticular nucleus** on their way to and from the amygdala.

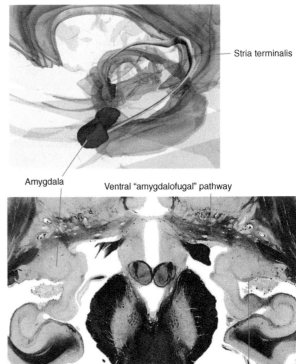

Stria terminalis

Amygdala

Ventral "amygdalofugal" pathway

Caudate nucleus

Stria terminalis

Thalamostriate (terminal) vein

Thalamus

Beginning of the stria terminalis

Figure 8.32 The hippocampus and fornix. (3D reconstruction provided by Dr. John Sundsten.)

The **hippocampus** has a much more massive output bundle, the **fornix**, that travels a similar C-**shaped course**. The fornix is a long, curved tract that starts out as fibers (the **alveus**) on the ventricular surface of the hippocampus. These fibers merge into the **fimbria** (literally "the fringe" of the hippocampus), which parts company with the dwindling hippocampus near the **splenium** of the **corpus callosum** and emerges from the temporal lobe as the **crus** of the fornix. Each crus then approaches its counterpart from the other hemisphere and continues traveling anteriorly, adjacent to the midline and at the inferior edge of the **septum pellucidum**, as the **body** of the fornix. The body diverges into the **columns** of the fornix, which travel through the **hypothalamus**, mostly on their way to the **mammillary bodies**. (The fornix also contains cholinergic afferents from the **septal nuclei** to the hippocampus.) Despite the size of the fornix, most hippocampal afferents and efferents actually take a more direct course to and from temporal lobe structures. These fibers, however, are distributed along the length of the hippocampus and do not form a discrete bundle.

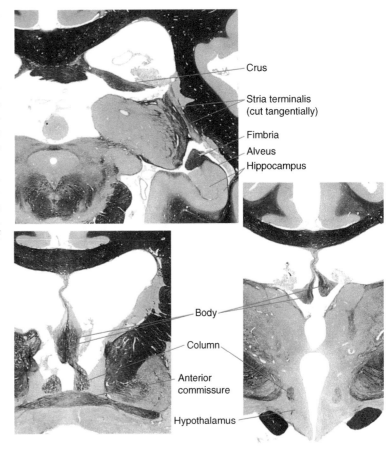

Crus

Stria terminalis (cut tangentially)

Fimbria

Alveus

Hippocampus

Body

Column

Anterior commissure

Hypothalamus

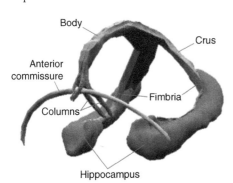

Body

Crus

Anterior commissure

Fimbria

Columns

Hippocampus

Figure 8.33 (A) Afferents to the amygdala.

The **amygdala**, one of the major constituents of the limbic system, is a collection of nuclei underlying the **uncus** of the medial temporal/limbic lobe. It is centrally involved in assessing and remembering the emotional and drive-related significance of stimuli—deciding, for example, whether to flee from something or eat it. As such, it has widespread connections with the cerebral cortex, thalamus, hypothalamus, a variety of brainstem locations, and other sites.

Afferents reach the amygdala from the cerebral cortex (through the white matter of the temporal lobe), the **olfactory bulb** (through the **lateral olfactory tract**), and from a variety of other subcortical sites (through the **stria terminalis** and **ventral "amygdalofugal" pathway**). Cortical afferents arise in **limbic areas**, especially **orbital** and **anterior cingulate cortex**, and in **association areas**, especially **sensory association areas**. Subcortical afferents arise in the **hypothalamus** (and nearby sites, such as the **septal nuclei**), multiple **thalamic nuclei,** and numerous brainstem sites, including the **periaqueductal gray**, **parabrachial nuclei**, and **nucleus of the solitary tract**.

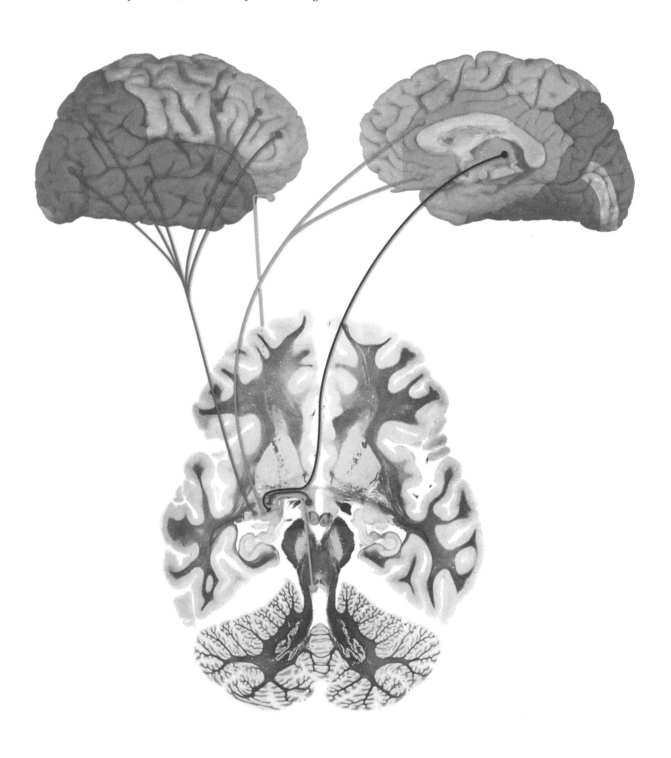

Figure 8.33 (Continued) **(B)** Afferents to the amygdala, continued.

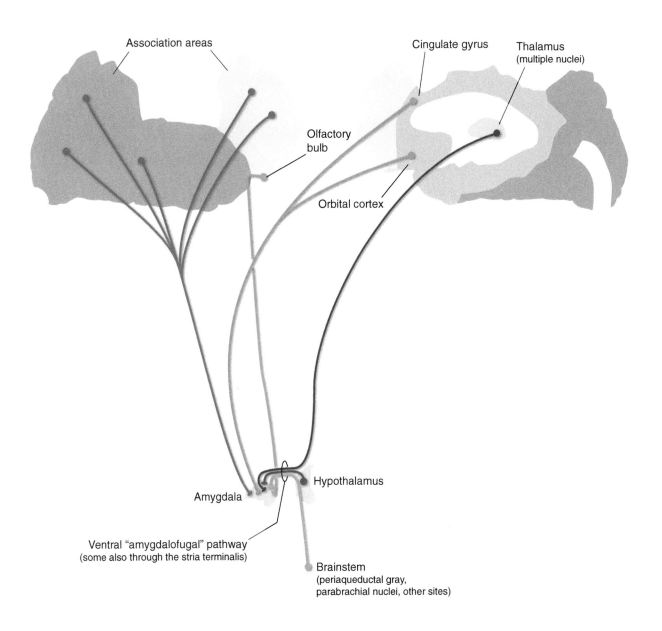

Figure 8.34 (A) Efferents from the amygdala.

The efferents from the **amygdala** for the most part reciprocate its afferents, although there are none to the **olfactory bulb**. Efferents reach more widespread cortical areas than those in which afferents to the amygdala arise, even extending to **primary sensory areas**. Projections to the **hippocampus** help ensure that emotionally significant events are remembered, and those to the **hypothalamus**, nearby regions such as the **septal nuclei**, and **brainstem nuclei** help regulate autonomic and behavioral responses to such events. In addition, efferents from the amygdala to **nucleus accumbens** and other parts of the **ventral striatum** are presumed to play a role in initiating behavioral responses to emotionally significant stimuli.

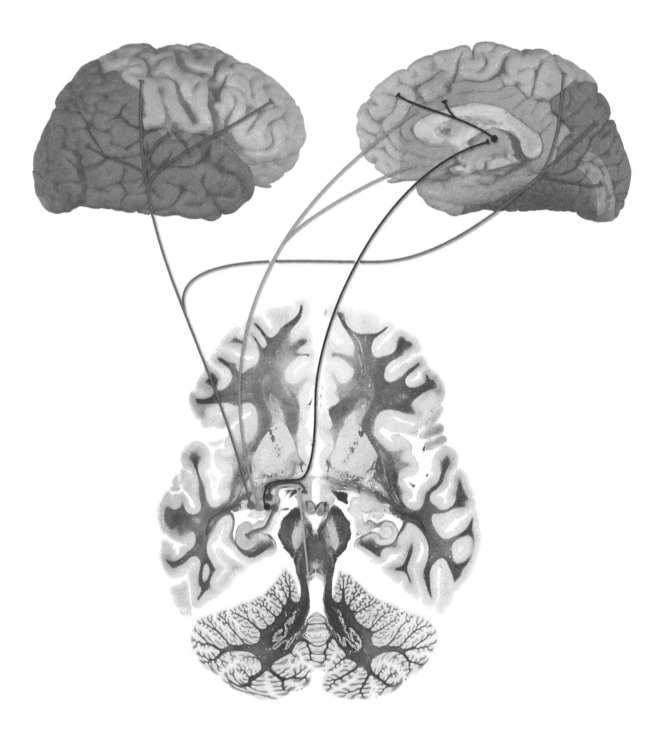

Figure 8.34 (Continued) **(B)** Efferents from the amygdala, continued.

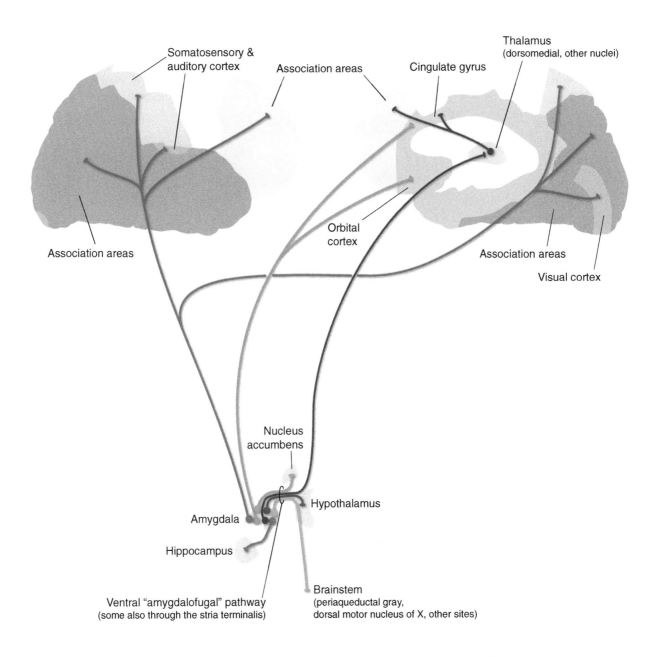

Figure 8.35 (A) Afferents to the hippocampus.

The **hippocampus** is a specialized area of cerebral cortex (see inset in *B*)—conceptually, the edge of the cortical sheet—rolled into the **medial temporal lobe**. It extends in the wall of the **lateral ventricle** from an enlarged anterior end that overlaps the **amygdala** underneath the **uncus** to a tapering posterior end near the **splenium** of the **corpus callosum**.[c] Formally, it consists of the **dentate gyrus**, the **hippocampus proper** (also called **Ammon's horn** or **cornu ammonis**), and the **subiculum**, which merges with the cerebral cortex of the **parahippocampal gyrus**.

[c]The hippocampus actually continues over the top of the corpus callosum as a thin, apparently rudimentary, band of tissue—the indusium griseum, which is not indicated in this atlas. Hence the hippocampus, strictly defined, extends along the entire edge of the cortical mantle.

As in the case of the amygdala, the hippocampus is connected anatomically like a bridge between the diencephalon and widespread areas of cerebral cortex, in this case as the substrate for its critical role in consolidation of new memories of facts and events.

Cholinergic afferents from the **septal nuclei** reach the hippocampus directly by traveling "backward" through the **fornix**, but most other inputs are relayed by adjacent parts of the anterior **parahippocampal gyrus** (the **entorhinal cortex**). Afferents to entorhinal cortex from posterior parts of the **cingulate gyrus** travel through the **cingulum**, a curved fiber bundle underlying the gyrus; those from **association areas** and the **amygdala** travel through the white matter of the temporal lobe. To simplify this figure, all cortical afferents are shown as projecting to entorhinal cortex, and all afferents from the amygdala as projecting directly to the hippocampus itself; in fact, each does both in complex patterns.

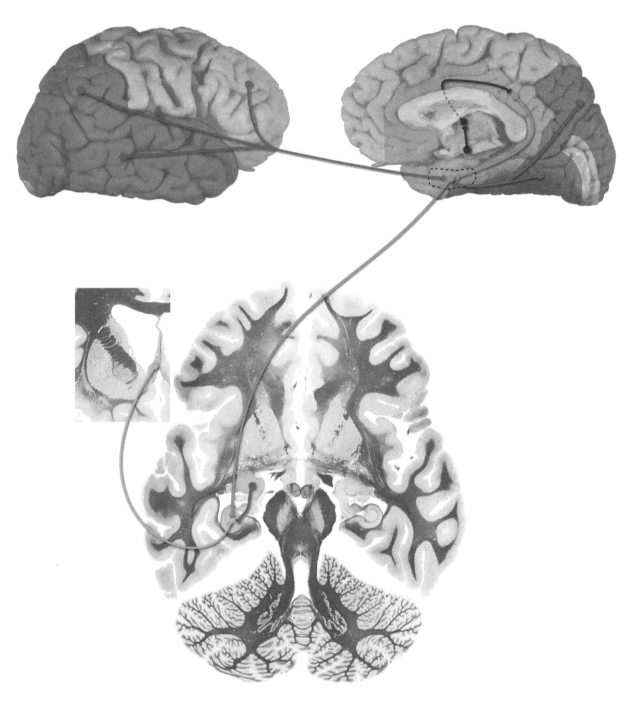

Figure 8.35 (Continued) **(B)** Afferents to the hippocampus, continued. (Inset provided by Pamela Eller, University of Colorado Health Sciences Center.)

In cross section, the hippocampus is made up of two interlocking C-shaped strips of cortex (the **dentate gyrus** and the **hippocampus proper**) and the **subiculum**, which is a transitional zone continuous laterally with the hippocampus proper and medially with **entorhinal cortex**. The hippocampus proper is itself further subdivided into four longitudinal strips called **CA fields** (*CA* for **cornu ammonis**). Abbreviations: C, Tail of the caudate nucleus; CA, hippocampus proper (cornu ammonis); D, dentate gyrus; F, fimbria; LGN, lateral geniculate nucleus; *LV*, inferior horn of the lateral ventricle; *ST*, stria terminalis; *Sub*, subiculum.

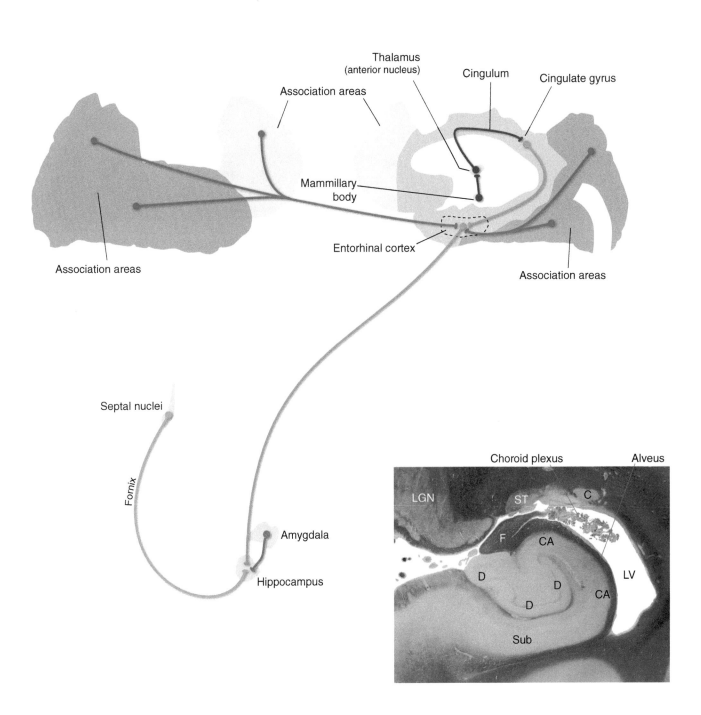

Figure 8.36 (A) Efferents from the hippocampus.

The anatomically most prominent efferent pathway from the hippocampus is the **fornix** (see Fig. 8.32), through which hippocampal pyramidal cells project to the **septal nuclei** and **subicular neurons** project to the **septal nuclei**, **mammillary bodies**, **ventral striatum**, and some cortical areas. At the level of the interventricular foramen, fornix fibers begin to splay out as they move toward their final destinations. Some pass in front of the **anterior commissure** (the **precommissural fornix**) to reach the septal nuclei and parts of the frontal lobe. Others turn posteriorly and end directly in the **anterior nucleus** of the **thalamus**. A large number descend through the hypothalamus in the **column** of the fornix, mostly directed toward the **mammillary body**.

Large numbers of subicular efferents, however, bypass the fornix and project directly to **entorhinal cortex** and other cortical areas.

(This is presumably part of the reason why bilateral damage to the hippocampus causes a much more severe memory deficit than does bilateral damage to the fornix.) As in the case of afferents to the hippocampus, more than one hippocampal component may project in parallel to the same structure (e.g., both subiculum and entorhinal cortex to other cortical areas).

The fundamental pattern of information flow in the hippocampus is unidirectional: afferents (mostly from entorhinal cortex) → granule cells of the **dentate gyrus → CA3 pyramidal cells → CA1 pyramidal cells** → pyramidal cells of the subiculum → output targets. Thus most of the output of the hippocampus comes from the subiculum, although some comes from hippocampal pyramidal cells.

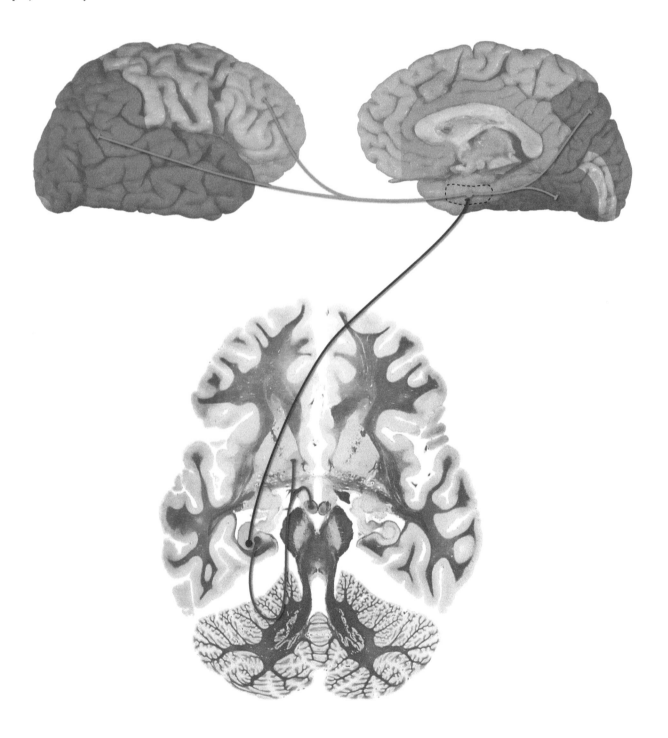

Figure 8.36 (Continued) **(B)** Efferents from the hippocampus, continued.

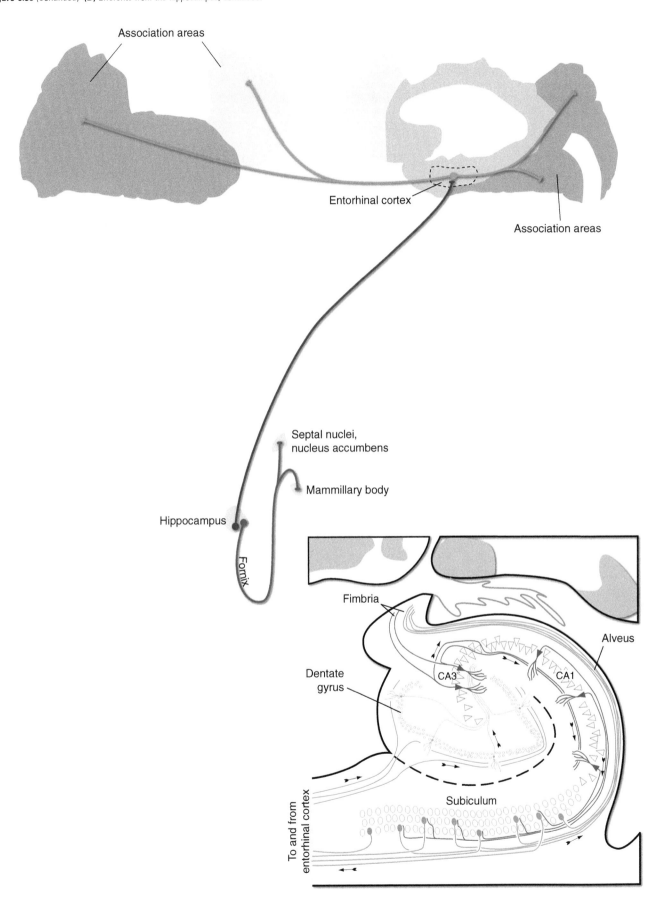

Figure 8.37 Neurons and pathways that use acetylcholine as a neurotransmitter.

Some neurotransmitters are found in neurons widely distributed in the nervous system. **Glutamate**, for example, is a common transmitter used by neurons throughout the brain at excitatory synapses. Similarly, **gamma-aminobutyric acid (GABA)** is a nearly ubiquitous transmitter used at inhibitory synapses. In contrast, some transmitters are found only in neurons in restricted locations (although the axons of these neurons may be distributed widely). **Acetylcholine**, the first neurotransmitter to be discovered, is a case in point.

Acetylcholine is of major importance in the peripheral nervous system, where it is the principal transmitter released by **motor neurons**, **preganglionic autonomic neurons**, **postganglionic parasympathetic neurons**, and a minority of **postganglionic sympathetic neurons**. Within the brain, its distribution is more restricted. Acetylcholine is used as a neurotransmitter by some interneurons of the **striatum** and by some parts of the **reticular formation**. However, the most prominent collection of cholinergic neurons in the brain is found in the **basal nucleus** (of **Meynert**), the **septal nuclei**, and nearby parts of the **basal forebrain**. Collectively these neurons project through the **cingulum** and the **external capsule** (the white matter between the **claustrum** and the **putamen**) and blanket the cerebral cortex and **amygdala** with cholinergic endings. In addition, some of the septal neurons send cholinergic axons through the **fornix** to the **hippocampus**.

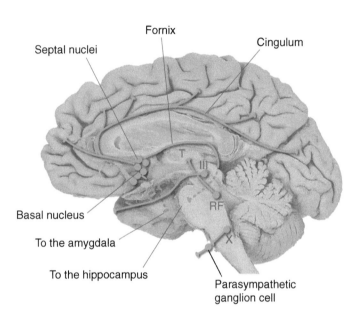

III, oculomotor nucleus (representing lower motor neurons in general)
X, dorsal motor nucleus of the vagus (representing preganglionic autonomic neurons in general)
RF, reticular formation
T, thalamus

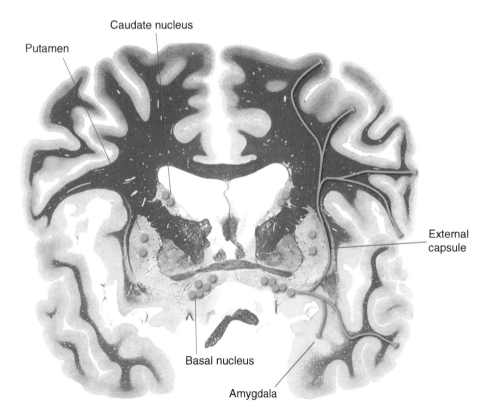

Figure 8.38 Neurons and pathways that use norepinephrine as a neurotransmitter.

Norepinephrine, one of the **catecholamine** neurotransmitters (so called because of the catechol group, shown in *red*, that forms part of the molecule) is the transmitter used by most **postganglionic sympathetic neurons**. Within the CNS, it is found in a series of pontine and medullary neurons with long, branching axons that collectively innervate most areas of the brain and spinal cord.

The majority of these **noradrenergic** neurons (noradrenaline is a synonym for norepinephrine) are located in the **locus ceruleus**, a column of pigmented cells in the rostral pons (see Fig. 3.14). Others are located in the **dorsal motor nucleus of the vagus**, the **nucleus of the solitary tract**, the medullary **reticular formation**, and a few other sites.

Ascending noradrenergic fibers (mostly from the locus ceruleus) travel through the brainstem in the **dorsal longitudinal fasciculus** and **central tegmental tract**. When they reach the cerebrum, many of them join the **medial forebrain bundle**, which travels longitudinally through the lateral **hypothalamus**. They then diverge to innervate practically all cerebral areas. Descending noradrenergic fibers (many from more caudally located neurons) similarly diverge to innervate the **cerebellum, brainstem,** and **spinal cord**.

These diffuse, nearly global projections are clearly unsuitable for mediating functions that depend on precise, point-to-point communication, and instead they are involved in regulating the overall level of activity in large areas of the brain (e.g., as levels of attention and vigilance vary).

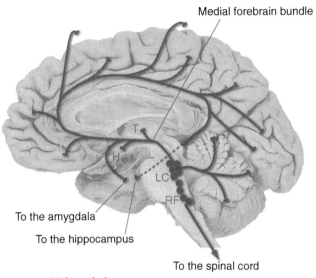

H, hypothalamus
LC, locus ceruleus
RF, reticular formation
T, thalamus

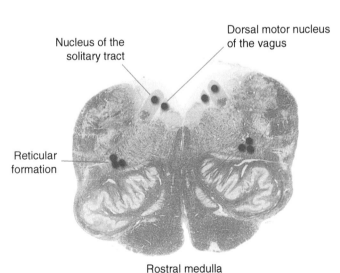

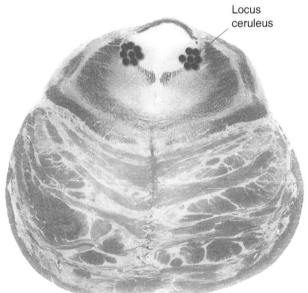

Figure 8.39 Neurons and pathways that use dopamine as a neurotransmitter.

Dopamine is a second major **catecholamine** neurotransmitter (so called because of the catechol group, shown in *red*, that forms part of the molecule). Most dopaminergic neurons are located in the midbrain, either in the **substantia nigra (compact part)** or in the medially adjacent **ventral tegmental area**. They project rostrally to most parts of the forebrain in three partially overlapping streams of fibers.

The first of these streams is the projection from the substantia nigra (compact part) to the **caudate nucleus** and **putamen** (see Fig. 8.17). Because of its origin in the midbrain, this **nigrostriatal** pathway is also referred to as the **mesostriatal** dopaminergic pathway (midbrain = mesencephalon).

Mesolimbic and **mesocortical** fibers originate mainly in the ventral tegmental area, medial to the substantia nigra, and project through the **medial forebrain bundle** to limbic-related subcortical structures (such as the **amygdala**, **septal nuclei**, and **ventral striatum**) and to cerebral cortex (especially **motor** and **limbic areas**).

Additional dopaminergic neurons are found in the **retina** and in the **hypothalamus**. The latter project to the **median eminence**, where dopamine released into capillaries of the **pituitary portal system** regulates the secretion of prolactin by the **anterior pituitary** (see Fig. 8.29).

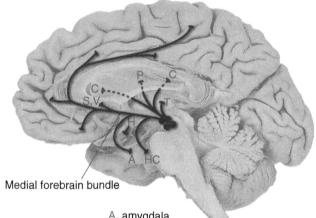

Medial forebrain bundle

A, amygdala
C, caudate nucleus
H, hypothalamus
HC, hippocampus
P, putamen
S, septal nuclei
T, thalamus
V, ventral striatum

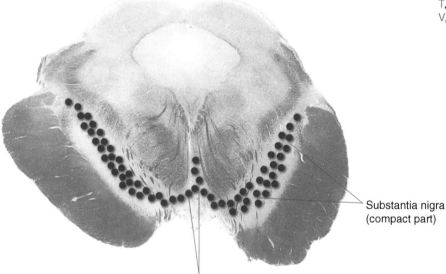

Substantia nigra
(compact part)

Ventral tegmental area

Figure 8.40 Neurons and pathways that use serotonin as a neurotransmitter.

Serotonin (shown below), a derivative of tryptophan, is used as a neurotransmitter by a collection of neurons located at most brainstem levels in a series of **raphe**[d] nuclei. Serotonergic neurons, like noradrenergic neurons, give rise to widely branched axons that innervate most parts of the CNS, including the **hypothalamus**, **striatum**, and **thalamus**. Serotonin, like norepinephrine, is thought to be involved in regulating the overall level of activity in the brain.

———————

[d]The Greek word *rhaphe* means "seam" and is used in this case to refer to the midline seam between the two halves of the brainstem.

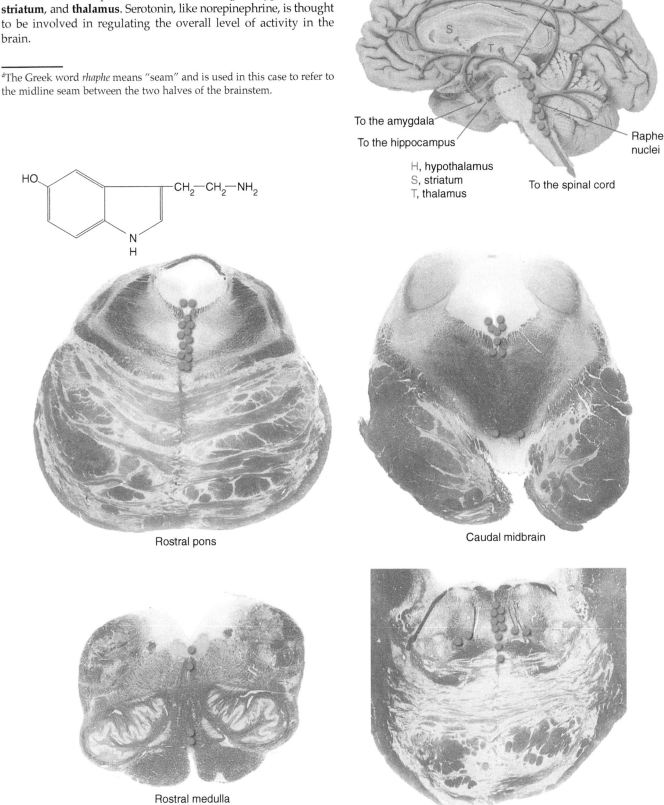

Medial forebrain bundle

To the amygdala
To the hippocampus

Raphe nuclei

H, hypothalamus
S, striatum
T, thalamus

To the spinal cord

Rostral pons

Caudal midbrain

Rostral medulla

Caudal pons

Figure 8.41 Modulatory outputs of the hypothalamus. Abbreviations: *C*, Caudate nucleus; *H*, hypothalamic histaminergic neurons; *LC*, locus ceruleus; *P*, putamen; *R*, raphe nuclei; *S*, septal nuclei; *T*, thalamus.

The **hypothalamus** projects back to cortical areas and the **hippocampus** by way of the **thalamus**, but it also contains two populations of neurons with widespread modulatory outputs directly to the cerebral cortex and to other CNS targets. These neurons play important roles in the sleep-wake cycle. Neurons of the first group (below right) are located near the **mammillary bodies** and use the monoamine **histamine** as a neurotransmitter. Much like the serotonergic neurons in Fig. 8.40, they essentially blanket the CNS with endings, including projections to brainstem components of the modulatory network. Neurons of the second group (below left) are located in the lateral hypothalamus, near the **fornix**, and use neuropeptides called **orexins** (also called **hypocretins**) as transmitters. Their projections to the striatum, globus pallidus, and cerebellum are limited, but otherwise are widely distributed to other parts of the CNS (including the histaminergic neurons).

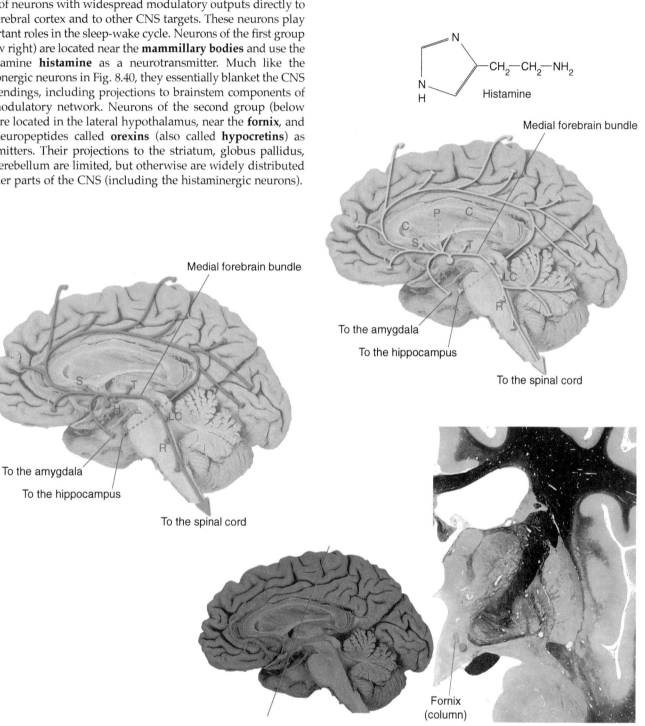

Histamine

Medial forebrain bundle

Medial forebrain bundle

To the amygdala

To the hippocampus

To the amygdala

To the hippocampus

To the spinal cord

To the spinal cord

Fornix
(column)

9

Clinical Imaging*

For many decades, the central nervous system (CNS) of living individuals could be examined only indirectly, for example by using **x-rays** to study changes in the bones surrounding the CNS or the blood vessels around or within it. In addition, these imaging studies involved projecting all the x-ray density under investigation in the head (a three-dimensional structure) onto a two-dimensional sheet of film. As a result, the images of structures actually separated in space (e.g., the middle cerebral and anterior cerebral branches in Fig. 9.17A) are superimposed on each other in these studies.

The past 40 years have seen revolutionary changes in clinical imaging, partly a result of the use of computers to reconstruct two-dimensional "slices" at various levels of a patient's head (i.e., **tomography**) and partly a result of the ability to construct images based on parameters other than x-ray density.

The most commonly used clinical imaging techniques at present are x-ray **computed tomography** (CT) and **magnetic resonance imaging** (MRI). CT provides images based on x-ray density, so structures that attenuate x-rays, such as bone, appear light; areas filled with air or cerebrospinal fluid, which do not attenuate x-rays as much, appear much darker. Appropriate techniques can accentuate brain, bone, or blood (Figs. 9.1 to 9.3). MRI (Fig. 9.4), in contrast, provides images based on chemical concentrations (most commonly emphasizing the concentration of free water). This chapter provides a series of examples of the use of CT and MRI to demonstrate normal anatomy in clinical imaging. In addition, although traditional **angiographic** techniques are no longer used very often, they still yield the most highly detailed images of the cerebral vasculature, so examples of **angiograms** are also provided.

---

*With gratitude for the images and assistance provided by Raymond F. Carmody, MD, Elena M. Plante, PhD, and Joachim F. Seeger, MD, my colleagues at The University of Arizona.

Figure 9.1 An axial (approximately horizontal) CT scan, demonstrating the relative x-ray densities of some cranial structures. The range of x-ray densities in the head, from bone through brain to air, is much greater than the human visual system can discriminate as a series of gray shades. In this case, the computer was adjusted so that the gray scale was applied to the x-ray density of brain and cerebrospinal fluid. Hence, bone is uniformly white, and fluid is black (as air would be); gray matter is very slightly more x-ray dense than white matter, so the two can be differentiated from each other. (Provided by Dr. Raymond F. Carmody.)

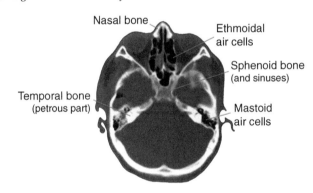

Figure 9.2 An axial (approximately horizontal) CT scan, adjusted so that the gray scale is distributed over the entire range of cranial and intracranial x-ray densities. Air is black, but little soft-tissue or fluid detail can be seen. However, the details and relative densities of different bones (e.g., sphenoid versus temporal) are apparent. (Provided by Dr. Raymond F. Carmody.)

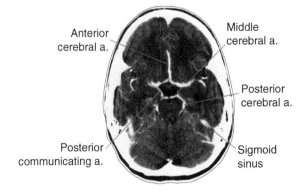

Figure 9.3 Blood flowing through arteries and veins can be seen more easily if an iodinated, x-ray dense contrast agent is injected intravenously before the CT scan. (Provided by Dr. Raymond F. Carmody.)

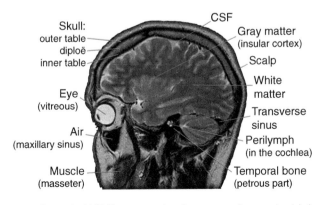

Figure 9.4 Parasagittal MRI. The concentration of water ranges from very low (air, bone) to intermediate levels (brain, muscle) to very high (cerebrospinal fluid [*CSF*], perilymph), allowing all of these to be differentiated. The lack of signal from certain spaces that contain a lot of water—blood vessels—is explained later. (Provided by Dr. Raymond F. Carmody.)

Figure 9.5 (A–D) A series of seven CT images at different levels of a normal brain. (Provided by Dr. Raymond F. Carmody.)

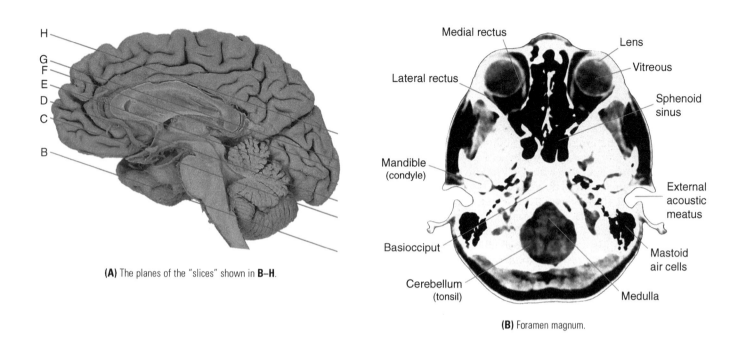

(A) The planes of the "slices" shown in **B–H**.

(B) Foramen magnum.

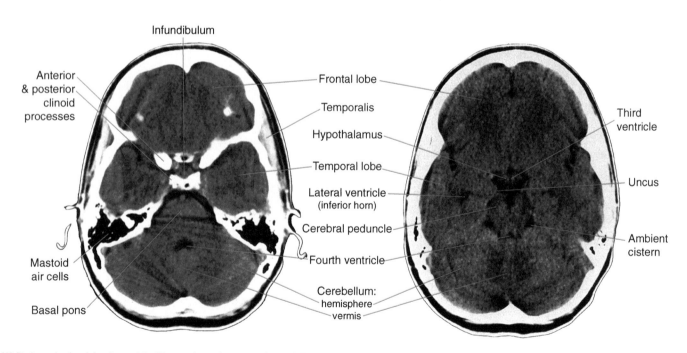

(C) Pituitary gland and fourth ventricle. (The streaks cutting across the cerebellum and pons are artifacts resulting from the presence of dense bone nearby. The density in each frontal lobe results from nearby bone in the orbital roofs.)

(D) Base of the diencephalon.

Figure 9.5 (Continued) **(E–H)** Normal CT images.

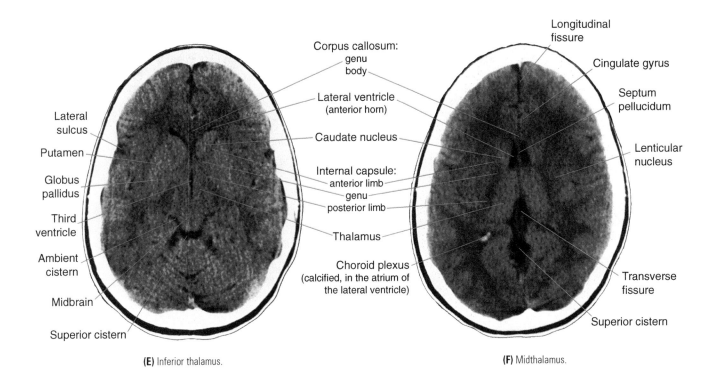

Corpus callosum:
genu
body

Lateral ventricle
(anterior horn)

Caudate nucleus

Internal capsule:
anterior limb
genu
posterior limb

Thalamus

Choroid plexus
(calcified, in the atrium of
the lateral ventricle)

Lateral
sulcus

Putamen

Globus
pallidus

Third
ventricle

Ambient
cistern

Midbrain

Superior cistern

(E) Inferior thalamus.

Longitudinal
fissure

Cingulate gyrus

Septum
pellucidum

Lenticular
nucleus

Transverse
fissure

Superior cistern

(F) Midthalamus.

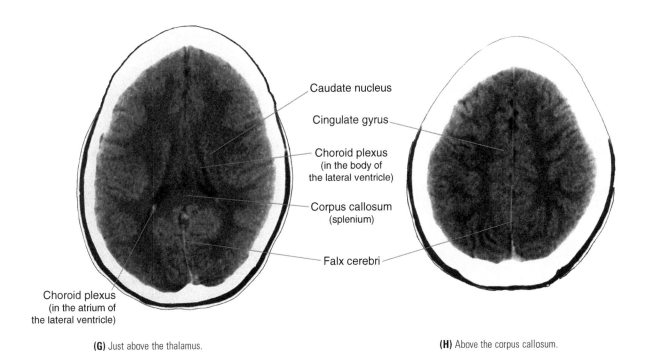

Caudate nucleus

Cingulate gyrus

Choroid plexus
(in the body of
the lateral ventricle)

Corpus callosum
(splenium)

Falx cerebri

Choroid plexus
(in the atrium of
the lateral ventricle)

(G) Just above the thalamus.

(H) Above the corpus callosum.

Figure 9.6 (A–D) A series of seven CT images from the same patient shown in Fig. 9.5. In this case an iodinated intravenous contrast agent was administered before the CT study, making blood vessels visible. (Provided by Dr. Raymond F. Carmody.)

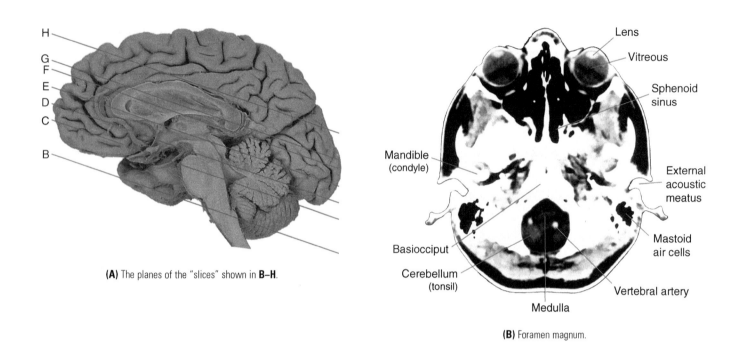

(A) The planes of the "slices" shown in **B–H**.

(B) Foramen magnum.

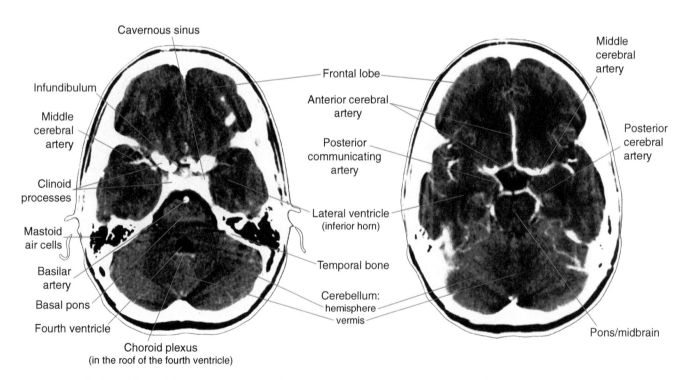

(C) Cavernous sinus. The infundibulum and choroid plexus appear x-ray dense because the blood–brain barrier is lacking at these sites, allowing the contrast agent to leak out.

(D) Circle of Willis.

Figure 9.6 (Continued) **(E–H)** Contrasted CT images.

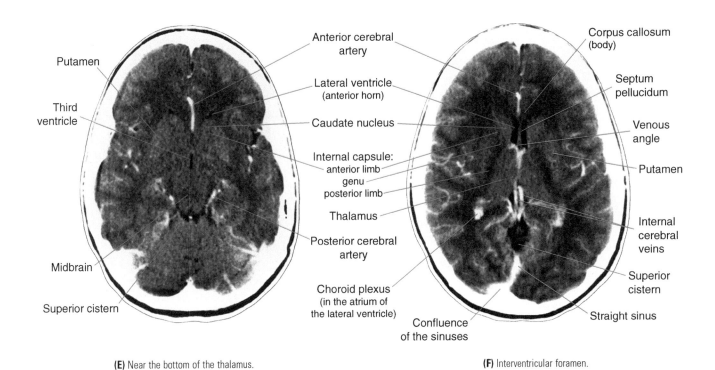

(E) Near the bottom of the thalamus.

Labels (left image): Putamen; Third ventricle; Midbrain; Superior cistern; Anterior cerebral artery; Lateral ventricle (anterior horn); Caudate nucleus; Internal capsule: anterior limb, genu, posterior limb; Thalamus; Posterior cerebral artery; Choroid plexus (in the atrium of the lateral ventricle); Confluence of the sinuses

(F) Interventricular foramen.

Labels (right image): Corpus callosum (body); Septum pellucidum; Venous angle; Putamen; Internal cerebral veins; Superior cistern; Straight sinus

(G) Just above the thalamus.

Labels (left image): Choroid plexus (in the atrium of the lateral ventricle); Caudate nucleus; Choroid plexus (in the body of the lateral ventricle); Corpus callosum (splenium); Great cerebral vein (of Galen); Straight sinus; Falx cerebri; Superior sagittal sinus

(H) Above the corpus callosum. The falx (dura mater) is outside the blood–brain barrier, so contrast agent leaks out here.

Figure 9.7 (A–F) The use of CT to demonstrate intracranial pathology. By convention, all axial scans (both CT and MRI) are oriented with anterior toward the top of the page and the patient's left on the right side, as though you were looking up from the patient's feet. (Provided by Dr. Raymond F. Carmody.)

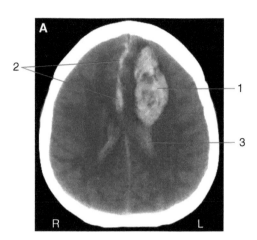

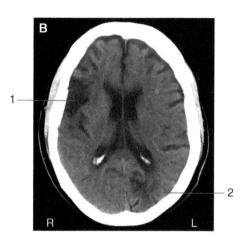

(A) CT measures x-ray density, so structures and substances more dense than brain stand out and are light. In this 31-year-old woman, blood in a recent left intracerebral hemorrhage *(1)* is apparent, spreading through subarachnoid space on either side of the falx cerebri *(2)* and through the lateral ventricle *(3)*.

(B) Structures and substances less dense than brain also stand out, but are dark. In this case, two old infarcts, one *(1)* in part of the right middle cerebral artery territory and another *(2)* in the left posterior cerebral territory, are apparent in this 67-year-old woman.

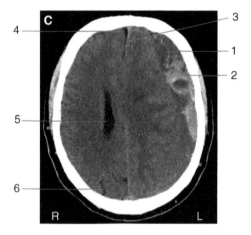

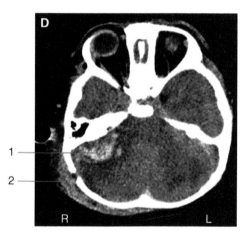

(C) Over a period of weeks, intracranial blood breaks down and becomes less dense than brain. The chronic left subdural hematoma in this 60-year-old man has re-bled and contains a mixture of old *(1)* and new *(2)* blood. Pressure from the hematoma bows the falx cerebri toward the right *(3)* and squeezes out CSF on the left, so that the subarachnoid space *(4, 6)* and lateral ventricle *(5)* apparent on the right can no longer be seen on the left.

(D) An epidural hematoma *(1)* in a 1-year-old boy with a head injury. Because dura mater adheres tightly to the skull, these hematomas usually have a characteristic convex shape (versus the long crescent shape of subdural hematomas such as the one in **C**). Contused and swollen tissue *(2)* can also be seen at the site of injury.

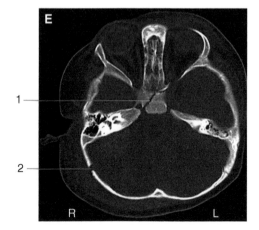

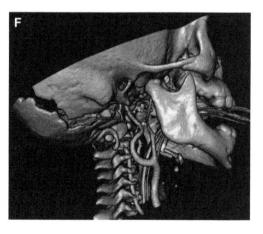

(E) The same patient as in **(D)** but with the CT contrast window set to show bone detail. Now the basal and occipital skull fractures *(1, 2)* are visible, but the hematoma is not.

(F) The same patient as in **D**. Multiple bone-window images such as that in **E** were combined to make a three-dimensional reconstruction of the skull, showing the occipital fracture in detail.

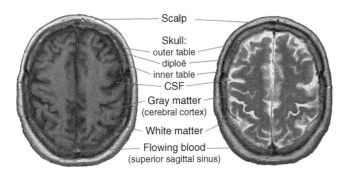

Figure 9.8 In T1-weighted images *(left)*, white matter is lighter than gray matter and cerebrospinal fluid *(CSF)* is dark. Conversely, in T2-weighted images *(right)*, white matter is darker than gray matter, and CSF is bright and prominent. In both, air and dense bone, which contain relatively few hydrogen nuclei, are dark. The appearance of flowing blood depends on a number of technical parameters, but in many instances (e.g., the T2-weighted image on the right), perturbed nuclei have left the area before the imaging measurement is made, so the blood vessel appears dark, as though no hydrogen nuclei were present. (Provided by Dr. Raymond F. Carmody.)

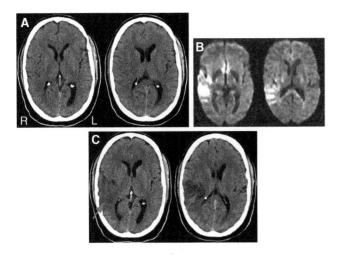

Figure 9.9 Use of diffusion-weighted imaging for early detection of stroke damage. **(A)** On the day of a stroke, CT images fail to reveal significant damage. **(B)** On the same day, diffusion-weighted MRI shows areas of edema and restricted diffusion in part of the right middle cerebral artery distribution. **(C)** Three days later, damage in the edematous areas shows up in CT images. (Provided by Dr. Raymond F. Carmody.)

Figure 9.10 Use of diffusion tensor imaging in planning a neurosurgical procedure. **(A)** A 20-year-old man was found to have a tumor (glioblastoma multiforme) in his left temporal lobe *(1)*. Because part of the optic radiation travels in this part of the temporal lobe (see Fig. 8.9), diffusion tensor imaging was used before surgery to study the relationship between the tumor and the optic radiation. **(B)** In this axial slice through the body of the corpus callosum, fibers traveling in different directions can be distinguished. By convention, areas where it is easier for water to diffuse in an anterior-posterior direction are *green*, here including fibers traveling to or from the frontal *(1)* or occipital *(3)* lobes and fibers in long association bundles *(2)*. Areas with fibers traveling in an inferior-superior direction are *blue*, here including those in the corona radiata *(4)*. Areas with fibers traveling in a side-to-side direction are *red*, here including those in the corpus callosum *(5)*. **(C)** At the level of the anterior commissure *(1)*, the right optic radiation *(2)* has a normal course back toward the occipital lobe. The left optic radiation *(3)* is bowed laterally by the tumor *(4)* but is outside it. (Provided by Dr. Raymond F. Carmody.)

CT reconstructs images based on spatial variations in x-ray density, so the relatively small density differences between gray and white matter limit its ability to differentiate between different areas of the brain. In addition, the much greater x-ray density of bone can overwhelm these small gray-white differences and cause artifacts in bony areas such as the posterior fossa (see Fig. 9.5C).

MRI overcomes these problems by being exquisitely sensitive to spatial variations in the concentration and physicochemical situation of particular atomic nuclei (almost always hydrogen nuclei). Nuclei with an odd number of protons or neutrons, such as hydrogen nuclei, behave like tiny magnets. Imposing a powerful magnetic field on something containing these nuclei (e.g., someone's head) causes a net tendency for the nuclei to align themselves with the external field. Once so aligned, the nuclei preferentially absorb and then emit electromagnetic energy at a particular frequency (the resonant frequency for that kind of nucleus in that situation). Hence, applying radiofrequency pulses to a subject in a strong, static magnetic field and then measuring the spatial distributions of various time constants with which the absorbed energy is re-emitted can provide the data for construction of images based on different tissue properties.

Two time constants—T1 and T2—are particularly important in clinical imaging. T1 is the time constant with which nuclei return to alignment with the static field. T2 is the time constant with which nuclei, all perturbed at the same time by radiofrequency pulses, lose alignment with each other. T1- and T2-weighted images emphasize different tissue parameters in different ways (Fig. 9.8). T1-weighted images show anatomical detail more clearly and so are used in Figs. 9.11 through 9.13. T2-weighted images, on the other hand, are highly sensitive to small changes in water concentration and so are very useful for demonstrating pathology within the brain (see Fig. 9.14A and B).

MRI parameters can be adjusted in additional ways to emphasize other tissue properties. For example, diffusion-weighted images map the ease with which water can diffuse through different parts of the brain. Cells swell when their energy supply is interrupted, moving water from extracellular to intracellular spaces and making it less able to diffuse. As a result, diffusion-weighted images provide a very early indication of the areas damaged in a stroke (Fig. 9.9). Measurements can also be made of the ease with which water can diffuse in particular directions. Because it is easier for water molecules to diffuse in a direction parallel to axons than to snake their way between axons in a direction perpendicular to a tract, it is possible to use this technique to map out the locations of known pathways. Such diffusion tensor images are now commonly used in planning neurosurgical procedures (Fig. 9.10).

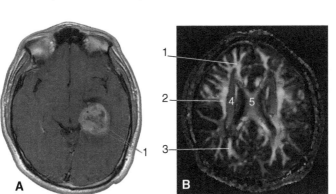

Figure 9.11 (A–O) T1-weighted coronal magnetic resonance (MR) images of the brain of a young man. The same brain is shown in different planes in Figs. 9.11 through 9.13, with the planes of "section" indicated in three-dimensional reconstructions. *The brain was remapped into Talairach space (i.e., morphed to match a standard brain), which is commonly done in preparation for functional imaging studies, making the data obtained from different subjects comparable. (Provided by Dr. Elena M. Plante.)

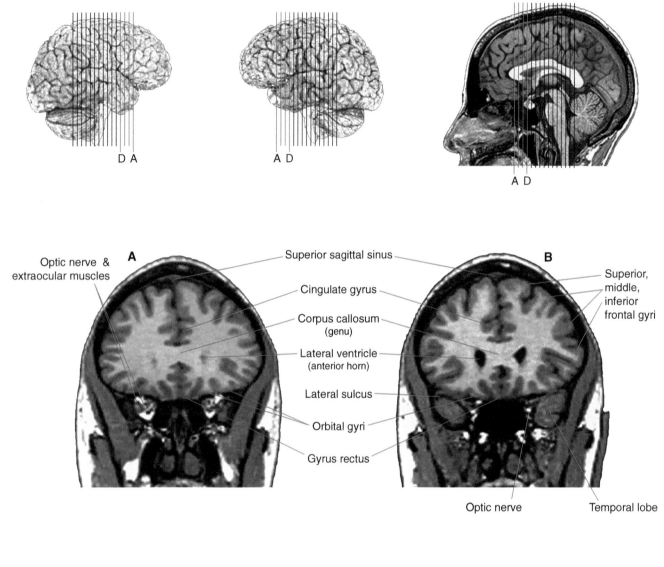

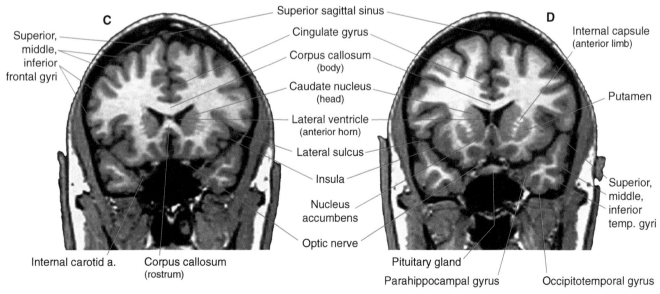

Figure 9.11 (Continued) T1-weighted coronal MR images.

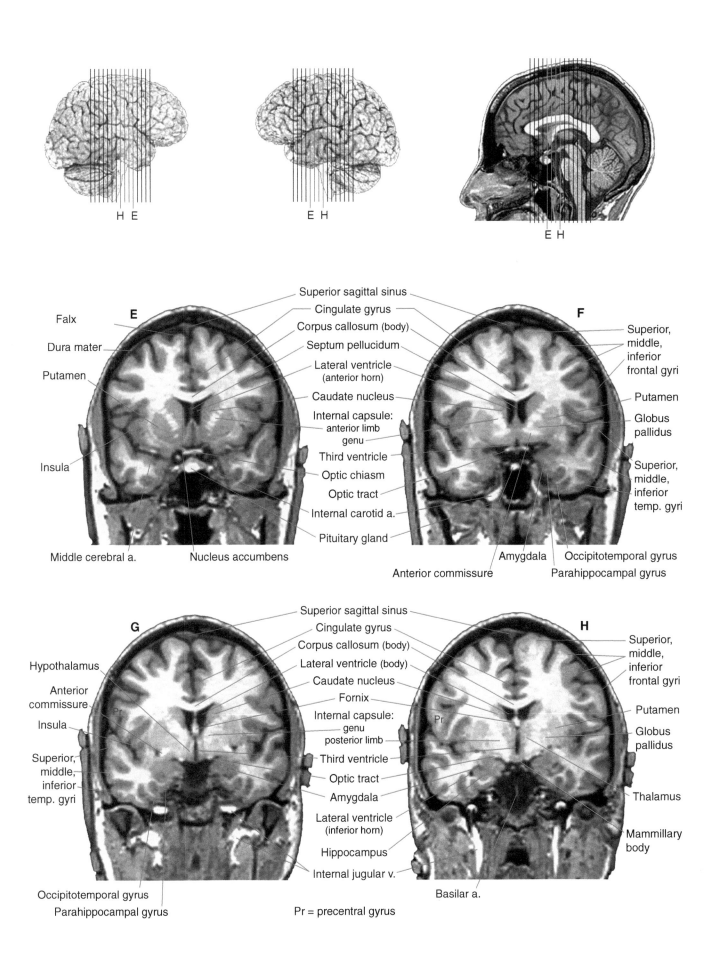

Superior sagittal sinus
Cingulate gyrus
Corpus callosum (body)
Septum pellucidum
Lateral ventricle (anterior horn)
Caudate nucleus
Internal capsule: anterior limb / genu
Third ventricle
Optic chiasm
Optic tract
Internal carotid a.
Pituitary gland

Falx
Dura mater
Putamen
Insula
Middle cerebral a.
Nucleus accumbens

E   F

Superior, middle, inferior frontal gyri
Putamen
Globus pallidus
Superior, middle, inferior temp. gyri
Occipitotemporal gyrus
Parahippocampal gyrus
Amygdala
Anterior commissure

Superior sagittal sinus
Cingulate gyrus
Corpus callosum (body)
Lateral ventricle (body)
Caudate nucleus
Fornix
Internal capsule: genu / posterior limb
Third ventricle
Optic tract
Amygdala
Lateral ventricle (inferior horn)
Hippocampus
Internal jugular v.

Hypothalamus
Anterior commissure
Insula
Superior, middle, inferior temp. gyri
Occipitotemporal gyrus
Parahippocampal gyrus

G   H

Superior, middle, inferior frontal gyri
Putamen
Globus pallidus
Thalamus
Mammillary body
Basilar a.

Pr = precentral gyrus

Figure 9.11 (Continued) T1-weighted coronal MR images.

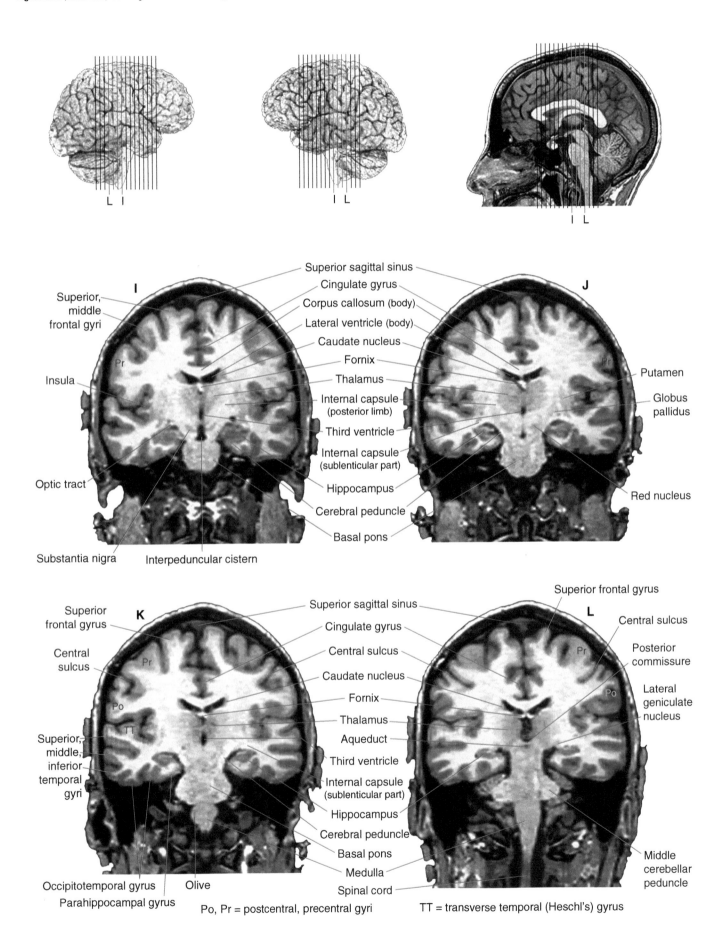

I

Superior sagittal sinus
Cingulate gyrus
Corpus callosum (body)
Lateral ventricle (body)
Caudate nucleus
Fornix
Thalamus
Internal capsule (posterior limb)
Third ventricle
Internal capsule (sublenticular part)
Hippocampus
Cerebral peduncle
Basal pons

Superior, middle frontal gyri
Insula
Optic tract
Substantia nigra
Interpeduncular cistern

J

Putamen
Globus pallidus
Red nucleus

K

Superior frontal gyrus
Central sulcus
Superior, middle, inferior temporal gyri
Occipitotemporal gyrus
Parahippocampal gyrus

Superior sagittal sinus
Cingulate gyrus
Central sulcus
Caudate nucleus
Fornix
Thalamus
Aqueduct
Third ventricle
Internal capsule (sublenticular part)
Hippocampus
Cerebral peduncle
Basal pons
Medulla
Spinal cord

Olive

L

Superior frontal gyrus
Central sulcus
Posterior commissure
Lateral geniculate nucleus
Middle cerebellar peduncle

Po, Pr = postcentral, precentral gyri   TT = transverse temporal (Heschl's) gyrus

Figure 9.11 (Continued) T1-weighted coronal MR images.

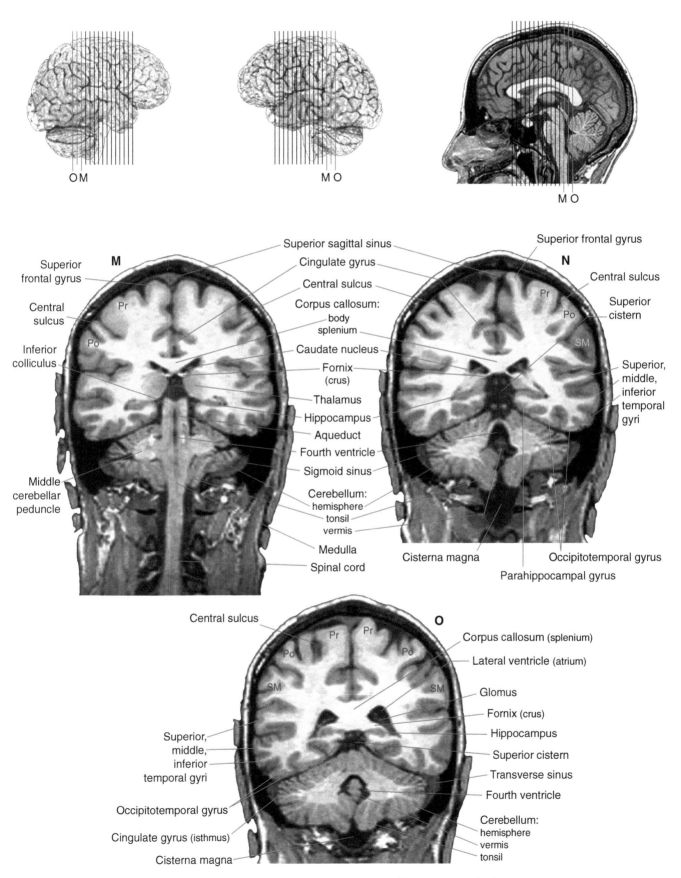

Po, Pr = postcentral, precentral gyri; SM = supramarginal gyrus

Figure 9.12 (A–O) T1-weighted axial (horizontal) MR images of the brain of a young man. The same brain is shown in different planes in Figs. 9.11 through 9.13, with the planes of "section" indicated in three-dimensional reconstructions. (Provided by Dr. Elena M. Plante.)

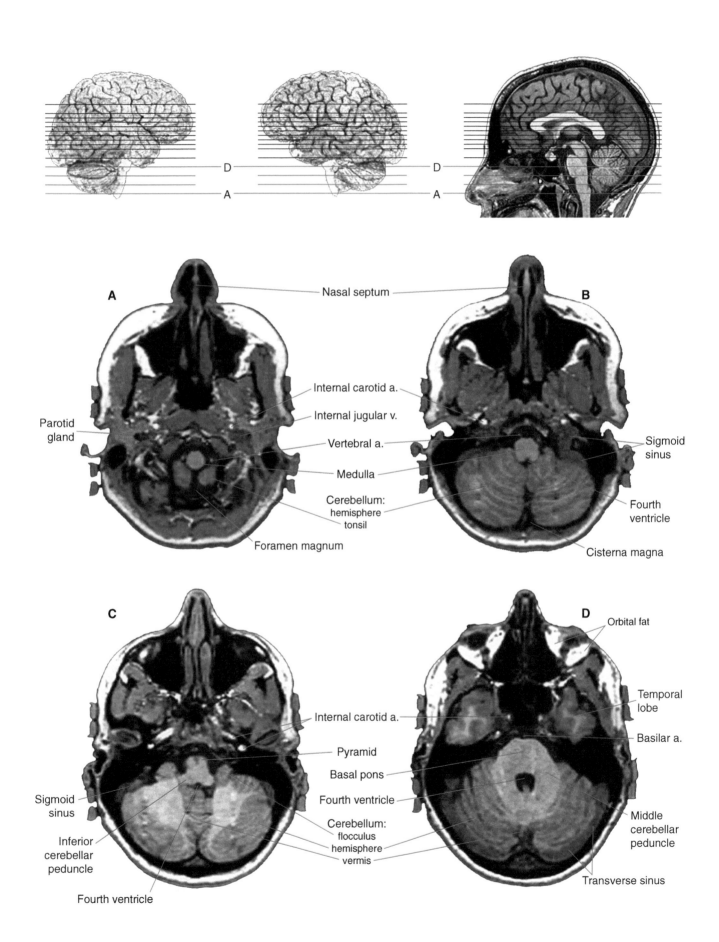

Figure 9.12 (Continued) T1-weighted axial (horizontal) MR images.

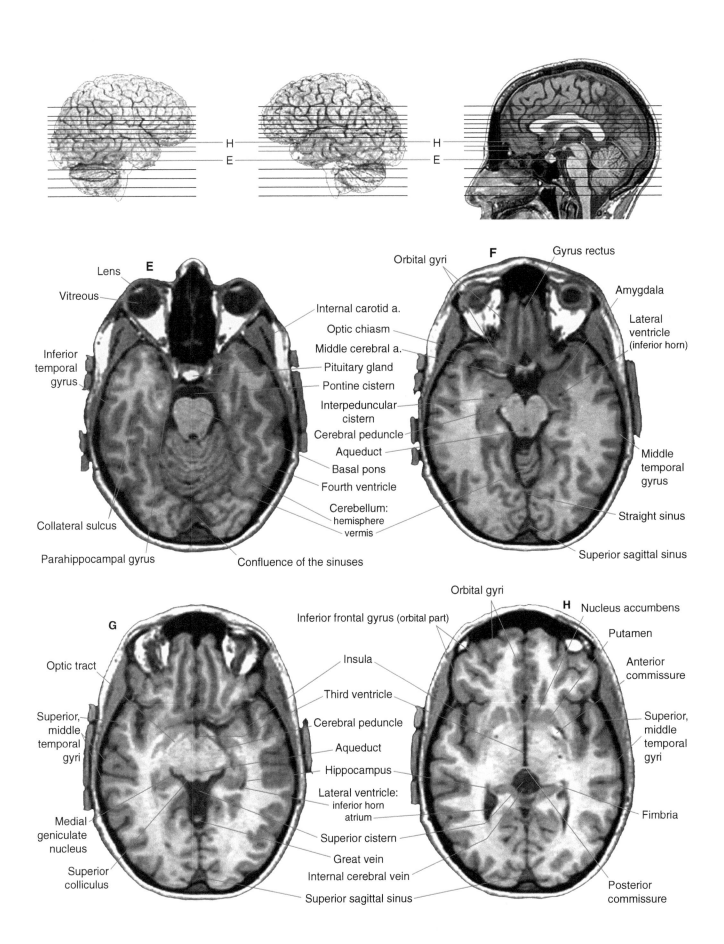

Figure 9.12 (Continued) T1-weighted axial (horizontal) MR images.

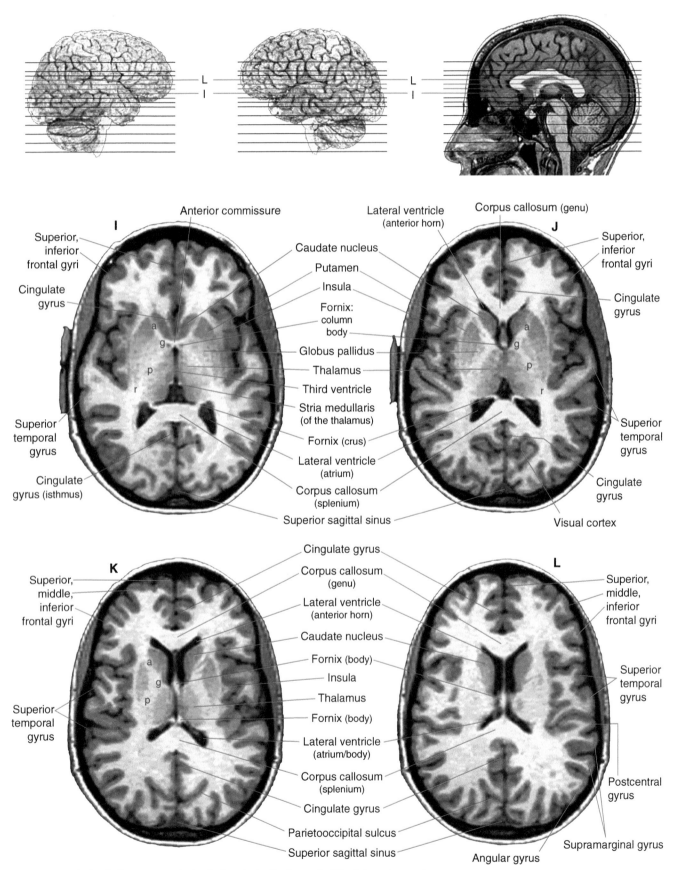

a, g, p, r = anterior limb, genu, posterior limb, retrolenticular part of the internal capsule

Figure 9.12 (Continued) T1-weighted axial (horizontal) MR images.

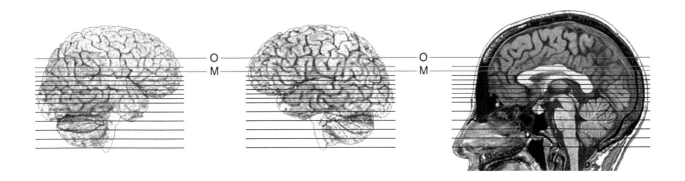

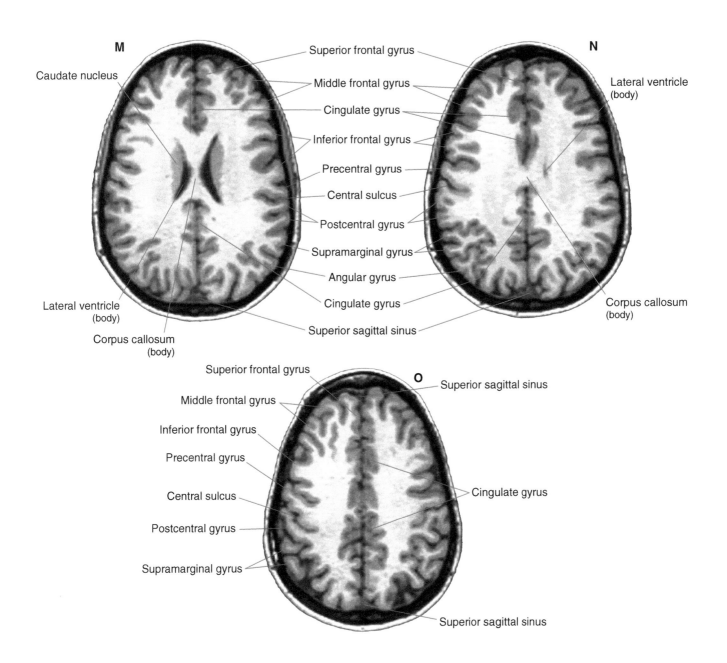

Figure 9.13 (A–G) T1-weighted sagittal and parasagittal MR images of the brain of a young man. The same brain is shown in different planes in Figs. 9.11 through 9.13, with the planes of "section" indicated in three-dimensional reconstructions. (Provided by Dr. Elena M. Plante.)

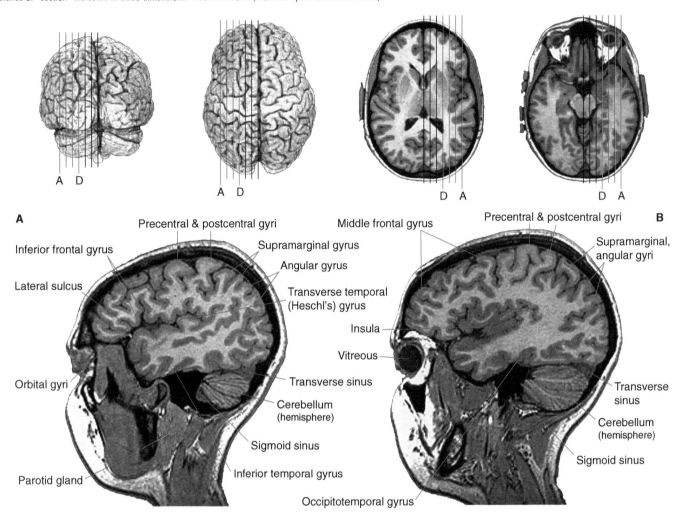

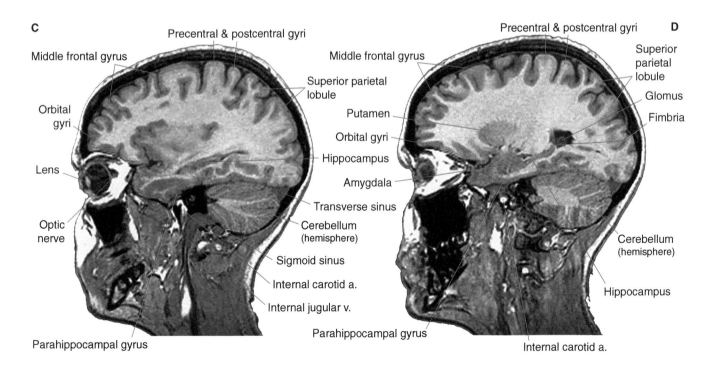

Figure 9.13 (Continued) T1-weighted sagittal and parasagittal MR images.

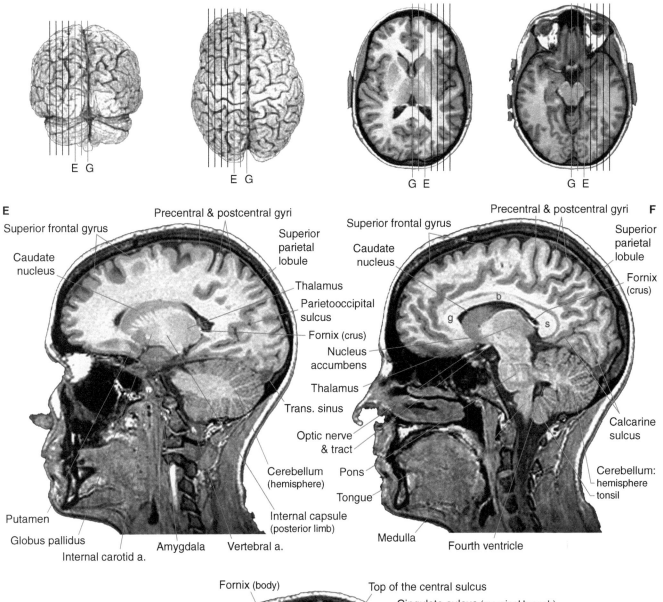

E

Superior frontal gyrus

Caudate
nucleus

Precentral & postcentral gyri

Superior
parietal
lobule

Thalamus

Parietooccipital
sulcus

Fornix (crus)

Nucleus
accumbens

Thalamus

Trans. sinus

Optic nerve
& tract

Cerebellum
(hemisphere)   Pons

Tongue

Internal capsule
(posterior limb)

Putamen

Globus pallidus

Internal carotid a.   Amygdala   Vertebral a.

F

Superior frontal gyrus

Caudate
nucleus

Precentral & postcentral gyri

Superior
parietal
lobule

Fornix
(crus)

Calcarine
sulcus

Cerebellum:
hemisphere
tonsil

Medulla   Fourth ventricle

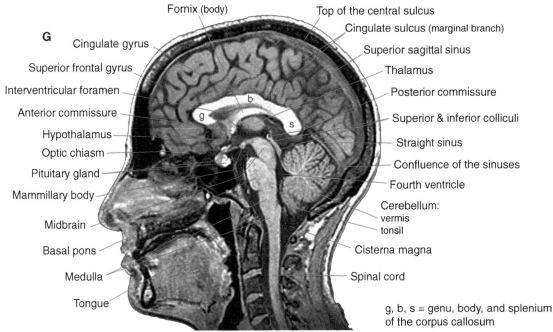

G

Fornix (body)

Cingulate gyrus

Superior frontal gyrus

Interventricular foramen

Anterior commissure

Hypothalamus

Optic chiasm

Pituitary gland

Mammillary body

Midbrain

Basal pons

Medulla

Tongue

Top of the central sulcus

Cingulate sulcus (marginal branch)

Superior sagittal sinus

Thalamus

Posterior commissure

Superior & inferior colliculi

Straight sinus

Confluence of the sinuses

Fourth ventricle

Cerebellum:
vermis
tonsil

Cisterna magna

Spinal cord

g, b, s = genu, body, and splenium
of the corpus callosum

Figure 9.14 (A–F) The use of MRI to show intracranial pathology. (Provided by Dr. Raymond F. Carmody.)

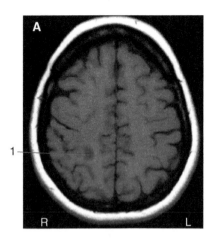

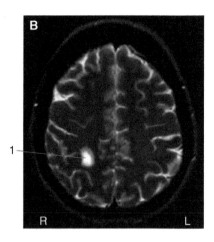

(A) This T1-weighted image shows a slight change in signal in the cerebral white matter *(1)* of a patient with multiple sclerosis (MS).

(B) In a T2-weighted image of the same patient as in *(A)*, the MS plaque in the white matter *(1)* is much more apparent.

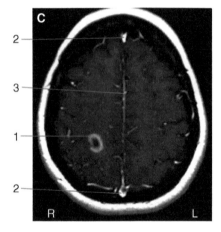

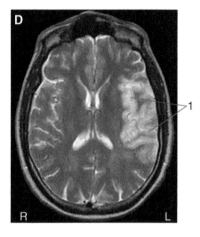

(C) The same patient as in *(A)* and *(B)*. A contrast agent (gadolinium) effective in MRI studies was injected intravenously before this MRI, revealing a rim around the edge of the plaque *(1)* where the blood–brain barrier had broken down. Blood vessels, including the superior sagittal sinus *(2)*, can also be seen, as can the falx cerebri *(3)* (because the dura mater is outside the blood–brain barrier).

(D) This T2-weighted image demonstrates the results of a stroke in the territory of the left middle cerebral artery. The damaged cerebral cortex *(1)* is edematous, and the increased water concentration makes it appear lighter than the neighboring cortex.

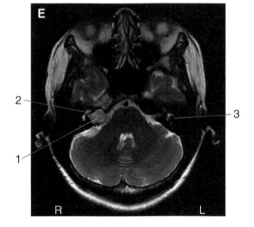

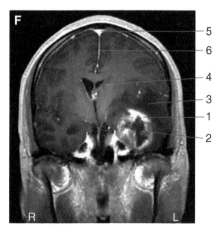

(E) A T2-weighted image showing a tumor *(1)* of the eighth nerve (a vestibular schwannoma, often referred to as an acoustic neuroma). Because fluids are bright in T2-weighted images, the cochlea *(2)* and semicircular canals *(3)* can also be seen.

(F) A T1-weighted image of a patient with a tumor (*1* and *2*, a glioblastoma multiforme) in the left temporal lobe. The tumor has a disrupted blood–brain barrier around its edges that allows contrast material to leak into it *(1)*, and a necrotic core *(2)*. Adjacent areas *(3)* appear darker than normal because of edema. The tumor has compressed the left lateral ventricle *(4)* and shifted parts of the left hemisphere to the right. Structures normally made visible by contrast agents include the superior sagittal sinus *(5)* and the falx cerebri *(6)*.

Blood vessels can be visualized with most imaging techniques by finding a way to make the blood contained within them differ in some way from surrounding structures. Traditional cerebral angiography uses the intravenous injection of iodinated dyes to make blood much more opaque than brain to x-rays (Fig. 9.15). More recently, MRI techniques that depend on the intrinsic properties of flowing blood have been developed (Fig. 9.16). MR angiography (MRA) has the advantage of being completely noninvasive—no intravenous contrast material is required—but the resulting images are not as detailed as those produced by traditional angiography.

An x-ray–based cerebral angiogram is typically produced by introducing a catheter into the femoral artery, threading it (under fluoroscopic control) up the aorta and into the aortic arch, then steering the catheter tip into the artery of interest. In this way, the contrast material can be introduced into a single vertebral or internal carotid artery. Once the dye has been introduced, a rapid series of radiographs can follow it as it flows through the artery, into capillaries, and then into veins (Fig. 9.15). Finally, photographic (as in Fig. 9.15) or digital (Fig. 9.21) techniques can be used to remove bone images and reveal blood vessels in relative isolation.

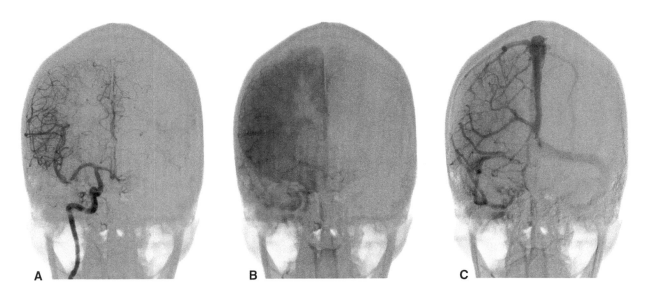

Figure 9.15 Movement of contrast material through the intracranial vasculature, as seen in a series of anterior-posterior (AP) views (as though you were looking at the patient's forehead) after injection of the right internal carotid artery. **(A)** About 2 seconds after injection, the arteries are filled. **(B)** About 5 seconds after injection, the contrast agent has moved out of arteries and into capillary beds. **(C)** About 7 seconds after injection, the contrast agent has moved into veins and venous sinuses. (Provided by Dr. Joachim F. Seeger.)

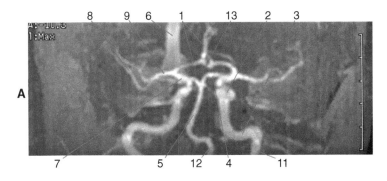

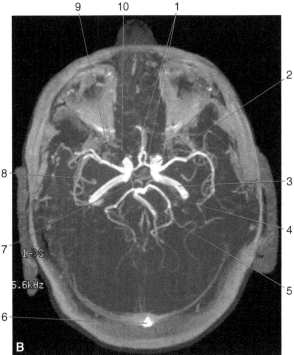

Figure 9.16 Magnetic resonance angiography uses some of the intrinsic properties of flowing blood to create images of parts of the vasculature; appropriate adjustments of technical parameters can emphasize arteries or veins. The views in these images are as though you were looking from the front **(A)** or looking up from below **(B)** at the entire arterial supply of the brain. The internal carotid artery can be seen ascending through the neck *(11)*, traversing the temporal bone *(3)*, and passing through the cavernous sinus *(2)*. The other arteries of the circle of Willis can also be seen—the anterior cerebral *(1)*, posterior cerebral *(4)*, and anterior *(13)* and posterior *(7)* communicating arteries—in addition to the middle cerebral artery *(9)*, its branches on the surface of the insula *(8)*, the vertebral *(12)* and basilar *(5)* arteries, the superior sagittal sinus *(6)*, and even the ophthalmic artery *(10)*. (Provided by Dr. Raymond F. Carmody.)

Figure 9.17 The arterial phase of a right internal carotid angiogram. **(A)** A lateral view; the patient's face is to the right. **(B)** An anterior-posterior projection; the view is as though you were looking at the patient's forehead.

A

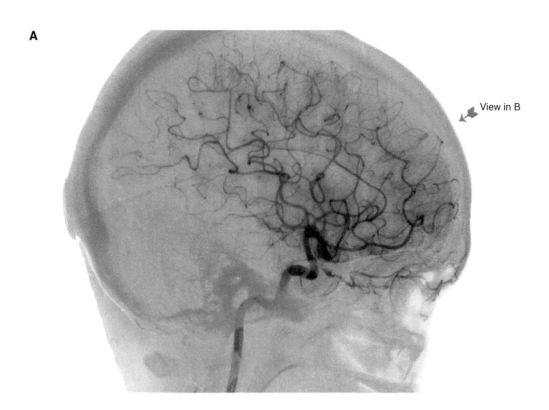

View in B

B

View in A

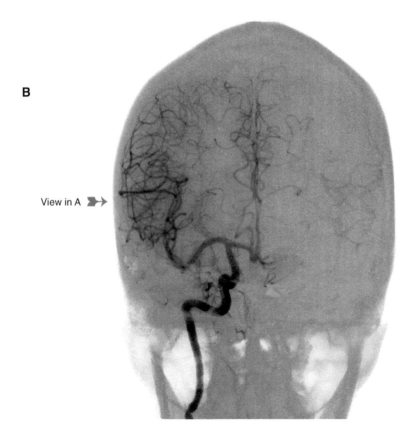

Figure 9.17 (Continued) **(C)** The internal carotid artery bifurcates into the anterior and middle cerebral arteries. The anterior cerebral artery in turn gives rise to two prominent branches, the pericallosal *(dark blue arrows)* and callosomarginal *(green arrows)* arteries, which curve around above the corpus callosum and supply most of the medial surface of the cerebral hemisphere. Branches of the middle cerebral artery traverse the insula *(light blue arrows)*, emerge from the lateral sulcus (⬤), and supply the lateral surface of the hemisphere. **(D)** In an anterior-posterior projection, the separation between anterior and middle cerebral territories can be seen more easily. (Provided by Dr. Joachim F. Seeger.)

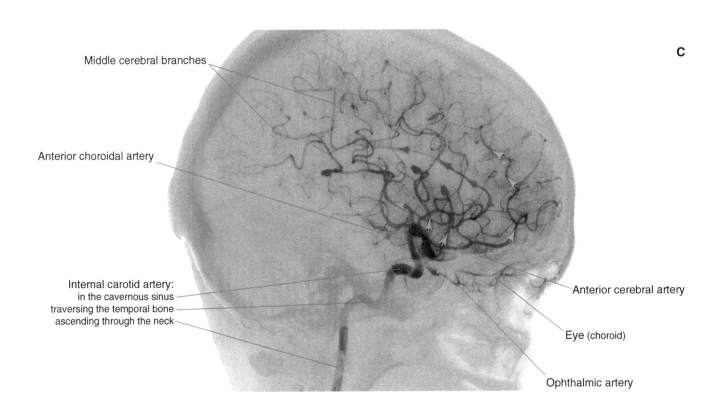

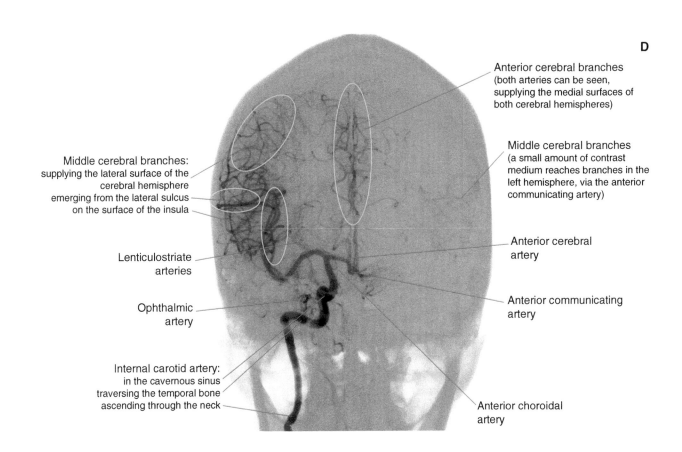

Figure 9.18 The venous phase of a right internal carotid angiogram. **(A)** A lateral view; the patient's face is to the right. **(B)** An anterior-posterior projection; the view is as though you were looking at the patient's forehead. Flow into the transverse sinuses is typically asymmetrical; in this patient, most blood from the superior sagittal sinus flows into the left transverse sinus (more commonly it flows to the right).

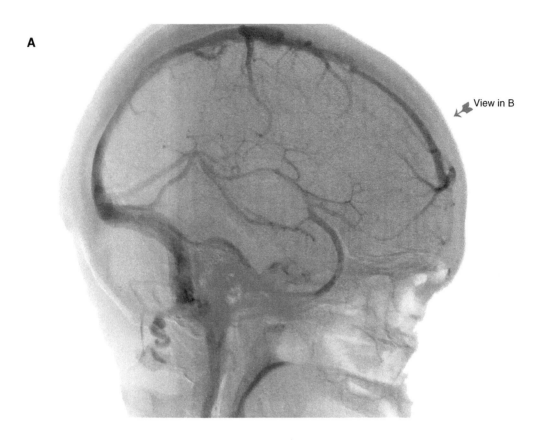

A

View in B

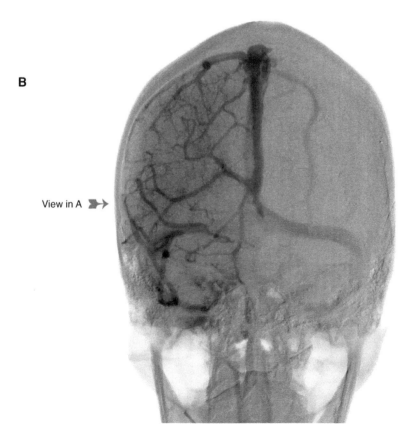

B

View in A

Figure 9.18 (Continued) **(C)** Blood flows through a system of deep veins *(dark blue arrows)* to the straight and transverse sinuses and through a system of superficial veins *(light blue arrows)* mostly into the superior sagittal sinus; both systems meet at the confluence of the sinuses. **(D)** In an anterior-posterior view, the superior sagittal sinus occupies much of the midline, obscuring other vessels. (Provided by Dr. Joachim F. Seeger.)

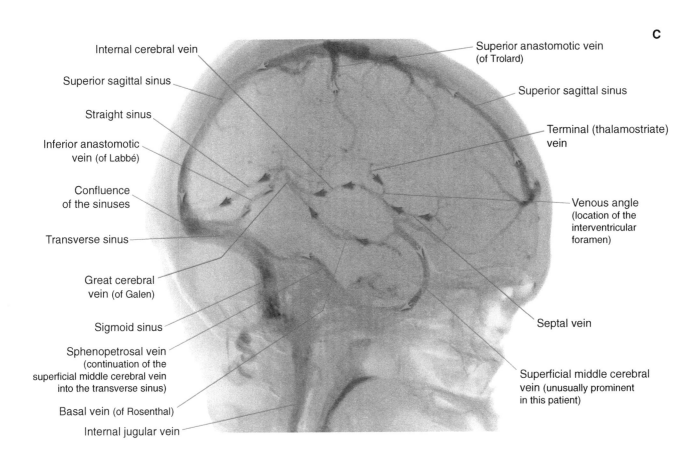

C

Internal cerebral vein

Superior sagittal sinus

Straight sinus

Inferior anastomotic vein (of Labbé)

Confluence of the sinuses

Transverse sinus

Great cerebral vein (of Galen)

Sigmoid sinus

Sphenopetrosal vein (continuation of the superficial middle cerebral vein into the transverse sinus)

Basal vein (of Rosenthal)

Internal jugular vein

Superior anastomotic vein (of Trolard)

Superior sagittal sinus

Terminal (thalamostriate) vein

Venous angle (location of the interventricular foramen)

Septal vein

Superficial middle cerebral vein (unusually prominent in this patient)

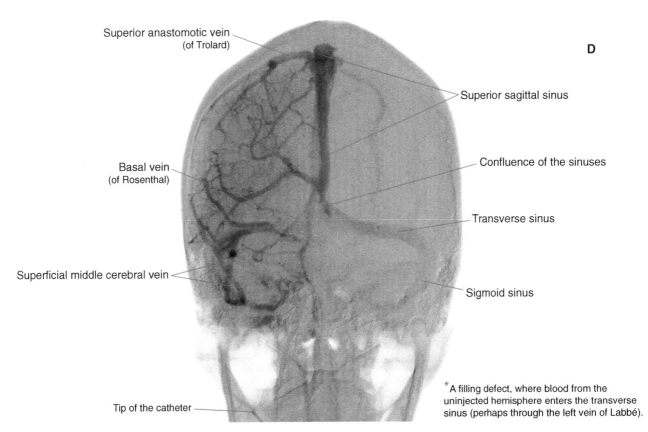

D

Superior anastomotic vein (of Trolard)

Basal vein (of Rosenthal)

Superficial middle cerebral vein

Tip of the catheter

Superior sagittal sinus

Confluence of the sinuses

Transverse sinus

Sigmoid sinus

*A filling defect, where blood from the uninjected hemisphere enters the transverse sinus (perhaps through the left vein of Labbé).

Figure 9.19 The arterial phase of a left vertebral-basilar angiogram. **(A)** A lateral view; the patient's face is to the right. **(B)** An anterior-posterior projection; the view is as though you were looking at the patient's forehead. The basilar artery appears shorter than it really is because of the angle of view—you are looking almost longitudinally along it. (The right vertebral artery is visible because the pressure of the injection propelled some contrast material into it.)

A

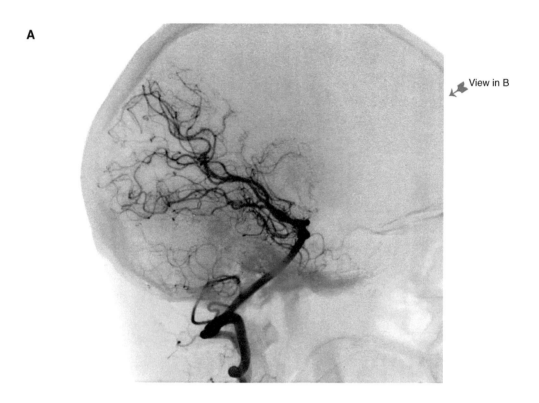

View in B

B

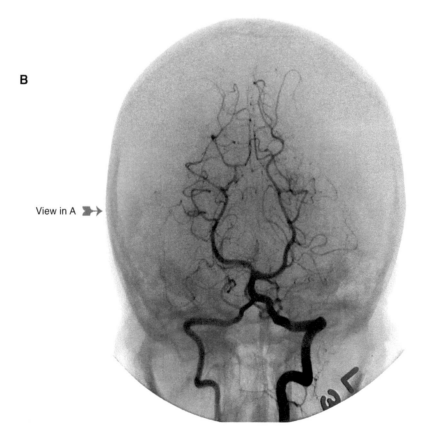

View in A

Figure 9.19 (Continued) **(C)** The vertebral and basilar arteries and their branches supply areas below the tentorium cerebelli (location of the tentorium indicated by *), and the posterior cerebral arteries supply parts of the midbrain and supratentorial structures (including much of the thalamus). **(D)** The two vertebral arteries *(green arrows)* join to form a single, midline basilar artery *(light blue arrow)*, which gives rise to a series of branches as it courses along the anterior surface of the pons, finally bifurcating at the level of the midbrain to form the two posterior cerebral arteries *(orange arrows)*. (Provided by Dr. Joachim F. Seeger.)

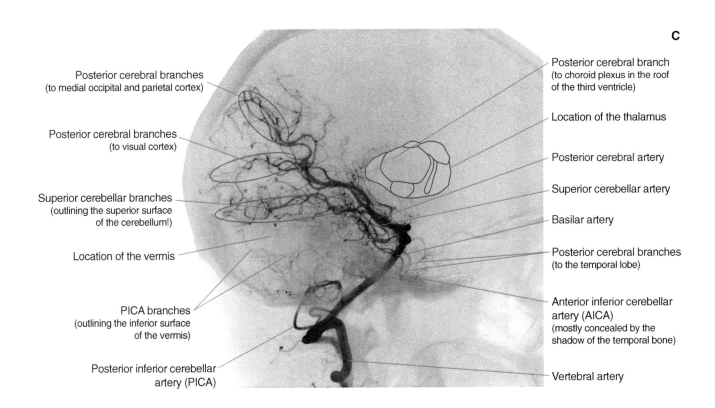

C

Posterior cerebral branches
(to medial occipital and parietal cortex)

Posterior cerebral branches
(to visual cortex)

Superior cerebellar branches
(outlining the superior surface
of the cerebellum!)

Location of the vermis

PICA branches
(outlining the inferior surface
of the vermis)

Posterior inferior cerebellar
artery (PICA)

Posterior cerebral branch
(to choroid plexus in the roof
of the third ventricle)

Location of the thalamus

Posterior cerebral artery

Superior cerebellar artery

Basilar artery

Posterior cerebral branches
(to the temporal lobe)

Anterior inferior cerebellar
artery (AICA)
(mostly concealed by the
shadow of the temporal bone)

Vertebral artery

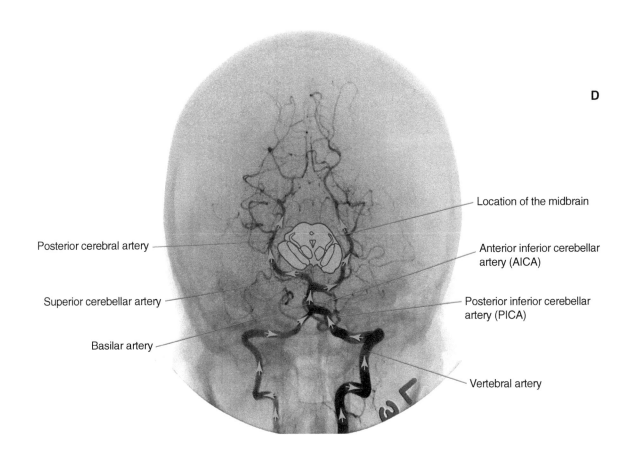

D

Posterior cerebral artery

Superior cerebellar artery

Basilar artery

Location of the midbrain

Anterior inferior cerebellar
artery (AICA)

Posterior inferior cerebellar
artery (PICA)

Vertebral artery

Figure 9.20 The venous phase of a vertebral angiogram. **(A)** A lateral view; the patient's face is to the right. **(B)** An anterior-posterior projection; the view is as though you were looking at the patient's forehead.

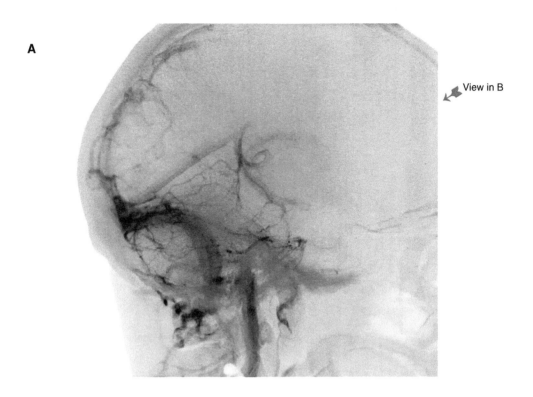

A

View in B

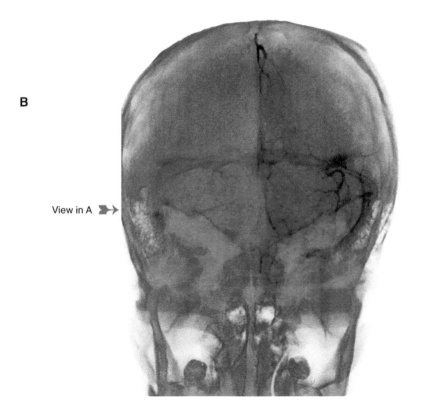

B

View in A

Figure 9.20 (Continued) **(C)** A network of veins drains from the cerebellum and brainstem into the great vein or straight sinus *(dark blue arrows)*, or into the transverse or petrosal sinuses. The medial surface of the occipital lobe drains into the superior sagittal sinus *(light blue arrows)*. **(D)** In an anterior-posterior view, the straight sinus is seen almost end-on. (Provided by Dr. Joachim F. Seeger.)

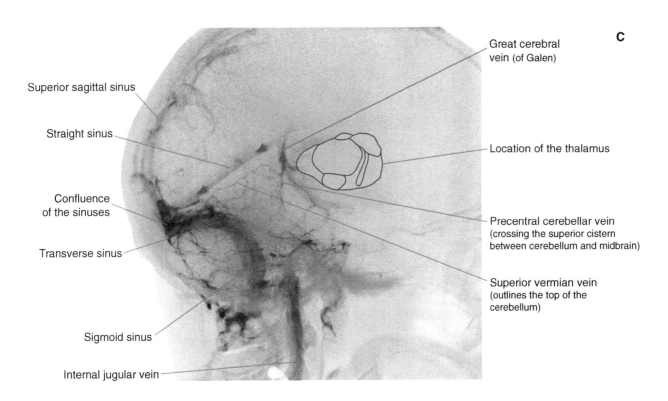

C

Superior sagittal sinus

Straight sinus

Confluence of the sinuses

Transverse sinus

Sigmoid sinus

Internal jugular vein

Great cerebral vein (of Galen)

Location of the thalamus

Precentral cerebellar vein (crossing the superior cistern between cerebellum and midbrain)

Superior vermian vein (outlines the top of the cerebellum)

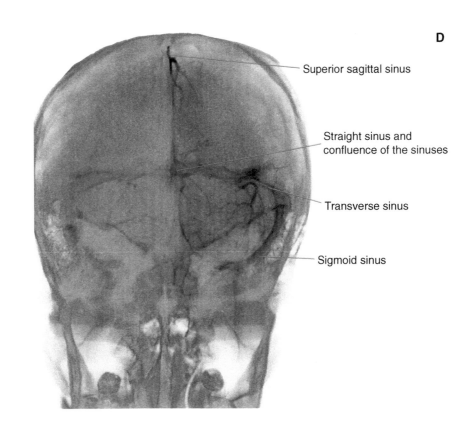

D

Superior sagittal sinus

Straight sinus and confluence of the sinuses

Transverse sinus

Sigmoid sinus

Figure 9.21 (A–F) The use of angiography to show intracranial pathology. (Provided by Dr. Raymond F. Carmody.)

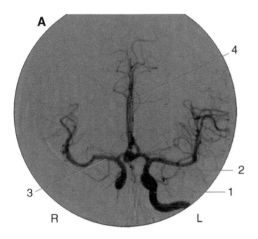

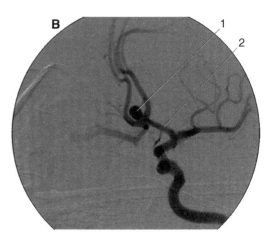

(A) An anterior-posterior view of a patient who had subarachnoid bleeding from a ruptured aneurysm (a balloon-like swelling of the wall of an artery). The internal carotid artery *(1)* was injected, and the left *(2)* and right *(3)* middle cerebral arteries and the anterior cerebral arteries *(4)* can be seen.

(B) The same patient as in **A**. Rotating the point of view by about 45 degrees makes the aneurysm *(1)* apparent, at a branch point of the anterior cerebral artery *(2)*.

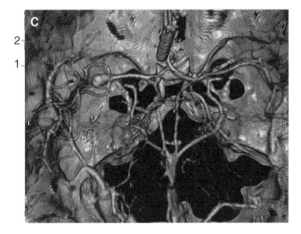

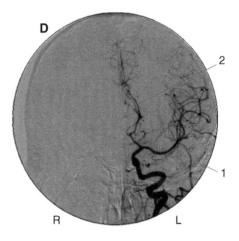

(C) A 38-year-old woman with an aneurysm. A three-dimensional reconstruction based on contrast-enhanced CT scans shows the aneurysm *(1)*, at a branch point of the middle cerebral artery *(2)*.

(D) An angiogram of a 78-year-old man who complained of a headache reveals that the left middle *(1)* and anterior *(2)* cerebral arteries were bowed outward, as though something were distorting them.

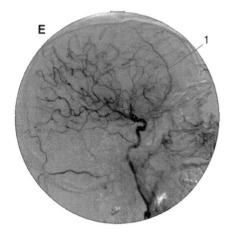

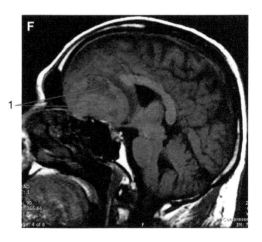

(E) The same patient as in **D**. A lateral view shows a forward bowing of the middle meningeal artery *(1)*.

(F) The same patient as in **D**. A T1-weighted MRI reveals a large meningioma *(1)*.

10

An Introduction to Neuropathology

The different diagnoses of diseases and disorders within the nervous system are made using neuropathology in coordination with clinical signs/symptoms and imaging. The imaging techniques discussed in Chapter 9, coalesced with biopsies, the use of selective antibodies to identify cellular markers, and particular stains to highlight cellular structures, are all used to make a diagnosis. This chapter will present some common neuropathological diseases/disorders.

Stains used to help identify the different cells of the central nervous system (CNS) include hematoxylin and eosin (H&E), Nissl stain, Luxol-fast blue stain, and silver stains. H&E stains are the most commonly used, with the cytoplasm of cells being more acidic (eosinophilic) and staining red, whereas the nuclei and nucleoli are more basic (hematoxylinophilic) and are stained blue. Nissl bodies, which are the rough endoplasmic reticulum of neurons, are basophilic, and the use of a Nissl stain (cresyl violet) results in a dark purple highlight of the rough endoplasmic reticulum. Axons and dendrites cannot be distinguished unless there are swelling-related changes. Astrocytes lack an eosinophilic cytoplasm and have nuclei that appear large and quite clear. When astrocytes react to tissue damage, they appear eosinophilic because their cytoplasm becomes more abundant as a result of an increase in fibrous components, which also accumulate in the nerve processes. Oligodendroglia are smaller than astrocytes, with basophilic densely staining nuclei and a barely visible cytoplasm. The nuclei of microglia present with basophilic club-shaped terminations and are thus easily distinguished. Luxol-fast blue stains the myelin sheath (lipids) blue and is often used to help diagnose demyelinating diseases.

Silver stains (i.e., Bodian staining) use silver, copper, and gold to stain neuronal cell bodies and nerve processes dark brown. Parts of the cells that take up the "silver" stain (called argentaffin parts) can include areas of localized axonal swelling, dendritic lesions, and Alzheimer neurofibrillary degeneration (neurofibrillary tangles [NFTs]). Other silver staining procedures enable clear visualization of amyloid components of senile plaques; immunostained images of β-amyloid proteins show similar results.

PRIMARY BRAIN TUMORS

Tumors of the brain include astrocytomas, oligodendrogliomas, and ependymomas, medulloblastomas as well as several others. Originally these primary brain tumors were thought to originate from glial cells, hence the name (gliomas); recent evidence suggest that they may not only come from glial cells but also from neural stem cells and are characterized based on the expression of particular cell markers. Primary brain tumors are classified not only using stains, selective antibodies, and/or their location (i.e., intra-axial = within the brain parenchyma, or extra-axial = outside of the brain parenchyma) but also based on how well defined the borders of the tumor are (i.e., well circumscribed vs. diffuse). In addition, there are tests, such as KI67 staining for identifying mitotic activity, performed in order to detect how rapidly the cancer is dividing, and the majority of tumors are given a "grade" (grades I-IV from slow to fast) for growth aggressiveness.

ASTROCYTOMAS

Astrocytomas are thought to develop from astrocytes and may arise anywhere in the brain or spinal cord *(intra-axial)*, yet they most often occur in the cerebrum. Astrocytomas are the most common primary CNS tumors and can be further divided based on their ability to either remain localized or diffusely infiltrate.

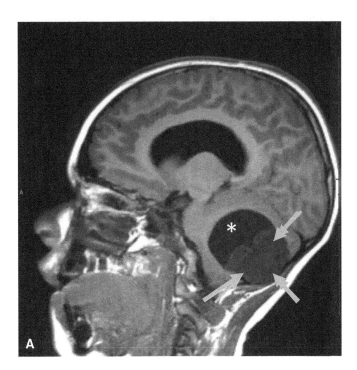

Figure 10.1 (A) Pilocytic astrocytoma MRI-T1, parasagittal view and **(B)** MRI-T1 gadolinium enhanced axial view *(arrows)*. The more localized, slow growing astrocytomas (i.e., grade I) are called **pilocytic astrocytomas**. These typically well-circumscribed tumors are found more often in children and young adults in areas like the cerebellum, but they are not limited to the cerebellum. These tumors are highly vascular and enhance well with contrast injection. They are often cystic *(*)* with a protruding solid nodule.

Illustration continued on following page

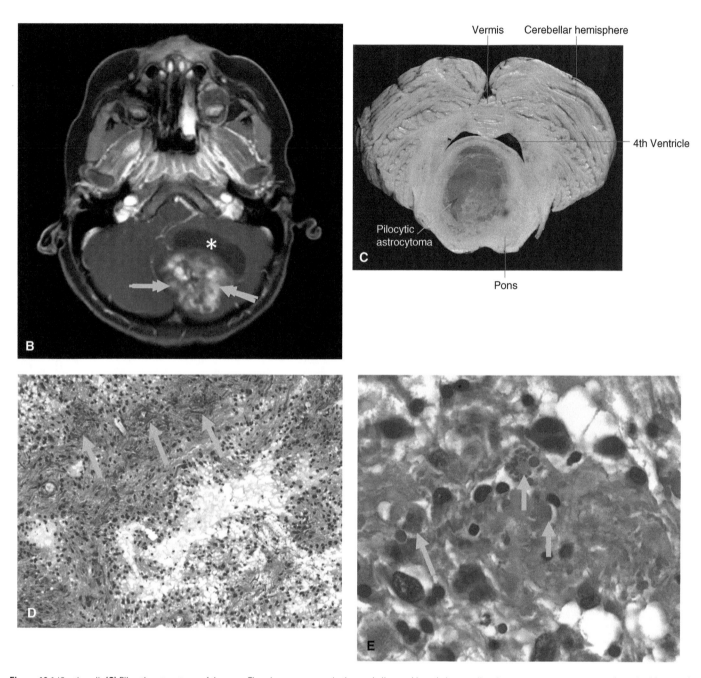

Figure 10.1 (Continued) **(C)** Pilocytic astrocytoma of the pons. Though more common in the cerebellum and hypothalamus, pilocytic astrocytoma may occur anywhere. As this example illustrates, pilocytic astrocytoma is frequently grossly cystic. Many cystic pilocytic astrocytomas have a solid mural nodule. **(D)** Biphasic (cystic and solid) pilocytic astrocytoma with numerous Rosenthal fibers *(arrows)*. These are cytoplasmic inclusions composed of GFAP (glial fibrillary acidic protein—a marker of neural glial cells), the intermediate filament protein of astrocytes. These types of tumors tend to lack signs of necrosis and mitotic figures with very limited infiltration of surrounding brain. **(E)** Granular eosinophilic bodies *(arrows)* are another cellular marker of pilocytic astrocytoma in addition to Rosenthal fibers. (**[A-B]** Provided by Dr. Raymond Carmody. **[C-E]** Provided by Dr. Dimitri P. Agamanolis.)

INFILTRATING ASTROCYTOMAS

Infiltrating astrocytomas are the most common adult primary CNS *(intra-axial)* tumor; they are often found in the cerebrum but can also appear in the cerebellum, brainstem, and spinal cord. These types of tumors can range from diffuse astrocytoma (grade II), to anaplastic astrocytoma (grade III), to glioblastoma (grade IV), depending on markers and their speed of proliferation (tumor aggression).

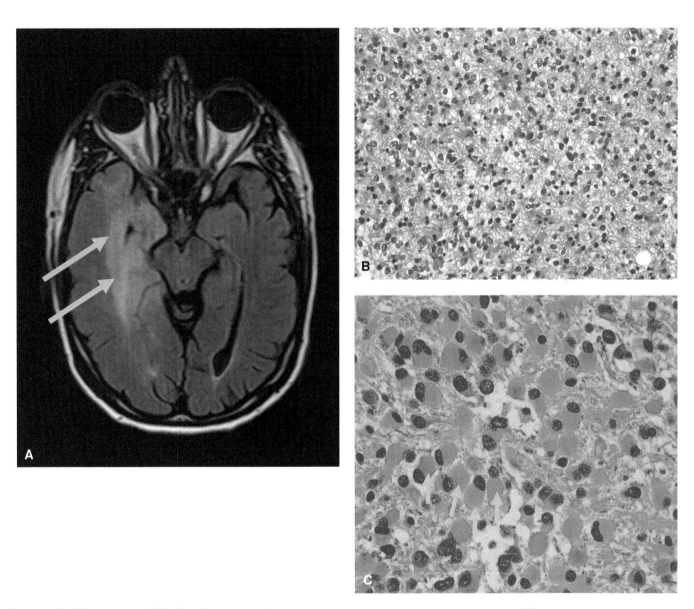

Figure 10.2 (A) Diffuse astrocytoma MRI-FLAIR axial view of the brainstem *(arrows* indicating low-grade astrocytoma in temporal lobe). Diffuse astrocytomas are poorly defined and tend to not be well demarcated, but unlike pilocytic astrocytomas they can show signs of infiltration of surrounding brain but often do not enhance using gadolinium. They have a cellular density that is greater than normal white matter with GFAP staining but not as dense as the anaplastic or glioblastoma stages. **(B)** Diffuse astrocytoma. Low grade cellularity, no atypia or mitoses. The tumor cells show mild atypia and rare mitoses and spread in a diffuse fashion. Diffuse astrocytoma corresponds to WHO grade II. **(C)** Gemistocytic astrocytoma. The tumor cells are plump with a large eosinophilic cytoplasmic mass *(arrows)*, similar to certain reactive astrocytes. This is also a WHO grade II tumor. They tend to have some nuclear pleomorphism (i.e., variability in the size, shape, and staining of cell nuclei). (**[A]** Provided by Dr. Raymond Carmody. **[B-C]** Provided by Dr. Dimitri P. Agamanolis.)

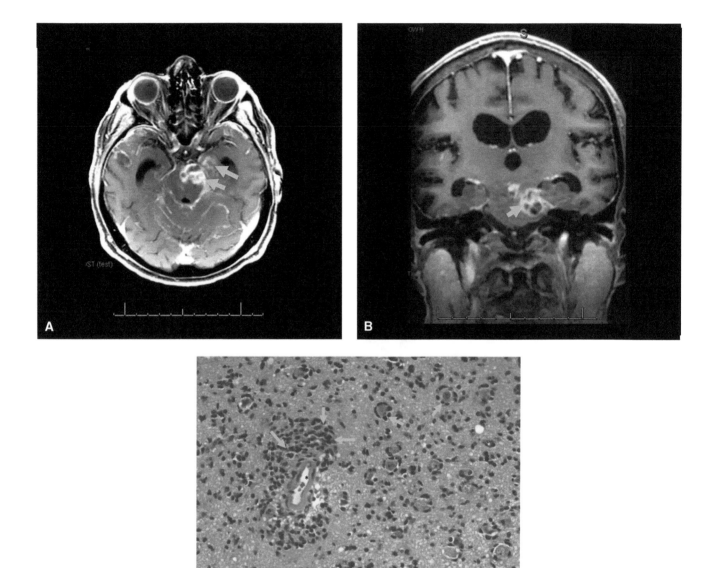

Figure 10.3 Anaplastic astrocytomas. MRI-T1 gadolinium-enhanced images of the temporal lobe as well as the midbrain of the brainstem (**[A]** axial view, **[B]** coronal view). *Arrows* indicate enhancing tumor in cerebral peduncle, mesial temporal lobe, and CSF spaces (extensive CSF "seeding" of tumor). The CSF spread is also causing communicating hydrocephalus. **(C)** Gliomatosis cerebri. Poorly differentiated glial cells infiltrate the brain and aggregate around blood vessels and neurons. Anaplastic astrocytomas demonstrate dense cellularity, have mitotic figures present demonstrating active proliferation, and have advanced nuclear pleomorphism as compared to the diffuse astrocytomas. Most anaplastic astrocytoma cases are composed of poorly differentiated glial cells, probably astrocytes, that infiltrate the brain diffusely and crowd around neurons and blood vessels *(*)* and under the pia. (**[A–B]** Courtesy Dr. Raymond Carmody. **[C]** Courtesy Dr. Dimitri P. Agamanolis.)

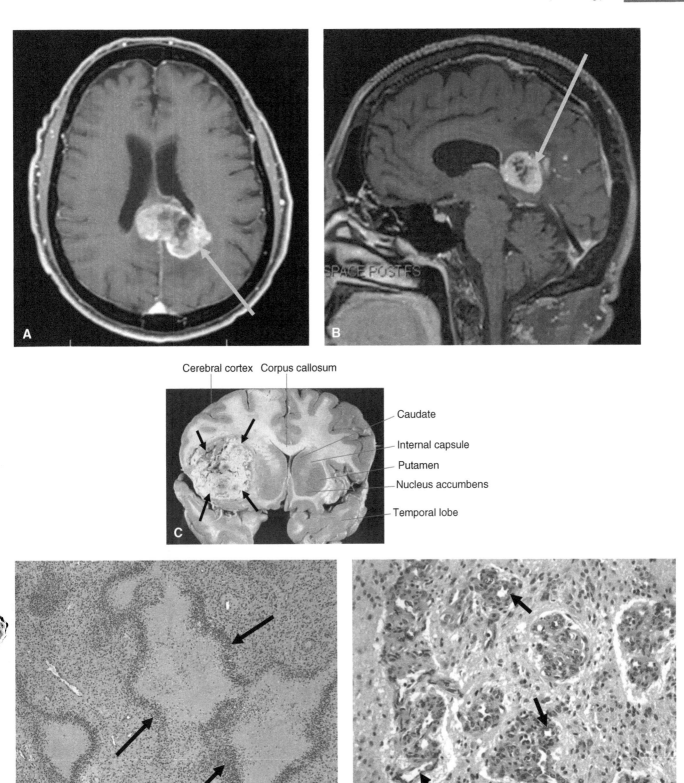

Figure 10.4 Glioblastoma *(previously called glioblastoma multiforme [GBM])*. **(A)** Grade IV, MRI-T1 with Gadolinium axial view of the tumor crossing via the corpus callosum *(arrow)*. **(B)** MRI-T1 with Gadolinium sagittal view *(arrow)*. These are aggressively growing tumors of the glial cells (i.e., astrocytes, oligodendrocytes) with recent suggestions that neural stem cells may also be a possible origin. Glioblastoma will have mitotic figures displaying rapidly dividing cells that often exhibit nearby necrosis and/or microvascular proliferation. Glioblastomas commonly exhibit a "butterfly appearance" since they can infiltrate through the white matter tracts of the corpus callosum, spreading to both hemispheres. **(C)** Glioblastoma of the frontal lobe. A large tumor with a variegated appearance due to necrosis and old hemorrhage *(arrows)*. This is the basis of the term glioblastoma multiforme. Glioblastoma. **(D)** Viable tumor cells are arranged in a perpendicular (pseudopalisading) fashion around serpiginous necrotic areas *(arrows)*. Glioblastoma. **(E)** Microvascular proliferation. The new vessels are often arranged in glomeruloid formations *(arrows)* and lack a blood–brain barrier. This contributes to cerebral edema and accounts for contrast enhancing in imaging studies. Glioblastomas can be stained for isocitrate dehydrogenase 1 (IDH1) as an important marker for GBM prognosis (IDH1w = poor prognosis [0.8–1.1 years]; IDH1m = better prognosis [2.0–3.8 years]). (**[A-B]** Provided by Dr. Raymond Carmody. **[C-E]** Provided by Dr. Dimitri P. Agamanolis.)

OLIGODENDROGLIOMAS

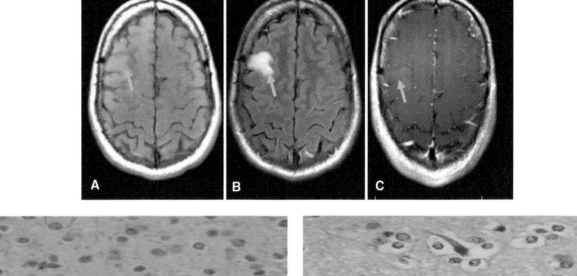

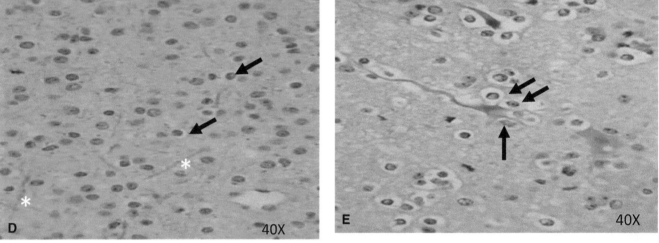

Figure 10.5 Oligodendroglioma. **(A)** T1-MRI axial image of an oligodendroglioma in the right frontal cortex, **(B)** MRI-FLAIR image and **(C)** MRI-T1 with Gadolinium image *(arrows)*. Oligodendrogliomas are subtle, slowly growing, abnormal proliferations of oligodendrocytes that can be found anywhere in the central nervous system *(intra-axial)*, yet they are most often found in the frontal and temporal lobes of the cerebral cortex. These tumors often arise in middle-aged adults. Oligodendrogliomas are more circumscribed than astrocytomas. **(D)** An H&E stained biopsy of a grade II oligodendroglioma demonstrating a blue (hematoxylin stained) nucleus and the appearance of the "fried egg" in which the oligodendroglioma lacks extensions *(arrows)*. Notice also the rich capillary network *(*)*, another feature of this neoplasm. **(E)** Example of perineuronal satellitosis (the accumulation of the oligodendroglial cells encircling a neuron; *arrows*). This particular biopsy is classified as grade II (low grade) due to no mitotic figures observed. (Provided by Dr. Raymond Carmody.)

EPENDYMOMAS

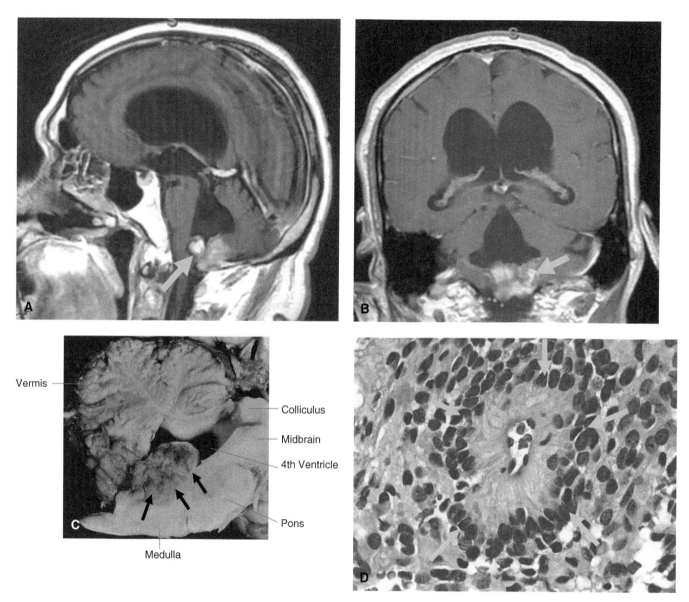

Figure 10.6 Ependymoma. **(A)** A sagittal MRI-T1 Gadolinium enhanced of an ependymoma within the fourth ventricle *(arrow)*. Ependymomas typically occur in or next to the ventricular system within the brain and the central canal of the spinal cord. **(B)** A coronal MRI-T1 Gadolinium enhanced of the ependymoma *(arrow)* demonstrating the blockage of CSF fluid resulting in a noncommunicating hydrocephalus. Notice in both **(A)** and **(B)** the increased ventricle sizes. **(C)** Ependymoma arising from the floor of the fourth ventricle. These solid tumors tend to grow in an exophytic fashion *(tending to grow outward beyond the surface epithelium from which it originates)*, protruding into and out of the fourth ventricle. Ependymoma. **(D)** Perivascular pseudorosette *(arrows)*. A tissue pattern characteristic of ependymoma in which the tumor cell nuclei are located at some distance from a central vessel with delicate cytoplasmic processes that radiate toward the vessel wall. Nuclei of an ependymoma are round-to-oval with abundant granular chromatin. Ependymomas can be classified from grade II to IV depending on the mitotic activity, cellular density, and necrosis. (**[A-B]** Provided by Dr. Raymond Carmody. **[C-D]** Provided by Dr. Dimitri P. Agamanolis.)

MEDULLOBLASTOMAS

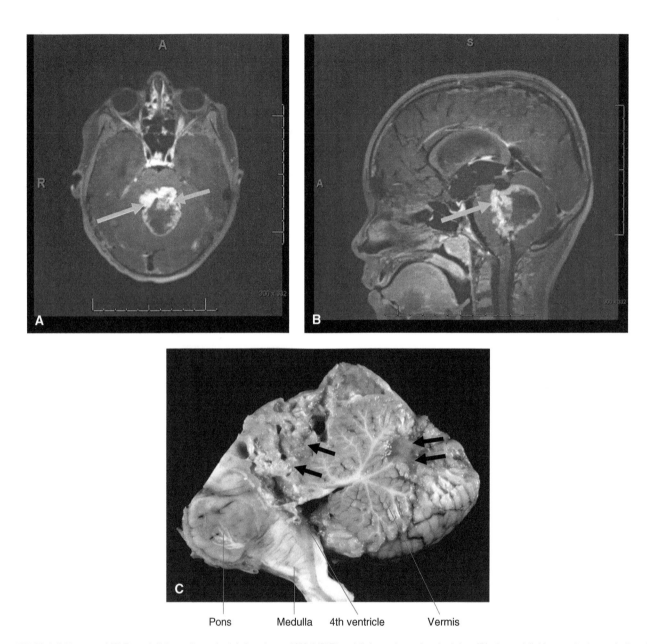

Pons   Medulla   4th ventricle   Vermis

Figure 10.7 Medulloblastoma. MRI-T1, gadolinium enhanced axial view *(arrows)* **(A)**. MRI-T1 gadolinium enhanced sagittal view **(B)** of a medulloblastoma in the cerebellum *(arrow)* pushing into the brainstem. Medulloblastomas are defined as an embryonal tumor of the brain that appears in the cerebellum, often in children, but that can appear in adults as well. This malignant, intra-axial, embryonal tumor, when in the midline, often blocks CSF flow through the ventricular system, resulting in noncommunicating hydrocephalus. These tumors may spread to other parts of the CNS via the CSF. Fortunately, they are very responsive to radiation. **(C)** Medulloblastoma as a midline cerebellar tumor *(arrows)* that is necrotic following previous treatments with radiation and chemotherapy.

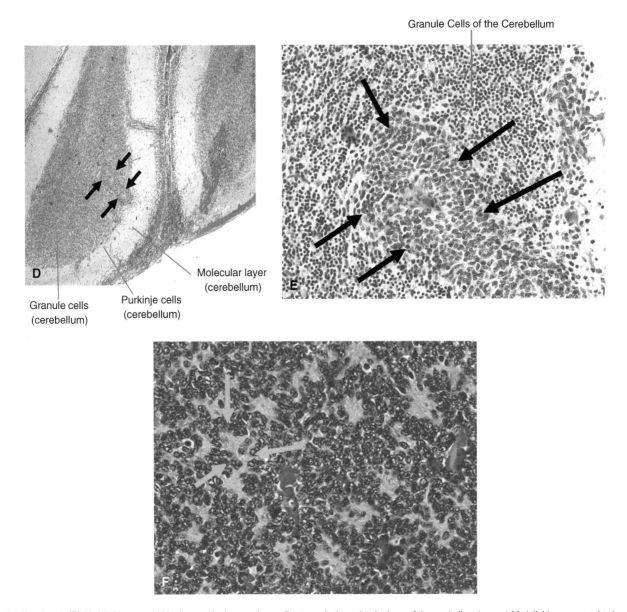

Figure 10.7 (Continued) **(D)** Medulloblastoma within the granular layer and extending towards the molecular layer of the cerebellum *(arrows)*. Medulloblastomas tend to be cellularly dense **(E)**, have hyperchromatic nuclei *(arrows)*, and have abundant mitotic figures with high Ki67 staining. These tumors are composed of diffuse masses of small, undifferentiated oval or round cells. Medulloblastoma. **(F)** Homer-Wright rosettes (groups of tumor cells arranged in a circle around a fibrillary center). Similar rosettes are seen in adrenal neuroblastoma. (**[A-B, D-E]** Provided by Dr. Raymond Carmody. **[C, F]** Provided by Dr. Dimitri P. Agamanolis.)

MENINGIOMA

Typically meningiomas have round to oval nuclei, dispersed chromatin (demonstrating active proliferation) with inconspicuous nucleoli. These tumors are also graded with a range from I to III based on brain invasion and mitoses. Grade I is a more benign tumor whereas a grade III is anaplastic/malignant.

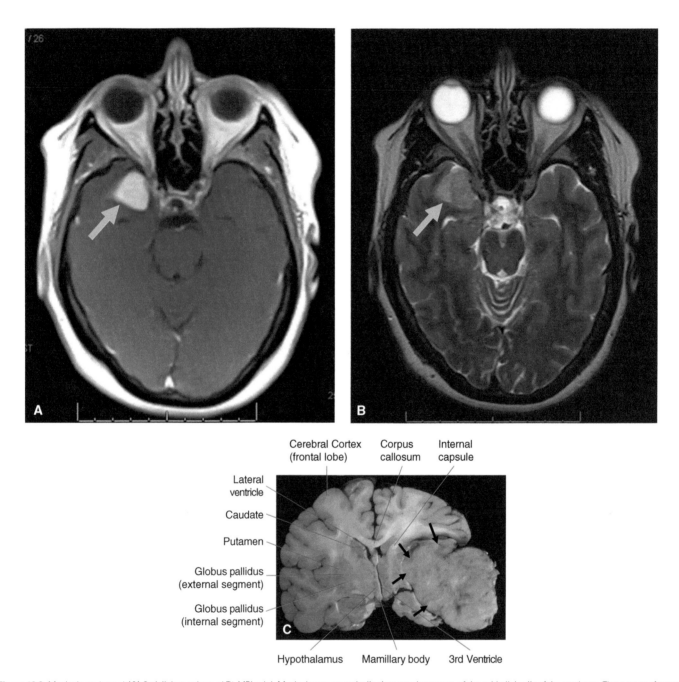

Cerebral Cortex (frontal lobe)
Corpus callosum
Internal capsule
Lateral ventricle
Caudate
Putamen
Globus pallidus (external segment)
Globus pallidus (internal segment)
Hypothalamus
Mamillary body
3rd Ventricle

Figure 10.8 Meningioma *(arrow)*. **(A)** Gadolinium-enhanced T1-MRI axial. Meningiomas are typically slow-growing tumors of the epithelial cells of the meninges. These types of tumors are extra-axial *(outside of the brain)* and well circumscribed. **(B)** T2-MRI axial view. They are most often benign, hard tumors with a grayish color. Meningioma. **(C)** An extra-axial tumor that usually displaces brain tissue without invading the parenchyma *(arrows)*. Notice how the ventricular system is compressed.

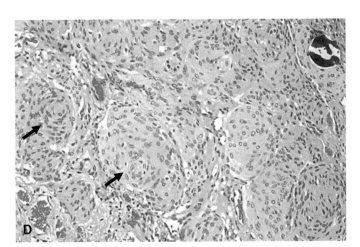

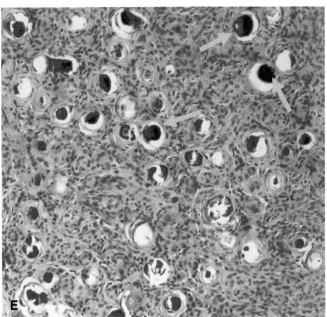

Figure 10.8 (Continued) **(D)** Meningiomas have characteristic whorls in H&E stains *(arrows).* **(E)** Psammomatous meningioma. A pattern of meningioma in which tumor cells are arranged in whorls with hyalinized and calcified centers that are called psammoma (sand) bodies because they resemble tiny grains of sand *(arrows).* (**[A-B, D]** Provided by Dr. Raymond Carmody. **[C, E]** Provided by Dr. Dimitri P. Agamanolis.)

DETECTION OF AN ABSCESS

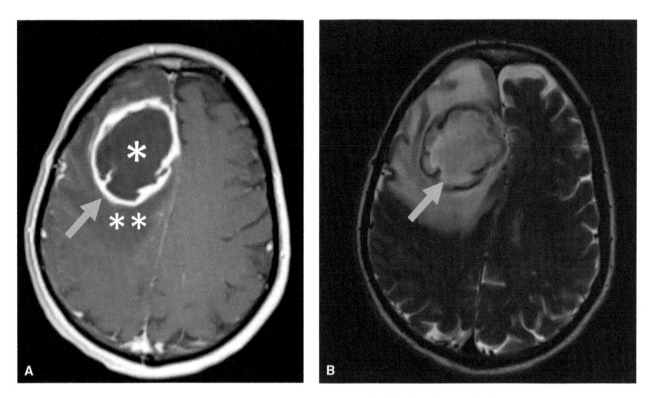

Figure 10.9 Abscess. Differentiating a CNS abscess from a tumor using imaging can at first be a bit tricky. **(A)** A T1-MRI enhanced with gadolinium demonstrating the ring-enhancing effect. A T1-MRI of an abscess will present with the central portion as being hypointense *(*)*, with vasogenic edema surrounding the abscess *(**)*. The wall of an abscess typically shows ring enhancement after gadolinium administration *(arrow)*. **(B)** A T2-MRI demonstrating the pathology often seen with T2 imaging *(arrow)*. The abscess center will demonstrate restricted diffusion using a DWI imaging technique (not shown), and as the abscess matures the capsule will show decreased low T2 signal. Typically abscesses are categorized into a four-stage model of disease development with the first stage of bacteria inoculation of the brain parenchyma that causes focal inflammation and edema (1 to 3 days after inoculation). On days 4 to 9 there is neutrophil accumulation, edema, and some tissue necrosis. Macrophages and lymphocytes predominate in the infiltrate. The third stage (days 10 to 14) is characterized by the development of a capsule that is vascularized and ring enhancing. In the fourth stage, the host immune response causes the capsule to wall off with destruction of surrounding healthy brain tissue in an attempt to sequester the infection. (Provided by Dr. Raymond Carmody.)

DEMYELINATING SYNDROMES

Demyelinating diseases of the central nervous system affect the oligodendrocytes. These types of disease are characterized by damage to the myelin (i.e., white matter) with preservation of the neuron itself, resulting in difficulties in conduction properties. There are many different types of infections that may cause the loss of myelin, while in some cases the immune system itself may attack the myelinating cells of the nervous system.

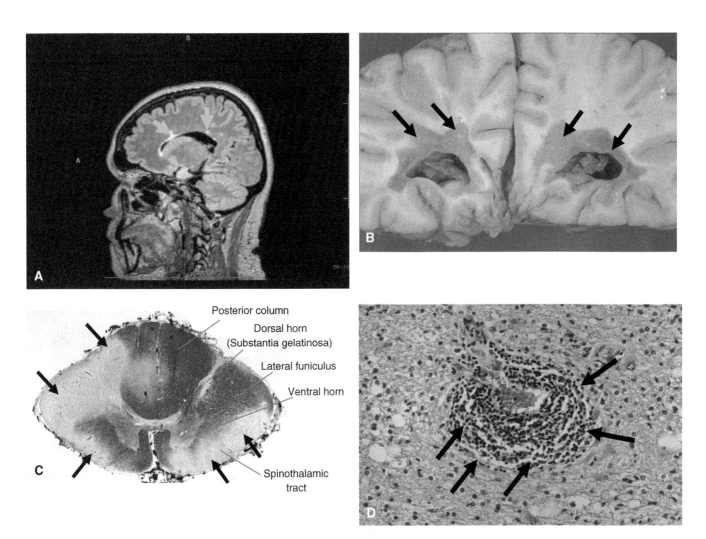

Figure 10.10 Multiple sclerosis (MS), a common demyelinating disease, is a CNS autoimmune demyelinating disorder that **(A)** presents with multiple lesions (often lateral to the ventricles, *arrows*) that are typically well circumscribed but often irregular in shape and referred to as plaques (MRI-FLAIR sagittal view). Clinical features include distinct episodes that may wax-and-wane over time. In the case of MS, autoantibodies attack components of the myelin made by oligodendrocytes in which distinct gray-tan spots in normally white matter tract areas within the CNS are observed. MS. **(B)** Periventricular plaques. MS plaques are randomly distributed *(arrows)*. They have a predilection for the periventricular white matter, optic nerves, and spinal cord but spare no part of the CNS. MS of the spinal cord. **(C)** The pale lesions are plaques *(arrows)*. The deep blue areas are normal myelin. Unlike neurodegenerative (ALS) or nutritional disorders (subacute combined degeneration), plaques have an irregular anatomical distribution. **(D)** Perivascular lymphocytes in an active MS plaque *(arrows)*. In the acute phase (active plaque), activated mononuclear cells, including lymphocytes, microglia, and macrophages destroy myelin and, to a variable degree, oligodendrocytes. (**[A]** Provided by Dr. Raymond Carmody. **[B-D]** Provided by Dr. Dimitri P. Agamanolis.)

Progressive multifocal leukoencephalopathy (PML) is a deadly demyelinating disease of the CNS due to lytic infection of oligodendrocytes by the ubiquitous opportunistic polyomavirus JC (JCV). Most persons acquire this virus at a young age but the virus remains latent. The virus is reactivated when cellular immunity is suppressed. Most PML cases occur in patients with AIDS, cancer, inflammatory disorders, and organ transplant recipients due to suppressive-immune medications. PML presents clinically as a variety of neurologic deficits (visual loss, paralysis, dementia) evolving rapidly towards death. Unlike MS, inflammation is minimal in PML.

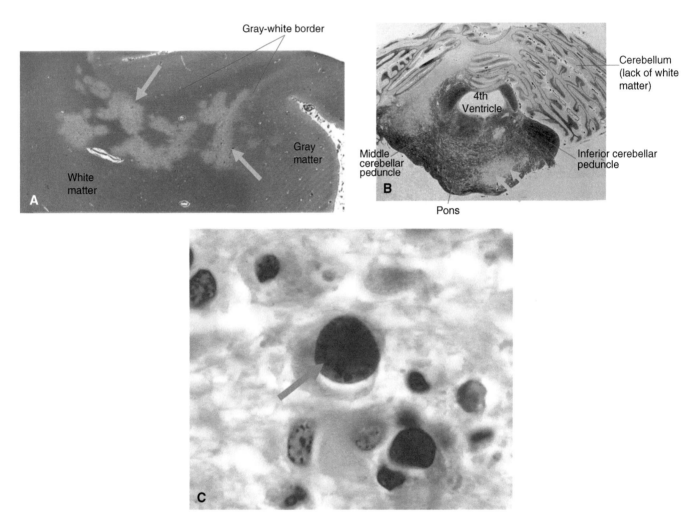

Figure 10.11 (A) Progressive multifocal leukoencephalopathy (PML) myelin stain. PML begins with small demyelinative foci at the cortex-white matter junction *(arrows)*. Confluence of these foci results in large irregular white matter lesions that involve the cerebrum, cerebellum, and brainstem. PML. **(B)** Demyelination of the cerebellum and pons *(arrows)*. PML. **(C)** Enlarged homogeneous oligodendrocyte nucleus with inclusion *(arrow)*. The nuclei of infected oligodendrocytes are packed with viral particles that cause them to enlarge and have a ground glass appearance. (Provided by Dr. Dimitri P. Agamanolis.)

Central Pontine Myelinolysis (CPM) is characterized as a loss of myelin on neurons within the base and tegmentum of the pons of the brainstem. Although the name suggests that this occurs only in the pons, it can also be extended to the cerebellum, cerebrum, and spinal cord (extrapontine myelinolysis). There is loss of myelin while axons are typically spared with very little to no inflammation.

Clinically, symptoms can vary from no symptoms to severe cases in which there can be spastic bulbar paralysis, quadriplegia, stupor, coma, or the locked-in syndrome. CPM is often caused by fluid and electrolyte imbalance precipitated by a rapid electrolyte influx in hyponatremia patients. CPM can be regarded as an osmotic-induced demyelination syndrome.

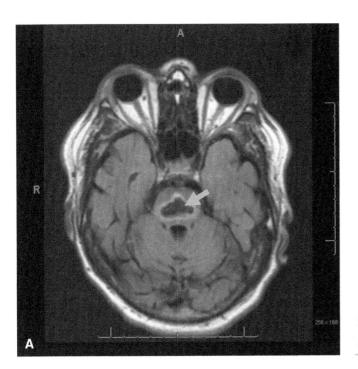
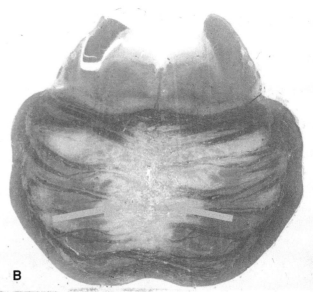

Figure 10.12 (A) MRI-T2 FLAIR axial view of a patient with central pontine myelinolysis (CPM) and the loss of the brainstem tissue *(arrow)*. CPM. **(B)** CPM is a degeneration of a symmetrical midline patch of the basis pontis *(arrows)*. There is loss of myelin and less severe loss of axons. Neurons of the nuclei pontis are relatively spared. No inflammation is seen. There is no selective involvement of fiber systems. (**[A]** Provided by Dr. Raymond Carmody. **[B]** Provided by Dr. Dimitri P. Agamanolis.)

NEURODEGENERATIVE DISEASES

Alzheimer Disease (AD) is the most common cause of global dementia that can be diagnosed based on the accumulation of two proteins—amyloid-Aβ and tau. Typically the likelihood of AD diagnosis is based on cognitive impairment over time along with CNS imaging. On imaging studies, the degree of cortical atrophy, based on expansion of sulci and enlargement of the ventricles (ex vacuo hydrocephalus), can be used along with clinical signs to make the diagnosis. Moreover, imaging studies are used to rule out treatable causes of dementia, such as unsuspected tumor.

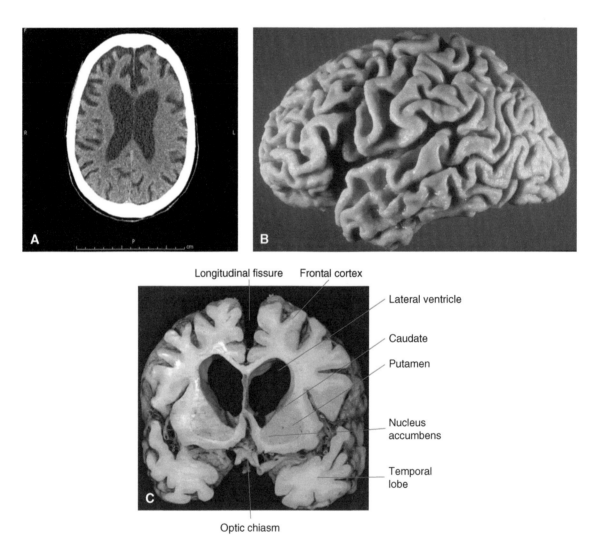

Figure 10.13 Alzheimer Disease (AD). **(A)** CT scan, axial view of a patient with AD demonstrating large sulci and ventricles. **(B)** Cortical atrophy in advanced AD. Notice the larger than normal sulci and reduced size of gyri. AD. **(C)** Cortical atrophy and dilatation of the lateral ventricles due to loss of brain tissue (hydrocephalus ex vacuo).

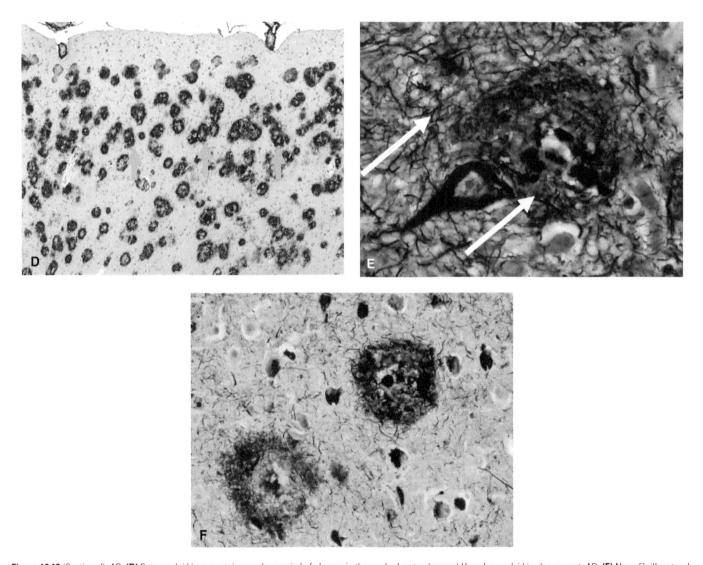

Figure 10.13 (Continued) AD. **(D)** Beta amyloid immunostain reveals a myriad of plaques in the cerebral cortex *(arrows)*. Vascular amyloid is also present. AD. **(E)** Neurofibrillary tangle and neuritic plaque. Bielschowsky silver stain. There are two main lesions in AD: senile plaques (also called Alzheimer plaques, neuritic plaques) and neurofibrillary tangles. Neuritic plaques are amyloid deposits containing degenerating neuronal processes with tau paired helical filaments *(arrows)*. AD. **(F)** Two senile plaques and multiple neurofibrillary tangles (the small dark objects around the plaques). Bielschowsky silver stain. (**[A]** CT image provided by Dr. Raymond Carmody. **[B-F]** Provided by Dr. Dimitri P. Agamanolis.)

Plaques are characterized as aggregates of Aβ peptide within the neuropil, while tangles are aggregates of tau, a microtubule binding protein. The amyloid Aβ protein within a plaque can be stained using Congo red and viewed under polarized light. The NFTs are tau-containing bundles of filaments that surround the nucleus of the neurons. Within the pyramidal cells they give a "flame-like" appearance using a silver stain and immunohisto-chemistry towards tau protein.

Parkinson Disease (PD) is a neurodegenerative disease that results in a decrease in the initiation of movements and a resting tremor. It is characterized by a loss of the dopaminergic neurons of the substantia nigra (in the midbrain of the brainstem). The confirmation of the diagnosis upon autopsy is the whiteness (pallor) of the substantia nigra *(Latin for black substance)*.

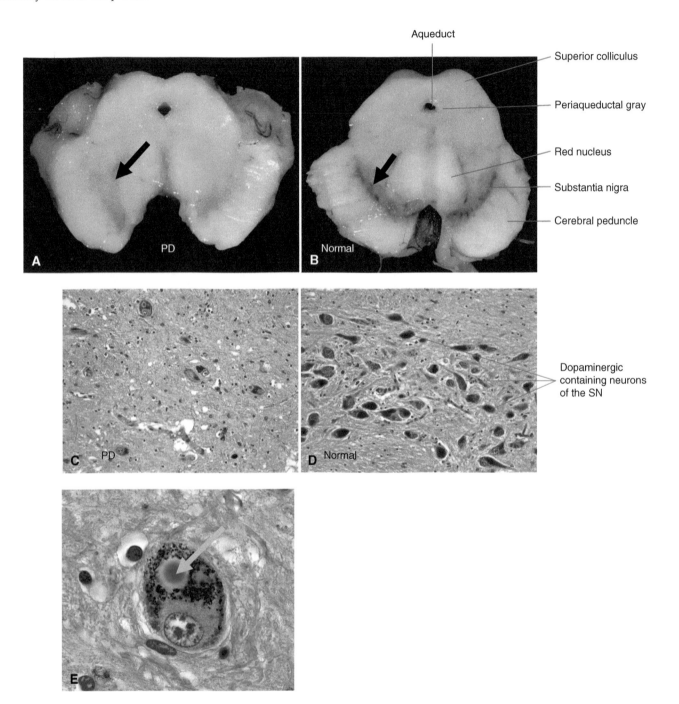

Figure 10.14 Parkinson disease (PD) **(A)** and **(B)** normal. Depigmentation of the substantia nigra (SN) of the zona compacta in PD *(arrow)* **(A)**. Normal SN *(arrow)* **(B)**. The pathology of PD affects the dopamine-producing neurons of the SN. In advanced PD, loss of pigmented neurons results in gross depigmentation of the SN. Micro of PD pathology **(C)** and **(D)** normal. The mid-section of the SN (zonal compacta) is involved earliest and most severely. Loss of SN neurons in the zona compacta **(C)**. Normal SN in the same area **(D)**. PD. **(E)** Lewy body in an SN neuron. The melanin granules are red-brown. The key pathology in PD is α-synuclein accumulation. Lewy bodies are large α-synuclein aggregates in the neuronal body forming round lamellated eosinophilic cytoplasmic inclusions *(arrow)*. (Provided by Dr. Dimitri P. Agamanolis.)

Huntington Disease (HD) is an autosomal dominant disease characterized by the progressive loss of selective neurons in the basal ganglia. Unlike in PD, patients with HD experience more erratic, hyperkinetic movements. HD is due to a polyglutamine trinucleotide repeat expansion in which the protein, huntingtin, is made with an excess of glutamine that can result in protein aggregation and neuronal loss. Protein aggregates of huntingtin can be found in neurons of the striatum. On CT or MR imaging there is prominent atrophy of the caudate nucleus with secondary atrophy of the putamen and clear signs of lateral ventricular expansion (hydrocephalus ex vacuo).

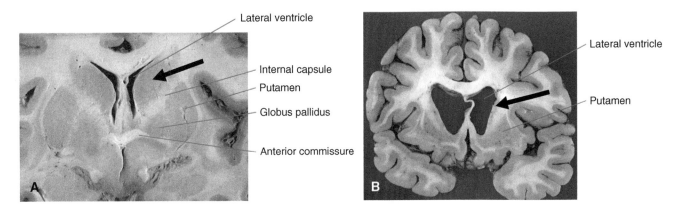

Figure 10.15 Huntington disease control. **(A)** Normal caudate nuclei *(arrow)*, small lateral ventricles. **(B)** Huntington disease. Gross examination of the brain reveals atrophy of the caudate nucleus *(arrow)* and putamen and dilatation of the anterior horns of the lateral ventricles, which are obvious on MRI in advanced cases. (Provided by Dr. Dimitri P. Agamanolis.)

Amyotrophic lateral sclerosis (ALS) is a progressive disease that affects both the upper and lower motor neurons, resulting in the denervation of muscle and the advance of weakness over time. ALS is thought to be caused by the accumulation of toxic proteins. At autopsy patients with ALS have a lack of gray matter in the anterior horns of the spinal cord, as well as atrophy of the precentral (primary motor cortex) gyrus.

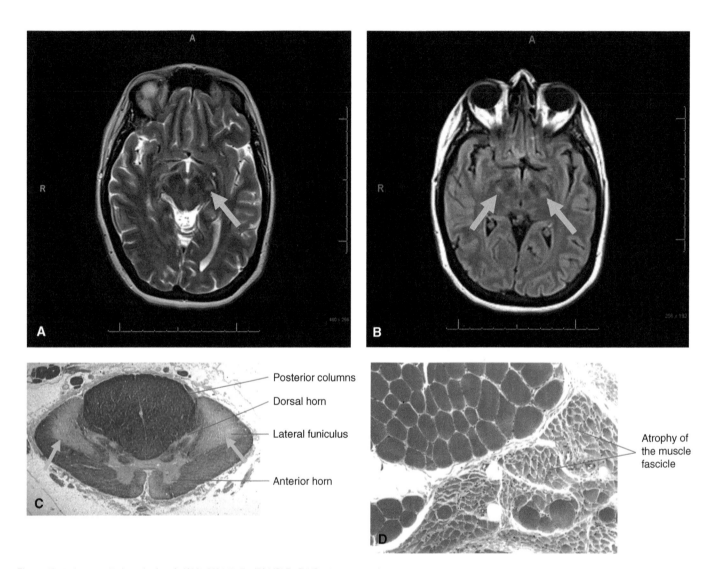

Figure 10.16 Amyotrophic lateral sclerosis (ALS). **(A)** MRI-T2, **(B)** MRI-T2 FLAIR axial views in the loss of motor fibers running though the descending corticospinal tract of the cerebral peduncle *(arrows)*. ALS. **(C)** Degeneration of the corticospinal tracts *(arrows)* (the axons of the upper motor neurons). Myelin stain. In ALS there is also degeneration and loss of motor neurons in the anterior horns of the spinal cord and motor nuclei of the brainstem (not illustrated in this picture). Remaining neurons will contain eosinophilic cytoplasmic inclusions called Bunina bodies (remnants of vacuoles) (not illustrated here). **(D)** Muscle, ALS. Denervation atrophy indicating chronic denervation. (**[A-B]** Images provided by Dr. Raymond Carmody; **[C-D]** Provided by Dr. Dimitri P. Agamanolis.)

This glossary provides brief descriptions and definitions of the neuroanatomical structures labeled in the preceding chapters (except for the bones and muscles indicated in Chapter 9). Within each entry, terms discussed further in their own entries elsewhere in the glossary are *italicized*.

Although these definitions were written specifically for this atlas, many are adapted from passages in **Nolte's The Human Brain, seventh edition.**[a] Some others derive, with modifications, from a text by Jay B. Angevine Jr. (with Carl W. Cotman), **Principles of Neuroanatomy.**[b] We thank Jeffrey House of Oxford University Press for permission to draw on the latter source.

We have illustrated most of the glossary terms, placing adaptations of figures from the atlas and some from **Nolte's The Human Brain**[a] after relevant entries. Space did not permit doing this for all entries, however, so alternative terms that may be consulted for an illustration are indicated by an asterisk (*).

Abducens nerve. The 6th cranial nerve, which emerges anteriorly from the *brainstem* between the *pons* and *medulla*. It innervates the lateral rectus of the ipsilateral eye, producing abduction (hence its name).

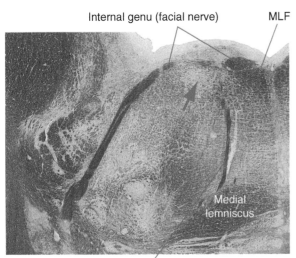

Internal genu (facial nerve)   MLF

Medial lemniscus

Abducens nerve fibers

Abducens nucleus. Contains the motor neurons for the ipsilateral lateral rectus, as well as interneurons that project through the contralateral *medial longitudinal fasciculus* (MLF) to medial rectus motor neurons. Activating the motor neurons and interneurons simultaneously provides for conjugate horizontal eye movements.

Accessory nerve. The 11th cranial nerve, which emerges laterally from the upper cervical *spinal cord* and innervates the sternocleidomastoid and trapezius muscles to mediate turning the head and elevating the shoulder. (The accessory nerve used to be described as having both cranial and spinal parts. The spinal part corresponded to the accessory nerve as defined here, and the cranial part to a series of rootlets that emerge laterally from the caudal *medulla*, join the *vagus nerve*, and run to the palate, pharynx, and larynx.)

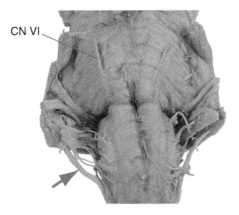

CN VI

Accessory nucleus. A column of motor neurons for the ipsilateral sternocleidomastoid and trapezius, extending from the midcervical *spinal cord* into the caudal *medulla*.

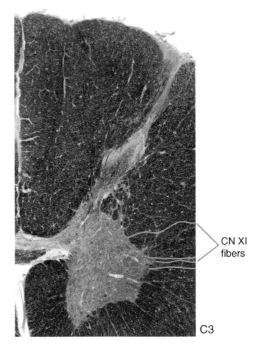

CN XI fibers

C3

Alveus. A layer of white matter on the ventricular surface of the *hippocampus**, mostly conveying hippocampal efferents.

[a]Nolte J: *The human brain*, ed 9, Philadelphia, 2009, Mosby Elsevier.
[b]Angevine JB Jr, Cotman CW: *Principles of neuroanatomy*, New York, 1981, Oxford University Press.

Ambient cistern. The combination of the *superior cistern* and sheetlike extensions from it that partially encircle the *midbrain*.

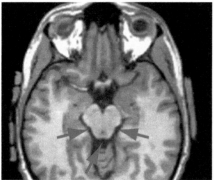

Provided by
Dr. Elena Plante,
University of Arizona

Amygdala. A collection of nuclei in the anteroinferior part of the *limbic lobe*, just beneath the *uncus*, forming the core of one of the two major limbic circuits. (The core of the other is the *hippocampus*.)

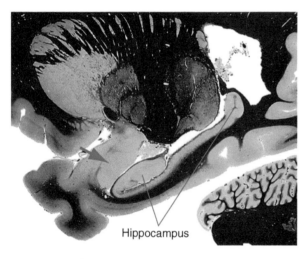

Hippocampus

Angular gyrus. The part of the *inferior parietal lobule** formed by the cortex surrounding the upturned end of the superior temporal sulcus; although variable in size and shape, this region (usually on the left) is important in language functions.

Ansa lenticularis. Part of the projection from the *globus pallidus* to the *thalamus*. It has fewer axons than the other part (the *lenticular fasciculus*). It forms a compact, conspicuous cable of myelinated fibers running beneath the *internal capsule* and hooking around its medial edge.

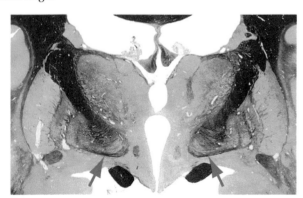

Anterior cerebral artery. The more anterior of the two terminal branches of the *internal carotid artery* (the other being the *middle cerebral artery*). It curves around the *corpus callosum* with branches

supplying *gyrus rectus* and *orbital gyri*, the medial surface of the *frontal* and *parietal lobes*, and an adjoining narrow band of cortex along their superior surfaces.

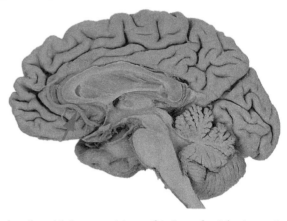

Anterior choroidal artery. A long, thin branch of the *internal carotid artery* that accompanies the *optic tract* and supplies many structures along the way: the *optic tract*, *choroid plexus* of the inferior horn of the *lateral ventricle*, part of the *cerebral peduncle*, deep regions of the *internal capsule*, and parts of the *thalamus* and *hippocampus*. The anterior choroidal artery is a particularly large example of the numerous penetrating arteries that arise from all arteries around the base of the brain and supply nearby deep structures.

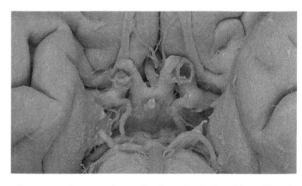

Anterior commissure. A small, sharply defined bundle of commissural fibers just beneath and behind the rostrum of the *corpus callosum*, to which it is closely related developmentally. A few inconspicuous anterior fibers interconnect olfactory structures, whereas the million or so posterior fibers interconnect the two *temporal lobes*.

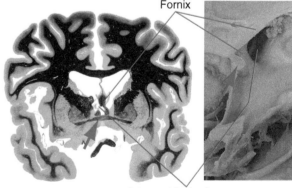

Fornix

Interventricular foramen

Anterior communicating artery. A short vessel at the anterior end of the *circle of Willis* interconnecting the two *anterior cerebral arteries* just anterior to the *optic chiasm*; a common site of aneurysm formation.

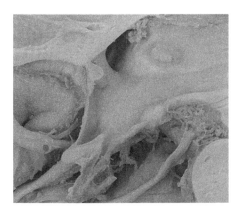

Anterior corticospinal tract. The smaller of the two *corticospinal tracts*. It consists of the fibers (about 15%) in each medullary *pyramid* that continue directly into the *anterior funiculus* of the *spinal cord* without decussating; many fibers eventually cross in the *anterior white commissure* of the cord before terminating, but some end ipsilaterally. Fibers of the anterior corticospinal tract end (mainly in the cervical and thoracic *spinal cord*) on spinal motor neurons or nearby interneurons.

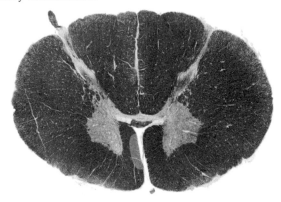

Anterior funiculus. One of the three major divisions of the spinal white matter, the others being the *lateral* and *posterior* funiculi. (Funiculus is Latin for "string" or "cord," as in the term "funicular" for "cable car.") The anterior funiculus is located between the anterior median fissure and the exiting *ventral roots* and contains various tracts (mostly descending), including the *anterior corticospinal tract*.

Anterior horn. One of the three general divisions of the spinal gray matter, the others being the *posterior horn* and the *intermediate gray*; contains numerous local-circuit neurons, cell bodies of alpha motor neurons, axons of which enter *ventral roots* and end on skeletal muscle, and cell bodies of gamma motor neurons that regulate muscle spindles.

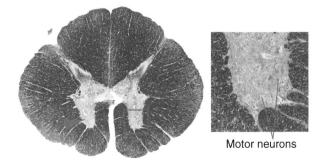

Motor neurons

Anterior inferior cerebellar artery. A long, circumferential branch of the *basilar artery* arising just above the union of the two *vertebral arteries*. It supplies anterior regions of the inferior surface of the

cerebellum, including the *flocculus*, and lateral parts of the caudal *pons*; often referred to by the acronym AICA.

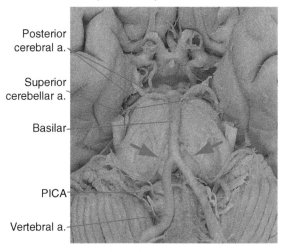

Posterior cerebral a.

Superior cerebellar a.

Basilar

PICA

Vertebral a.

Anterior nucleus. See *thalamus**.

Anterior perforated substance. The inferior surface of the forebrain, roughly between the *orbital gyri* and the *hypothalamus*. So named because numerous *lenticulostriate* and other small penetrating branches enter the brain here.

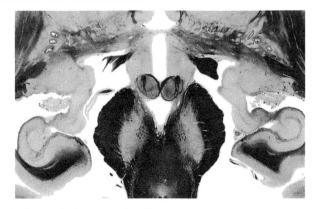

Anterior root. See *ventral root**.

Anterior spinal artery. A single midline vessel that originates rostrally as two arteries (one from each *vertebral artery*), which shortly join and then course within the anterior median fissure along the entire *spinal cord*. It receives additional blood from the thoracic/abdominal aorta through numerous anastomoses with radicular arteries below the upper cervical region and gives rise to hundreds of central and circumferential branches that supply the anterior two thirds of the cord.

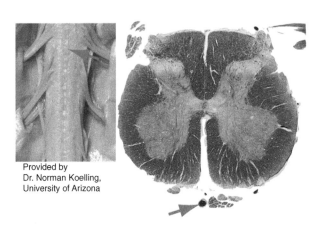

Provided by
Dr. Norman Koelling,
University of Arizona

Anterior spinocerebellar tract. Crossed fibers from lumbosacral spinal gray matter, carrying mechanoreceptive and other information related to leg movement. The anterior spinocerebellar tract stays in a lateral position along the *spinal cord* and *brainstem* until the rostral *pons* and there moves over the *superior cerebellar peduncle* and enters the *cerebellum*, where it largely recrosses before terminating.

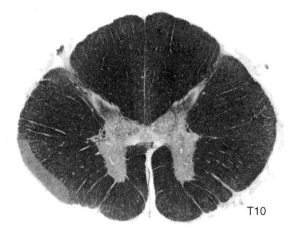

T10

Anterior white commissure. A thin sheet of spinal white matter between the *central canal* and the anterior median fissure, providing a route for fibers such as those of the *spinothalamic tract* to cross the midline in the *spinal cord*.

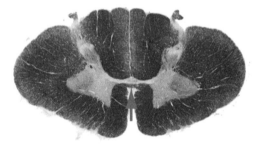

Anterolateral system. An umbrella term for the *spinothalamic tract* and closely related ascending fibers, all of which deal with pain, temperature, and to some extent tactile/pressure sensation. Many do not reach the *thalamus*, ending instead at higher spinal levels and/or in *brainstem* sites such as the *reticular formation*.

Aqueduct (of Sylvius). The narrow channel (a remnant of the lumen of the embryonic mesencephalon) through the *midbrain* connecting the *third* and *fourth ventricles*. The aqueduct lacks *choroid plexus* and serves only as a conduit for cerebrospinal fluid descending through the ventricular system (its stenosis or obstruction is the most common cause of congenital hydrocephalus).

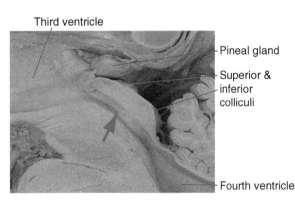

Third ventricle

Pineal gland

Superior & inferior colliculi

Fourth ventricle

Arachnoid. The middle layer of the three layers of meninges, named for its cobweb-like appearance. The arachnoid is loosely adherent to the *dura mater* and connected to the pia mater by fine strands of connective tissue (arachnoid trabeculae). The resulting subarachnoid space, between arachnoid and pia, provides a route for the distribution of blood vessels and the flow of cerebrospinal fluid over the surface of the CNS.

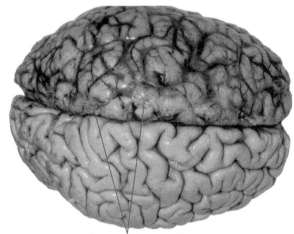

Arachnoid granulations

Arachnoid granulations. Small evaginations of the *arachnoid** protruding through a hiatus in dural connective tissue into the lumen of a dural sinus of the brain (especially the *superior sagittal sinus*), so that only loosely arranged arachnoid cells and endothelium intervene between subarachnoid space and venous blood. Arachnoid granulations are the major (but not exclusive) sites of reabsorption of cerebrospinal fluid into the venous system.

Area postrema. A small region at the caudal end of the *fourth ventricle* where the ventricular walls join at the *obex*. The area postrema is one of several circumventricular organs of the brain where cerebral capillaries are fenestrated and allow free communication between the blood and brain extracellular fluid ("holes" in the blood-brain barrier); it is thought to monitor blood for toxins and to trigger vomiting.

Basal forebrain. A loosely used umbrella term for an area at and near the inferior surface of the cerebrum between the *hypothalamus* and *orbital gyri*. It includes the *anterior perforated substance* superficially and extends superiorly into the *septal nuclei* and the adjacent oxymoronically named *substantia innominata* (see also *basal nucleus*).

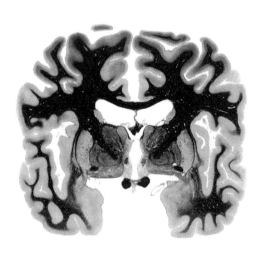

Basal ganglia. A group of subcortical nuclei, most prominently including the *striatum, globus pallidus, substantia nigra,* and *subthalamic nucleus,* that collectively modulate the output of frontal cortex. Basal ganglia damage has traditionally been thought to cause disorders characterized by involuntary movements, difficulty initiating movement, and alterations in muscle tone (e.g., Parkinson's disease). However, damage to certain parts of the basal ganglia can cause disturbances of cognition and motivation instead.

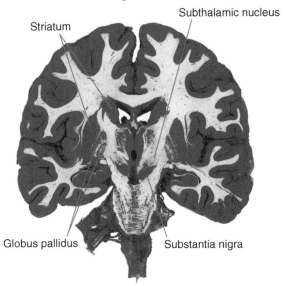

Striatum

Subthalamic nucleus

Globus pallidus

Substantia nigra

Basal nucleus (of Meynert). Groups of large cholinergic neurons in the *substantia innominata* of the *basal forebrain.* Widespread projections of these and nearby *septal* neurons blanket the neocortex, *hippocampus,* and *amygdala* with cholinergic endings, suggesting that it plays a role in general regulation of cerebral activity.

Basal pons. A mass of gray and white matter, straddling the anterior surface of the *pons* and filled with transversely and longitudinally coursing fibers. The basal pons looks like a bridge (thus the name *pons,* which is Latin for bridge) between the two *cerebellar hemispheres,* but in fact it is a key link between the cerebrum and *cerebellum:* *Corticopontine* fibers end in its scattered *pontine nuclei,* which in turn give rise to *pontocerebellar fibers* that project across the midline and enter the *cerebellum* via the *middle cerebellar peduncle.*

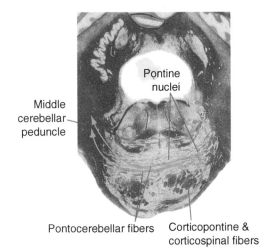

Middle cerebellar peduncle

Pontine nuclei

Pontocerebellar fibers

Corticopontine & corticospinal fibers

Basal vein (of Rosenthal). A deep cerebral vein whose tributaries drain the *insula* and some structures near the inferior surface of the forebrain. The basal vein then curves around the *midbrain* and joins the *great cerebral vein.*

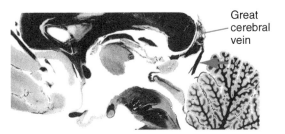

Great cerebral vein

Basilar artery. A large vessel formed by union of the two *vertebral arteries.* The basilar artery runs upward along the anterior median surface of the *pons* and gives rise to many branches that supply the *pons,* superior surface of the *cerebellum,* and caudal *midbrain;* it bifurcates at the level of the *midbrain* into the two *posterior cerebral arteries.*

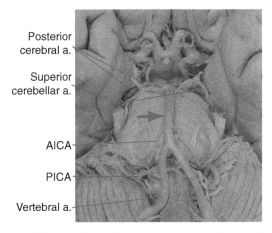

Posterior cerebral a.

Superior cerebellar a.

AICA

PICA

Vertebral a.

Brachium of the inferior colliculus. Auditory afferents from the *inferior colliculus* on their way to the *medial geniculate nucleus.*

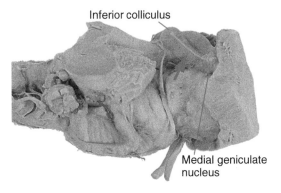

Inferior colliculus

Medial geniculate nucleus

Brachium of the superior colliculus. A bundle of fibers that passes over the *medial geniculate nucleus* to reach the *superior colliculus.* Contains afferents from the retina directly to the *superior colliculus* and *pretectal area,* as well as projections from cerebral cortex to the *superior colliculus* and from the *superior colliculus* to the *pulvinar.*

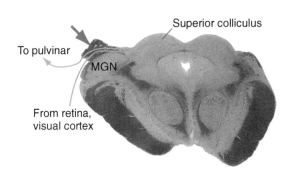

Superior colliculus

To pulvinar

MGN

From retina, visual cortex

Brainstem. In common medical usage, the *midbrain*, *pons*, and *medulla*. (Earlier definitions sometimes included various parts of the *diencephalon* and telencephalon as well [e.g., *thalamus*, *basal ganglia*].)

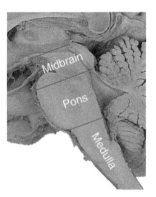

Calcarine sulcus. A prominent, deep cerebral infolding. It originates anteriorly in the *temporal lobe* near the splenium of the *corpus callosum* and continues posteriorly into the *occipital lobe*, where it terminates near the occipital pole. Its upper and lower banks contain the primary visual cortex. Anteriorly along this course, the *parietooccipital sulcus* branches off from it.

Parietooccipital
sulcus

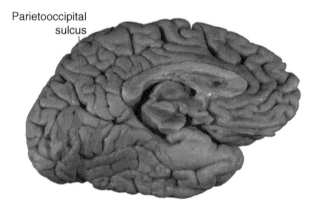

Callosomarginal artery. A branch of the anterior cerebral artery that follows the cingulate sulcus.

Cauda equina. A collection of *dorsal* and *ventral roots*, named for their collective resemblance to a horse's tail, descending from the caudal end of the *spinal cord* (at about vertebral level L1/L2) to the intervertebral foramina at which they exit the vertebral canal.

Filum terminale   Conus medullaris

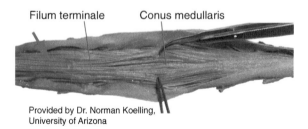

Provided by Dr. Norman Koelling,
University of Arizona

Caudate nucleus. The more medial part of the *striatum**, bulging into the *lateral ventricle* with its large head in the wall of the anterior horn, tapering body immediately behind, and long slender tail running posteriorly into the atrium and then anteriorly into the inferior horn. It is principally connected with prefrontal and other association areas of the cortex and is involved more in cognitive functions and less directly in movement.

Central canal. The narrow, functionless vestige of the lumen of the spinal part of the embryonic neural tube, lined by ependyma and usually obstructed by epithelial debris. It runs the length of the *spinal cord*, contains traces of cerebrospinal fluid, and opens into the *fourth ventricle* at the *obex* of the *medulla*.

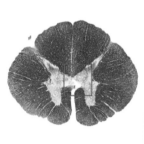
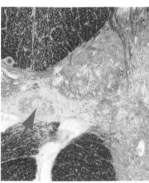

Central sulcus (of Rolando). An anatomically and functionally important infolding of the cerebral hemisphere, beginning just medial to its superior border, proceeding over its superior margin, and descending obliquely forward almost to the *lateral sulcus*. The central sulcus is the boundary between *frontal* and *parietal lobes* and the transition zone between primary motor and primary somatosensory cortex.

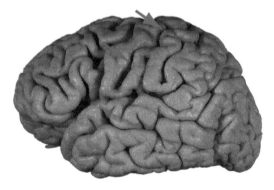

Central tegmental tract. A complex, heterogeneous tract running centrally through each side of the brainstem *reticular formation* and providing a major highway through which reticular afferents and efferents are distributed. It also contains a major projection from the *red nucleus* to the *inferior olivary nucleus*, axons intrinsic to the *reticular formation*, and undoubtedly other types of fibers that are not yet fully characterized.

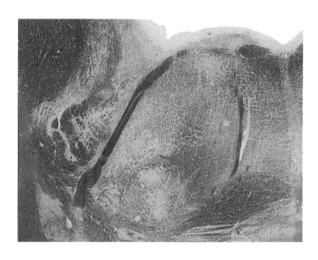

Centromedian nucleus. See *thalamus**.

Cerebellar cortex. The extensively folded, three-layered sheet of gray matter that covers the *cerebellum*.

Granular layer. The deepest layer, adjacent to the cerebellar white matter. Named for the enormous number of tiny granule cells that occupy it: about half of all the neurons in the CNS live in this layer.

Molecular layer. The most superficial layer, containing relatively few neurons. Mainly a layer in which the axons of granule cells and other cerebellar interneurons synapse on Purkinje cell dendrites.

Purkinje cell layer. A layer of relatively large neurons whose axons provide the output from cerebellar cortex.

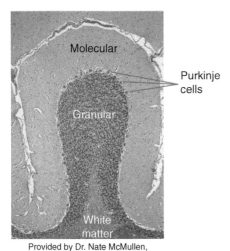

Provided by Dr. Nate McMullen, University of Arizona

Cerebellothalamic fibers. Efferent fibers from the deep cerebellar nuclei (mainly the *dentate nucleus*) that pass via the *superior cerebellar peduncle* and its decussation through or around the contralateral *red nucleus** to the *ventral lateral nucleus* of the *thalamus* (VL), which in turn projects to motor areas of cortex. This tract completes a long, doubly crossed circuit between each cerebral hemisphere and the contralateral *cerebellar hemisphere* that is crucial for the planning and coordination of skilled movements. Because most of these fibers arise in the *dentate nucleus*, they are sometimes referred to as the dentatothalamic tract.

Cerebellum. A large, convoluted subdivision of the nervous system (cerebellum literally means "little brain") that receives input from sensory systems, the cerebral cortex, and other sites and participates in the planning and coordination of movement.

Anterior lobe. All of the cerebellum anterior to the primary fissure (partly vermis, partly hemisphere).

Flocculus. The hemispheral component of the flocculonodular lobe, the part of the cerebellum particularly concerned with the vestibular system and eye movements.

Hemispheres. The large paired lateral parts, important for coordination of the limbs.

Nodulus. The vermal component of the flocculonodular lobe, the part of the cerebellum particularly concerned with the vestibular system and eye movements.

Posterior lobe. All of the cerebellum, except for the flocculonodular lobe, posterior to the primary fissure (partly vermis, partly hemisphere).

Primary fissure. Separates the anterior and posterior lobes of the cerebellum.

Tonsil. A medial, inferior part of the posterior lobe hemisphere, adjacent to the *medulla* as it passes through the foramen magnum.

Vermis (Latin for "worm"). The most medial zone of the cerebellum, straddling the midline. Extends through the anterior, posterior, and flocculonodular lobes.

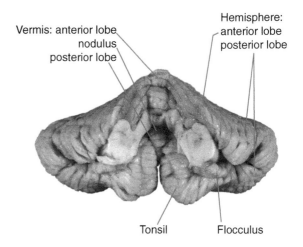

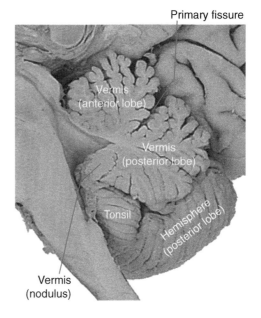

Cerebral peduncle. As the term is used in this book, a massive bundle of tightly packed *corticospinal*, *corticobulbar*, and *corticopontine* fibers traveling along the base of the *midbrain*. (Others use the term *cerebral peduncle* to refer to all of one side of the *midbrain* inferior to the *aqueduct*. In this terminology, the bundle of corticofugal fibers is called the pes pedunculi, basis pedunculi, or crus cerebri.)

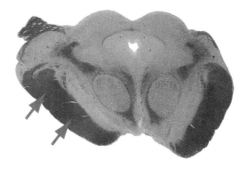

Choroid fissure. A C-shaped fissure on the medial surface of each cerebral hemisphere, leading into the *choroid plexus* of each *lateral ventricle*. Because of this C shape, coronal sections often cut through the choroid fissure in two places.

Choroid plexus

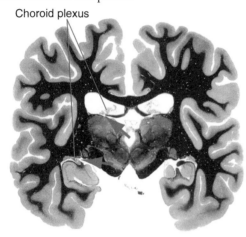

Choroid plexus. Long, highly convoluted, vascularized strands in the *lateral*, *third*, and *fourth ventricles* that produce most of the cerebrospinal fluid.

Choroidal vein. A tortuous vessel that joins the *terminal* (*thalamostriate*) *vein* near the *interventricular foramen* and drains the *choroid plexus* of the body of the *lateral ventricle*.

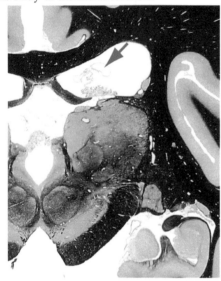

Cingulate gyrus. A broad belt of cortex partially encircling the *corpus callosum*. The cingulate gyrus forms the upper part of the *limbic lobe*, continuing through a narrow isthmus into the *parahippocampal gyrus*. It has extensive limbic connections, particularly in cortical circuits leading ultimately to or from the *hippocampus*.

Marginal branch   Cingulate sulcus

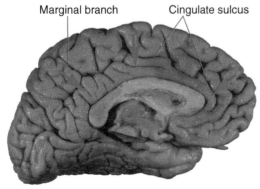

Cingulate sulcus. A more or less continuous, curved infolding of each cerebral hemisphere clearly demarcating the outer margin of the *cingulate gyrus**; posteriorly a branch (the marginal branch) ascends to the superior surface of the *parietal lobe* immediately behind the upper end of the *central sulcus*.

Cingulum. An association bundle located in the white matter underlying the *cingulate gyrus* and interconnecting limbic cortical areas.

Circle of Willis. The anastomotic arterial polygon at the base of the brain, consisting of parts of the *internal carotid*, *anterior cerebral*, and *posterior cerebral arteries*, interconnected by the *anterior* and *posterior communicating arteries*.

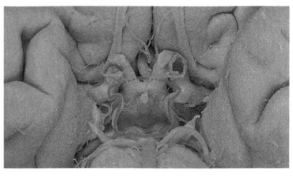

Cisterna magna. A large subarachnoid cistern between the *medulla* and the inferior *vermis*. Also referred to as the cerebellomedullary cistern.

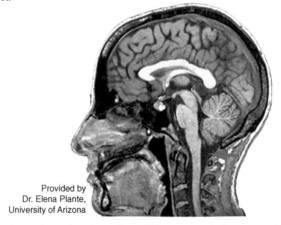

Provided by
Dr. Elena Plante,
University of Arizona

Clarke's nucleus (nucleus dorsalis). A rounded group of large cell bodies in the *intermediate gray* of the *spinal cord* near the medial edge of the base of the *posterior horn*, from about T1 through L2 or L3. Clarke's nucleus is the origin of the *posterior spinocerebellar tract*, through which stretch receptor and other mechanoreceptive input from the leg reaches the ipsilateral *cerebellar vermis* and medial part of the *cerebellar hemisphere*.

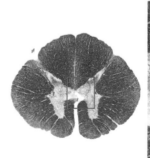
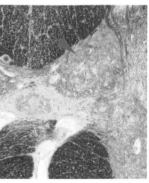

Claustrum. A thin but extensive layer of gray matter beneath the *insula*, separated from it and the underlying *putamen* by the *extreme* and *external capsules* respectively. The claustrum has reciprocal connections with cerebral cortex, but incompletely understood functions.

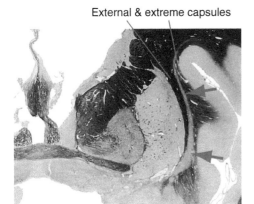

External & extreme capsules

Cochlear nuclei. The nuclei in which the primary auditory afferents of the *vestibulocochlear nerve* terminate. The dorsal and ventral cochlear nuclei form a continuous band of gray matter draped over the *inferior cerebellar peduncle** near the pontomedullary junction and project bilaterally to the *superior olivary nucleus* and into the *lateral lemniscus*.

Collateral sulcus. A deep infolding of the inferior surface of the *temporal lobe**, bulging into the wall of the inferior horn of the *lateral ventricle* as the collateral eminence. It separates the *occipitotemporal* (fusiform) *gyrus* from the *parahippocampal gyrus*.

Conus medullaris. The pointed caudal end of the spinal cord, at about vertebral level L1/L2, beyond which the pial covering of the spinal cord continues as the *filum terminale*, surrounded by the *cauda equina**.

Corpus callosum. Latin for "hard body," a massive curvilinear bridge of commissural fibers, shaped in sagittal sections like an overturned canoe. The corpus callosum interconnects most cortical areas of the two cerebral hemispheres and serves to join them functionally, providing an important substrate for a unitary consciousness.
    Body. The main arched part of the corpus callosum. Its fibers distribute extensively within each hemisphere.
    Genu. The kneelike sharp anterior bend, containing fibers to and from the *frontal lobes*.
    Rostrum. The slender, narrow part beneath the genu, resembling the prow of the (overturned) boat; interconnects *orbital gyri*.
    Splenium. The thick, rounded posterior bend (like a rolled bandage, for which it was named), containing fibers to and from the *occipital* and *temporal lobes*.

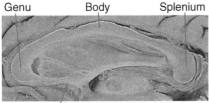

Genu   Body   Splenium

Rostrum

Corticobulbar tract. Strictly defined, a large collection of fibers originating in the cerebral cortex and descending through the *internal capsule* (immediately anterior to the closely related *corticospinal* fibers) to terminate (via numerous, often intricate routes) in the "bulb" (an old term for the *medulla* or, by extension, for the entire *brainstem*) on neurons of sensory relay nuclei, the *reticular formation*, and motor nuclei of cranial nerves. In common usage, the term refers only to the last fibers of this group. Basically the equivalent of the *corticospinal tract* for cranial nerve nuclei.

Corticopontine tract. A very large collection of fibers originating in the *frontal, parietal, occipital, temporal,* and even *limbic lobes* and descending through the *internal capsule* (anterior and posterior to the *corticospinal/corticobulbar* projections) to *pontine nuclei* of the *basal pons**, from which axons pass to the contralateral half of the *cerebellum* through the *middle cerebellar peduncle*.

Corticospinal tract. A collection of about a million axons that originate in the cerebral cortex, descend through the *internal capsule, cerebral peduncle, basal pons,* and medullary *pyramid*, then reach the *spinal cord,* where they terminate, via the *lateral* and *anterior corticospinal tracts*. Roughly a third of them originate in primary motor cortex, the rest arising from premotor and supplementary motor areas and the *parietal lobe* (especially somatosensory cortex). Corticospinal axons end in the *spinal cord* on cells of the *posterior horn, intermediate gray,* and *anterior horn,* where some synapse directly on alpha and gamma motor neurons. Although the corticospinal tract has multiple functions, the principal one is mediating voluntary movements.

Cuneate tubercle. A swelling on the dorsolateral aspect of the lower *medulla* overlying *nucleus cuneatus*, which contains the cells of origin of the part of the *medial lemniscus* carrying tactile and proprioceptive information from the arm and upper body.

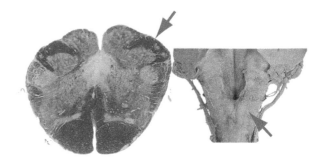

Cuneus. The wedge-shaped area of the medial surface of the *occipital lobe* between the *calcarine* and *parietooccipital sulci*. Includes the upper half of primary visual cortex and parts of visual association cortex.

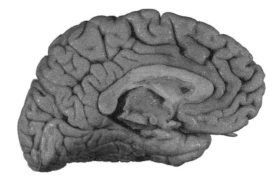

Dentate nucleus. The largest and most lateral of the deep cerebellar nuclei, featuring a highly convoluted narrow band of neurons arranged like a bag, with an anteriorly directed opening (hilus)

from which efferents emerge to form most of the *superior cerebellar peduncle*.

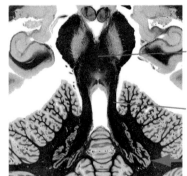

Decussation of superior cerebellar peduncles

Superior cerebellar peduncle

Denticulate ligament. A thickened, lateral, serrated sheet of pia mater on each side of the *spinal cord*, with periodic extensions that attach to the *arachnoid* and *dura mater*, supporting the weight and stabilizing the position of the cord within the dural sac.

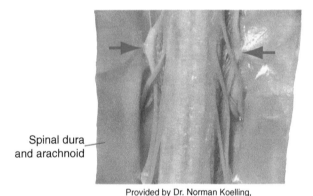

Spinal dura and arachnoid

Provided by Dr. Norman Koelling, University of Arizona

Diencephalon. Literally the "in-between brain," the caudal subdivision of the embryonic forebrain, giving rise to the *pineal gland, habenula, thalamus, subthalamic nucleus, retina, optic nerve* and *tract, hypothalamus, infundibulum* (pituitary stalk), and posterior lobe of the *pituitary gland*.

Dorsal cochlear nucleus. See *cochlear nuclei*.

Dorsal longitudinal fasciculus. Ascending and descending fibers connecting the *hypothalamus* directly and indirectly to visceral sensory neurons and preganglionic autonomic neurons, traveling through the *periaqueductal* and periventricular gray matter.

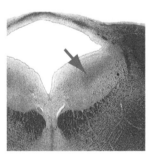
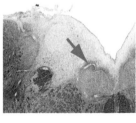

Dorsal motor nucleus of the vagus. A prominent autonomic efferent nucleus containing most of the preganglionic parasympathetic neurons for thoracic and abdominal viscera.

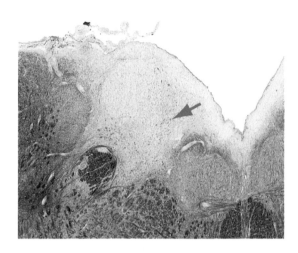

Dorsal raphe nucleus. See *raphe nuclei*.

Dorsal root. The posterior (sensory) root of a spinal nerve, which divides into a variable number of regularly spaced rootlets that enter the *spinal cord* along its posterolateral sulcus.

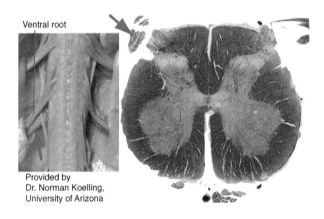

Ventral root

Provided by Dr. Norman Koelling, University of Arizona

Dorsomedial nucleus (DM). See *thalamus*.

Dura mater. The outermost of the three layers of meninges, providing critical mechanical support for the CNS. Cranial dura mater is continuous with the periosteum of the inner surface of the skull, whereas in the vertebral canal it forms a dural sac within which the *spinal cord* is suspended by *denticulate ligaments*.

Edinger-Westphal nucleus. A column of small nerve cell bodies near the midline of the *oculomotor nucleus*. Its neurons form the efferent limb of the direct and consensual pupillary light reflexes, through which preganglionic parasympathetic neurons (via postganglionic neurons in the ciliary ganglion) cause contraction of the pupillary sphincter. Also part of the efferent limb of the near reflex, through which it causes (again via postganglionic neurons in the ciliary ganglion) ciliary muscle contraction to thicken the lens and pupillary constriction to increase depth of focus.

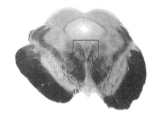
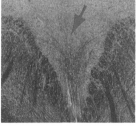

Entorhinal cortex. The cortex covering the anterior part of the *parahippocampal gyrus*, near the *uncus*. Entorhinal cortex receives inputs from the *amygdala, olfactory bulb*, the *limbic lobe*, and other cortical areas and in turn is the major source of afferents to the *hippocampus*.

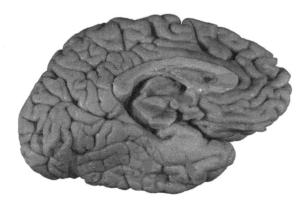

External capsule. A thin layer of white matter interposed between the *claustrum** and *putamen*, containing association fibers that interconnect various cortical areas and modulatory fibers from sites such as the *basal nucleus*.

External medullary lamina (of the thalamus). A thin, curved sheet of myelinated fibers (afferent and efferent), in places reticulated and in others dense, surrounding the lateral surface of the *thalamus**; enclosed by a thin shell of gray matter, the *reticular nucleus*, which intervenes between it and the *internal capsule*.

Extreme capsule. A thin layer of white matter interposed between the *claustrum** and *insula*. The extreme capsule is the subcortical white matter of the *insula* but also contains association fibers that interconnect various other cortical areas.

Facial colliculus. A swelling in the floor of the fourth ventricle, caused by the underlying internal genu of the *facial nerve* looping around the *abducens nucleus*.

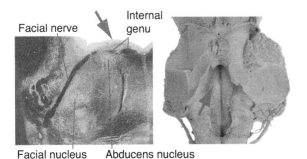

Facial nerve · Internal genu

Facial nucleus · Abducens nucleus

Facial nerve. The 7th cranial nerve, which emerges anterolaterally from the *brainstem* along the groove between the *basal pons* and the *medulla*.
 Motor root. Large, medial root containing axons of motor neurons for muscles of facial expression.
 Sensory root (intermediate nerve). The smaller of the two roots, emerging between the motor root and the vestibulocochlear nerve, containing afferents from taste buds, nasopharyngeal mucous membranes, and skin of the outer ear, as well as

preganglionic parasympathetic axons for submandibular, sublingual, and lacrimal glands.

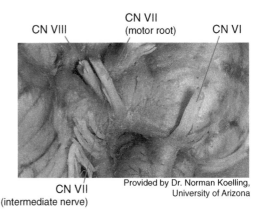

CN VIII · CN VII (motor root) · CN VI

CN VII (intermediate nerve)

Provided by Dr. Norman Koelling, University of Arizona

Facial nucleus. A group of motor neurons in the caudal pontine tegmentum that innervate muscles of the ipsilateral half of the face. Their axons loop around the *abducens nucleus* in the internal genu of the *facial nerve*, forming the *facial colliculus** in the floor of the *fourth ventricle*, before leaving the *brainstem*.

Fasciculus cuneatus. Uncrossed, large, myelinated, primary afferents entering the *posterior column* of the *spinal cord* rostral to T6 and carrying tactile and proprioceptive information from the ipsilateral arm; many of these fibers ascend to the *medulla* to terminate in *nucleus cuneatus*.

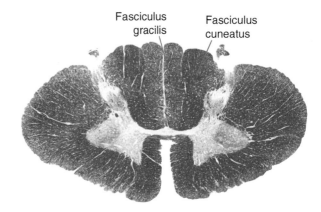

Fasciculus gracilis · Fasciculus cuneatus

Fasciculus gracilis. Uncrossed, large, myelinated, primary afferents entering the *posterior column* of the *spinal cord* caudal to T6 and carrying tactile and proprioceptive information from the ipsilateral leg; many of these fibers ascend to the *medulla*, medial to *fasciculus cuneatus**, to terminate in *nucleus gracilis*.

Fastigial nucleus. The most medial of the deep cerebellar nuclei. Its afferents come mainly from the *cerebellar vermis*, and its efferents project bilaterally to the *vestibular nuclei* and *reticular formation*.

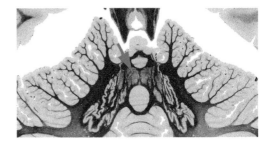

Filum terminale. A thin strand of connective tissue that anchors the caudal end of the *spinal cord* to the coccyx. It begins as a pial extension from the *conus medullaris*, extends through the lumbar cistern surrounded by the *cauda equina**, picks up a covering of *dura mater* at about vertebral level S2 (where the spinal dural sac ends), and merges with the periosteum of the coccyx.

Fimbria. Literally the "fringe," a prominent band of white matter along the medial edge of the *hippocampus**. The fimbria is an accumulation of myelinated axons (mostly efferent) that first collect on the ventricular surface of the *hippocampus* as the *alveus*. Near the splenium of the *corpus callosum* the fimbria separates from the *hippocampus* as the crus of the *fornix**.

Flocculus. The hemispheral component of the flocculonodular lobe, the part of the *cerebellum** particularly concerned with the vestibular system and eye movements.

Foramen of Monro. See *interventricular foramen**.

Fornix. A prominent paired fiber bundle, mostly containing hippocampal efferents, that interconnects the *hippocampus* of each cerebral hemisphere and the ipsilateral *septal nuclei* and *hypothalamus*.
   Body. Upper arched cable formed by the union of the crura beneath the *septa pellucida* in the midline.
   Column. One of the two bundles that diverge from the body, then pass down and back toward the *mammillary bodies*.
   Crus. One of the two origins ("legs") of the body, formed by detachment of the *fimbria* from the *hippocampus*.
   Fimbria. Hippocampal efferents that have assembled from the *alveus* on their way into the crus.
   Precommissural fornix. Fornix fibers that leave the columns just above the *anterior commissure*, bound for the *septal nuclei*, *ventral striatum*, and some nearby cortical areas.

Interventricular foramen

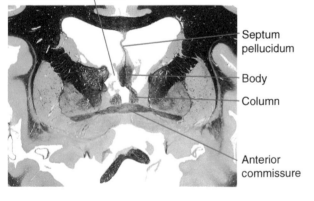

Septum
pellucidum

Body

Column

Anterior
commissure

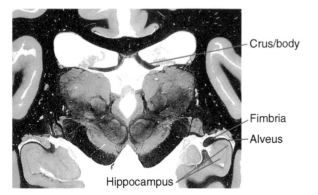

Crus/body

Fimbria

Alveus

Hippocampus

Fourth ventricle. The most caudal of the brain ventricles, shaped like a tent with a peaked roof protruding into the overlying *cerebellum* and a diamond-shaped floor formed by the dorsal surface of the *pons* and rostral *medulla*; continuous with the *third ventricle* via the cerebral *aqueduct* and open to the subarachnoid space through three foramina: one *median aperture* and two *lateral apertures*.

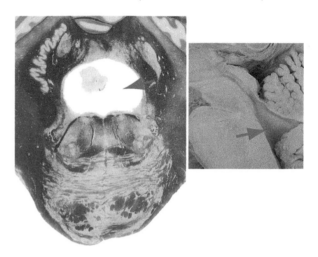

Frontal lobe. The most anterior lobe of each cerebral hemisphere. The frontal lobe includes motor, premotor, and supplementary motor cortex; an extensive prefrontal region; and a large expanse of *orbital* cortex. The latter two regions have access via long association fibers to all other lobes and also the limbic system; they are important (in ways still only partially understood) in working memory, decision making, and regulating emotional tone.

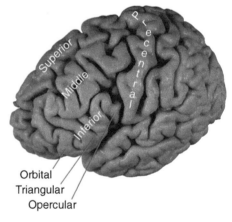

Orbital
Triangular
Opercular

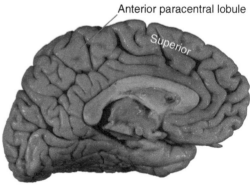

Anterior paracentral lobule

Fusiform gyrus. See *occipitotemporal gyrus**.

Globus pallidus. A wedge-shaped nucleus medial to the *putamen* that gives rise to most of the efferents from the *basal ganglia*.

External segment (GPe). Afferents from the *striatum*, efferents (via the *subthalamic fasciculus*) to the *subthalamic nucleus*.

Internal segment (GPi). Afferents from the striatum and subthalamic nucleus, efferents (via the ansa lenticularis and lenticular fasciculus) to the thalamus.

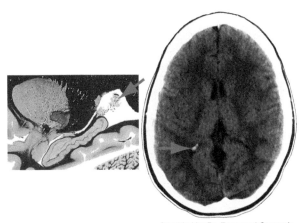

Glomus. An enlarged strand of *choroid plexus* in the atrium of the *lateral ventricle*. The glomus ("ball of thread") accumulates calcium deposits with age and so can often be seen in CT images.

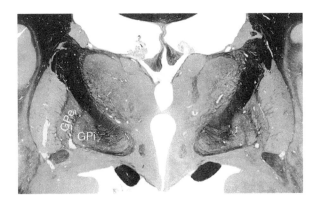

Provided by Dr. Raymond Carmody,
University of Arizona

Glossopharyngeal nerve. The 9th cranial nerve. Its rootlets emerge laterally from a shallow groove on the lateral surface of the *medulla* at the rostral end of the series of filaments that form the *vagus nerve*. The glossopharyngeal nerve contains afferents from taste buds, pharyngeal and middle ear mucous membranes, the carotid body and sinus, and skin of the outer ear; axons of motor neurons for a pharyngeal muscle (stylopharyngeus); and preganglionic parasympathetic axons for the parotid gland.

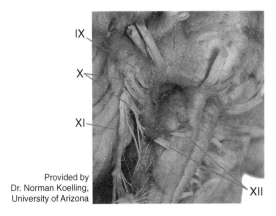

IX
X
XI
XII

Provided by
Dr. Norman Koelling,
University of Arizona

Gracile tubercle. A dorsomedial swelling on the caudal *medulla*, just caudal to the *obex*, overlying *nucleus gracilis*. Nucleus gracilis in turn gives rise to the part of the *medial lemniscus* that carries tactile and proprioceptive information from the leg and lower body.

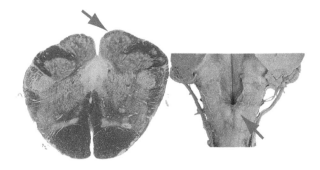

Great vein (great cerebral vein of Galen). A large unpaired vessel arising in the *superior cistern* by union of the two *internal cerebral veins*. During its short course it receives the *basal veins* (of Rosenthal), then turns superiorly around the splenium of the *corpus callosum* and joins the inferior sagittal sinus to form the *straight sinus*. The *great vein* is a key conduit in the deep venous drainage of the brain.

Internal cerebral vein

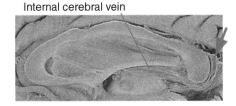

Gyrus rectus. A slender straight convolution, medial to the *orbital gyri** covering the rest of the inferior surface of the *frontal lobe*. Gyrus rectus has extensive limbic connections, particularly in circuits involving the *amygdala*.

Habenula. A small mound of neurons (derived from the embryonic *diencephalon*) on the dorsomedial surface of the posterior *thalamus*. The habenula receives diverse afferents from the ventral and medial forebrain (e.g., *septal nuclei, preoptic area*) that arrive through the *stria medullaris* of the thalamus. Habenular efferents descend to various paramedian *midbrain* reticular nuclei via the *habenulointerpeduncular tract*. Hence it is anatomically evident that the habenula is a relay in caudally directed limbic projections, although its exact role in primates is poorly understood.

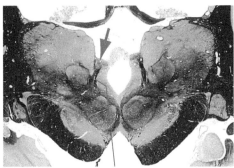

Habenulointerpeduncular tract

Habenulointerpeduncular tract. Also called *fasciculus retroflexus*, owing to its lordotic curvature, conveys outputs from the *stria* *medullaris/habenula** route precipitously down again to the paramedian *midbrain reticular formation* (where most other caudally directed limbic projections arrive more expediently by passing caudally through the *hypothalamus*).

Heschl's gyri. See *transverse temporal gyri**.

Hippocampus. A specialized cortical area rolled into the medial *temporal* (or *limbic*) *lobe*. The hippocampus plays a critical role in the consolidation of new memories of facts and events. Anatomically, it has three subdivisions (until recently, usually referred to collectively as the hippocampal formation rather than the hippocampus), from within outward as follows:

    Dentate gyrus. In cross section, one of two interlocking C-shaped strips of cortex (the hippocampus proper is the other). Afferents from *entorhinal cortex*, efferents to hippocampal pyramidal cells.

    Hippocampus proper (also called cornu ammonis, or Ammon's horn). Afferents from the dentate gyrus and *septal nuclei*, efferents to the subiculum and *septal nuclei*.

    Subiculum. A transitional zone between the hippocampus proper and *entorhinal cortex*, the subiculum receives afferents from the hippocampus proper and is the principal source of efferents from the hippocampus in general.

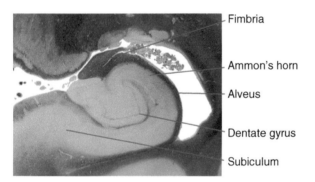

Fimbria

Ammon's horn

Alveus

Dentate gyrus

Subiculum

Hypoglossal nerve. The 12th cranial nerve, whose rootlets emerge from the *medulla* in an anterolateral sulcus between the *pyramid* and the *olive*. It innervates intrinsic and extrinsic skeletal muscles of the tongue.

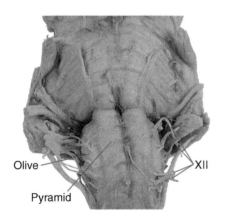

Olive

Pyramid

XII

Hypoglossal nucleus. A group of motor neurons that innervate muscles of the ipsilateral half of the tongue.

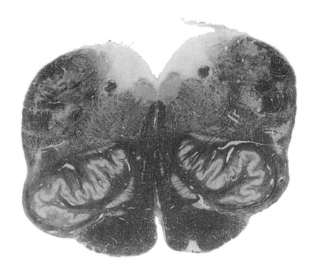

Hypoglossal trigone. A triangular elevation in the floor of the caudal *fourth ventricle* formed by the underlying *hypoglossal nucleus*.

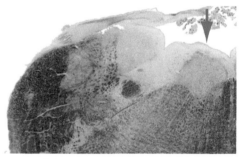

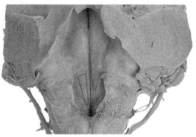

Hypothalamic sulcus. A shallow, curved indentation (convex side down) in the wall of the *third ventricle*, extending from the *interventricular foramen* to the opening of the cerebral *aqueduct*. The hypothalamic sulcus is the boundary between the *thalamus* and the *hypothalamus**.

Hypothalamus. The most inferior of the four divisions of the *diencephalon*, the hypothalamus plays a major role in orchestrating visceral and drive-related activities. It has three general zones:

    Anterior region. Includes the suprachiasmatic, supraoptic, and paraventricular nuclei and continues anteriorly into the *preoptic area*; projects axons to the posterior lobe of the *pituitary gland* and to caudal sites (including the *spinal cord*).

    Tuberal region. Includes the dorsomedial, ventromedial, and arcuate nuclei. The last secretes releasing hormones and inhibiting hormones into the *pituitary* portal system.

Posterior region. Includes the *mammillary* and posterior nuclei and projects to the *thalamus* and *midbrain tegmentum*.

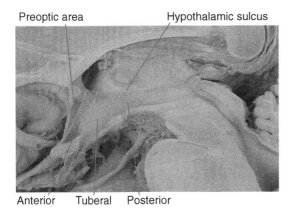

Preoptic area   Hypothalamic sulcus

Anterior   Tuberal   Posterior

Inferior brachium. See *brachium of the inferior colliculus**.

Inferior cerebellar peduncle. A major input route to the *cerebellum*, containing crossed olivocerebellar fibers, the uncrossed *posterior spinocerebellar* and cuneocerebellar tracts, vestibulocerebellar fibers, and other cerebellar afferents. Sometimes referred to as the restiform (Latin for "ropelike") body.

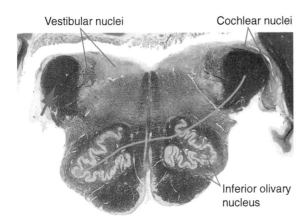

Vestibular nuclei   Cochlear nuclei

Inferior olivary nucleus

Inferior colliculus. A large, rounded mass of gray matter in the roof of the caudal *midbrain*. The inferior colliculus is a major link in the auditory system, receiving the *lateral lemniscus* and giving rise to the *brachium of the inferior colliculus**, which in turn conveys auditory fibers to the *thalamus* (medial geniculate nucleus).

Inferior frontal gyrus. The most inferior of three longitudinally oriented gyri in the anterior part of the *frontal lobe**. The opercular and triangular parts of this gyrus in the dominant hemisphere form Broca's area, which is a language area important for the production of spoken and written language.

Inferior olivary nucleus. A large nucleus in the anterolateral *medulla*, shaped like a bag, with a convoluted wall of gray matter (like a crumpled, pitted olive). Olivary afferents are diverse (from the *spinal cord*, *red nucleus*, deep cerebellar nuclei, etc.), but efferents are all olivocerebellar. They pour out of its medially facing mouth (or hilus), cross the midline as *internal arcuate fibers*, join the *inferior cerebellar peduncle**, and blanket the contralateral *cerebellum* as climbing fibers that powerfully excite Purkinje cells and other neurons.

Inferior parietal lobule. The lower part of the lateral surface of the *parietal lobe*, below the *intraparietal sulcus* and behind the *postcentral gyrus*. The inferior parietal lobule consists of the *angular* and *supramarginal gyri*, which (in the dominant hemisphere) are functionally related to Wernicke's area and thus important in the comprehension of language.

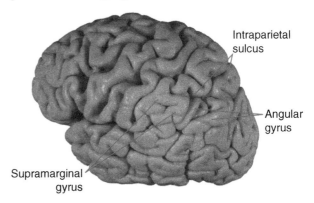

Intraparietal sulcus

Angular gyrus

Supramarginal gyrus

Inferior temporal gyrus. The most inferior of three longitudinally oriented convolutions visible on the lateral aspect of the *temporal lobe**. The inferior temporal gyrus is part of a large region of visual association cortex occupying most of the *occipital lobe* and much of the *temporal lobe*.

Inferior thalamic peduncle. A small bundle of fibers emerging anteriorly from the *thalamus* and curving down toward the *basal forebrain* (just anterior to the *ansa lenticularis*). Its fibers include interconnections between the dorsomedial nucleus and *orbital* cortex, but they do not traverse the *internal capsule* like other thalamic connections.

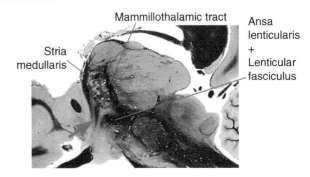

Mammillothalamic tract   Ansa lenticularis + Lenticular fasciculus

Stria medullaris

Inferior vestibular nucleus. See *vestibular nuclei*.

Infundibulum. The hollow, funnel-like stalk of the *pituitary gland* descending from the *median eminence* of the *hypothalamus* to the posterior lobe of the *pituitary gland*. The infundibulum arises during embryonic development as a ventral outgrowth of the floor of the *diencephalon* and is later joined by the anterior lobe derived from the roof of the oral cavity.

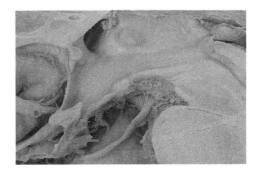

Insula. The original lateral surface of the embryonic telencephalic vesicle overlying an area of fusion with the *diencephalon*, forming in the adult a central lobe of the cerebral hemisphere, typically convoluted into about three short gyri (located more anteriorly) and two long gyri. With rapid cerebral expansion during fetal development, the insula is overgrown and by birth concealed by frontal, parietal, and temporal *opercula*. It includes limbic, gustatory, and autonomic areas but is less well understood than other cortical areas because of its hidden location.

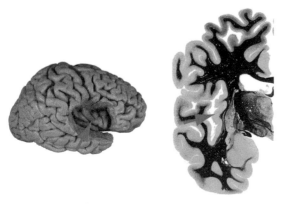

Intermediate gray. The spinal gray matter interposed between the *posterior* and *anterior horns*. It contains interneurons and tract cells of various sensory and motor circuits (including *Clarke's nucleus*), preganglionic sympathetic neurons in thoracic and upper lumbar segments, and preganglionic parasympathetic neurons in segments S2-S4.

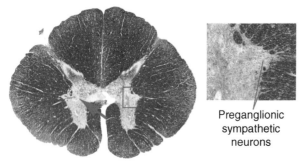

Preganglionic sympathetic neurons

Internal arcuate fibers. A general term for the large collection of axons that arch across the midline of the *medulla*. Many internal arcuate fibers are axons leaving the *posterior column nuclei* to form the contralateral *medial lemniscus*, some are trigeminothalamic fibers leaving the spinal *trigeminal nucleus* to join the contralateral *spinothalamic tract*, and most others are efferents from the *inferior olivary nucleus* to the contralateral half of the *cerebellum*.

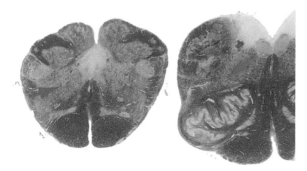

Internal capsule. A compact, curved sheet of thalamocortical, corticothalamic, and other cortical projection fibers shaped like part of a funnel. The internal capsule is divided into five regions, based on each region's relationship to the *lenticular nucleus*:

Anterior limb. Between the *lenticular nucleus* and the head of the *caudate nucleus*. Connections between the *thalamus* (dorsomedial and anterior nuclei) and prefrontal and anterior *cingulate* cortex, plus many frontopontine fibers.

Genu. At the junction between the anterior and posterior limbs, adjacent to the anterior end of the thalamus. Connections between the *thalamus* (VA, VL) and motor/premotor cortex, plus some frontopontine fibers.

Posterior limb. Between the *lenticular nucleus* and the *thalamus*. Connections between the *thalamus* (VA, VL, VPL/VPM) and motor, somatosensory, and other parietal cortex, plus *corticobulbar* and *corticospinal* fibers.

Retrolenticular part. Passing posterior to the *lenticular nucleus*. Connections between the *thalamus* (pulvinar, LP) and parietal-occipital-temporal association cortex, plus the upper part of the *optic radiation* (from the lateral geniculate nucleus).

Sublenticular part. Dipping under the posterior part of the *lenticular nucleus*. Projections to and from the *temporal lobe*, including the auditory radiation (from the medial geniculate nucleus) and the lower part of the *optic radiation* (from the lateral geniculate nucleus) before it turns posteriorly toward the *occipital lobe*.

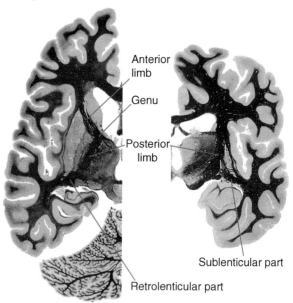

Anterior limb

Genu

Posterior limb

Sublenticular part

Retrolenticular part

Internal carotid artery. A large distributing artery, originating from the bifurcation of the common carotid artery and running cranially in the neck to enter the base of the skull and eventually the cranial vault. The internal carotid artery branches at the *circle of Willis* into *anterior* and *middle cerebral arteries*. The paired carotids account for about 80% of cerebral blood flow and thus supply most of the blood to the brain.

Anterior cerebral arteries

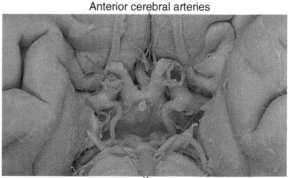

Middle cerebral arteries

Internal cerebral vein. The major deep vein of each cerebral hemisphere, formed at the *interventricular foramen* by the confluence of the smaller *septal* and *terminal* (thalamostriate) *veins* (the latter receiving the *choroidal vein*, which drains much of the *choroid plexus*). Immediately after its origin the internal cerebral vein bends sharply posteriorly (through the *venous angle*), proceeds posteriorly in the *transverse fissure*, and fuses with its counterpart in the *superior cistern* to form the unpaired *great vein**.

Internal medullary lamina (of the thalamus). A dense, curved sheet of myelinated fibers within the *thalamus** that divides it into medial and lateral compartments everywhere except posteriorly, where it does not enter the pulvinar, and anteriorly, where it forks into a V-shaped groove for the anterior nuclei. The internal medullary lamina contains several small and two large intralaminar nuclei (the centromedian and parafascicular nuclei).

Interpeduncular fossa. A depression on the anterior aspect of the *midbrain* between the two *cerebral peduncles*. Its surface is pierced by penetrating branches of the *basilar artery* and is therefore termed the posterior perforated substance. Rootlets of the *oculomotor nerve* exit here.

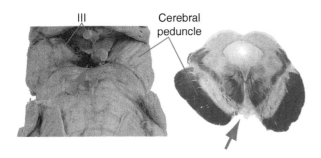

Interposed nucleus. The deep cerebellar nucleus interposed between the *dentate* and *fastigial nuclei*. The interposed nucleus has two distinct subdivisions, the globose nucleus medially and emboliform nucleus laterally (looks like an embolus in the hilus of the adjoining *dentate nucleus*). Both subdivisions receive input from the medial part of the ipsilateral *cerebellar hemisphere*; both project (via the *superior cerebellar peduncle*, like the *dentate nucleus*) to the *red nucleus* and the ventral lateral nucleus (VL) of the *thalamus*. (The projection of the interposed nucleus differs mainly in emphasis, favoring the *red nucleus* over VL, whereas the dentate projection is just the opposite.)

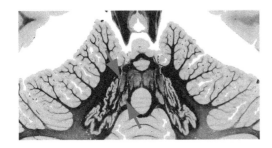

Interthalamic adhesion (massa intermedia). A small, ovoid area of continuity between the two *thalami* resulting from expansion and fusion of the walls of the *third ventricle* during development. The interthalamic adhesion is mainly gray matter, containing neurons and axonal and dendritic processes. (This structure is often reduced in size or absent, especially in the brains of older persons; however, in some mammals, such as rodents, it is massive, reducing the size

of the *third ventricle* but anatomically making the *thalamus* almost a single unpaired structure; see *third ventricle**.)

Interventricular foramen (of Monro). The narrow orifice between each *lateral ventricle* and the *third ventricle*.

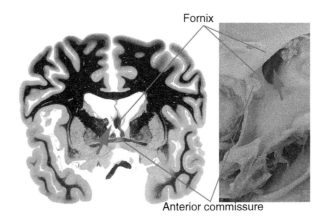

Intraparietal sulcus. A longitudinally oriented sulcus on the lateral aspect of the *parietal lobe*, separating it into a *superior parietal lobule* above and an *inferior parietal lobule** below.

Lamina terminalis. A thin membrane at the anterior end of the *third ventricle*, curving down from the rostrum of the *corpus callosum* to the *optic chiasm* and corresponding (roughly, if not precisely) to the rostral end of the neural tube. The lamina terminalis connects the two telencephalic vesicles of the embryonic forebrain and provides a route through which commissural fibers that will later make up the *anterior commissure* and *corpus callosum* begin to grow.

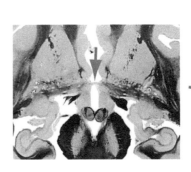
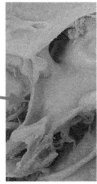

Lateral aperture. The aperture (also called the foramen of Luschka) at the end of each lateral recess of the *fourth ventricle*, through which this ventricle communicates with subarachnoid space.

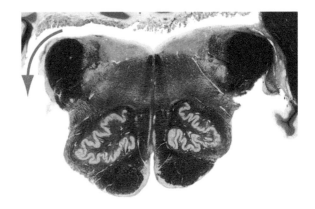

Lateral corticospinal tract. The larger of the two *corticospinal tracts*, comprising those fibers (about 85%) in each medullary *pyramid* that enter the *pyramidal decussation* and cross the midline to the opposite *lateral funiculus*. The axons of this tract end on spinal motor neurons or (more often) on smaller interneurons that in turn synapse on motor neurons. Its fibers are often said to be arranged somatotopically, with those passing to more caudal cord levels located more laterally, but anatomical evidence does not support this view.

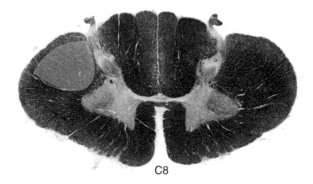

C8

Lateral cuneate nucleus. The equivalent for the arm of *Clarke's nucleus* for the leg. Proprioceptive primary afferents travel through *fasciculus cuneatus* to this nucleus, which then gives rise to uncrossed cuneocerebellar fibers that enter the *cerebellum* via the *inferior cerebellar peduncle*.

Lateral dorsal nucleus (LD). See *thalamus**.

Lateral funiculus. One of the three major divisions of the spinal white matter, the others being the *anterior* and *posterior** *funiculi*. The lateral funiculus contains various ascending and descending tracts, including the *anterior* and *posterior spinocerebellar*, *spinothalamic*, and *lateral corticospinal tracts*.

Lateral geniculate nucleus (LGN). See *thalamus**.

Lateral horn. A small, pointed lateral extension of the *intermediate spinal gray* from T1 through L2 or L3. The lateral horn contains the intermediolateral cell column, a long slender column of preganglionic sympathetic neurons supplying the entire body. Axons of these preganglionic sympathetic neurons leave through the *ventral roots*.

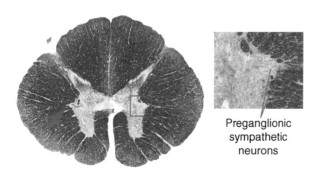

Preganglionic sympathetic neurons

Lateral lemniscus. A flattened ribbon of fibers on the lateral surface of the rostral pontine *tegmentum*, arising from the *cochlear* and *superior olivary nuclei*. The lateral lemniscus is part of the ascending auditory pathway, conveying information from both ears to the *inferior colliculus*.

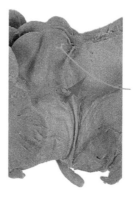
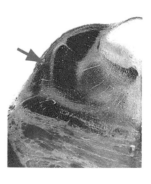

Lateral olfactory tract. A small tract in humans (although relatively much larger in animals that rely more extensively on the sense of smell) through which fibers that originated in the *olfactory bulb* and passed through the *olfactory tract* continue on their way by traveling across the surface of the *basal forebrain* to olfactory cortex and the *amygdala*.

Piriform cortex

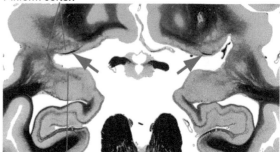

Periamygdaloid cortex

Lateral posterior nucleus (LP). See *thalamus**.

Lateral sulcus (Sylvian fissure). A long, deep indentation on the lateral aspect of each cerebral hemisphere resulting from downward and forward expansion of the *temporal lobe* during fetal development. The *insula* lies hidden within the depths of this sulcus, which separates the *temporal lobe* from the *frontal* and *parietal lobes* and provides a route by which the *middle cerebral artery* accesses the lateral convexity.

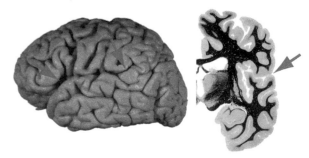

Lateral ventricle. The large central cavity of each cerebral hemisphere, following a C-shaped course through the hemisphere and derived from the lumen of the embryonic telencephalic vesicle.
   Anterior horn. The frontal horn, in the *frontal lobe* anterior to the *interventricular foramen*.
   Body. In the *frontal* and *parietal lobes*, extending posteriorly to the region of the splenium of the *corpus callosum*.
   Atrium (or trigone). The region near the splenium of the *corpus callosum* where the body and the posterior and inferior horns meet.

Inferior horn. The temporal horn, curving down and forward into the *temporal lobe.*

Posterior horn. The occipital horn, projecting backward into the *occipital lobe.*

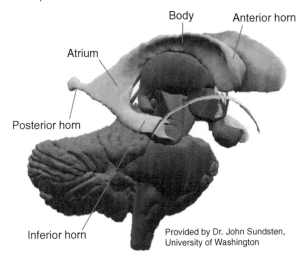

Provided by Dr. John Sundsten, University of Washington

Lateral vestibular nucleus. See *vestibular nuclei.*

Lenticular fasciculus. Part of the projection from the *globus pallidus* to the *thalamus.* It has more axons than the other part (see *ansa lenticularis*) and is more spread out, forming numerous conspicuous bundles of myelinated fibers running medially through the *internal capsule,* like the teeth of a comb. Medial to the *internal capsule,* the lenticular fasciculus is joined by the *ansa lenticularis* before both enter the *thalamus* through the *thalamic fasciculus.*

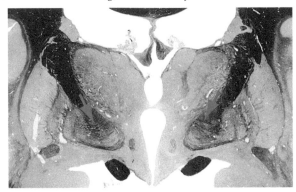

Lenticular nucleus. The *putamen* and *globus pallidus* considered as one anatomical structure.

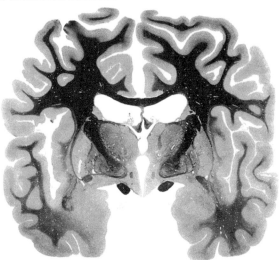

Lenticulostriate arteries. A collection of about a dozen small branches of the *middle cerebral artery* along its course toward the *lateral sulcus.* They penetrate the overlying brain near their origin and pass upward to supply deep structures (*internal capsule, globus pallidus, putamen*). The lenticulostriate arteries exemplify a large collection of small penetrating arteries that arise from all arteries around the base of the brain; these narrow, thin-walled vessels are involved frequently in strokes that deprive deep cerebral structures of blood and thus cause neurological deficits out of proportion to their size.

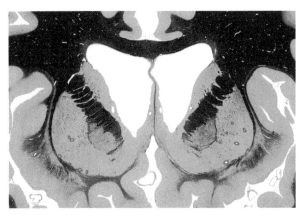

Limbic lobe. The most medial lobe of the cerebral hemisphere, facing the midline and visible grossly only in sagittal sections. The limbic lobe consists of a continuous border zone of cortex around the *corpus callosum,* comprising the *cingulate* and *parahippocampal gyri* and their narrow connecting isthmus; this lobe and its many connections, cortical and subcortical, make up a large part of the limbic system and give the latter its name.

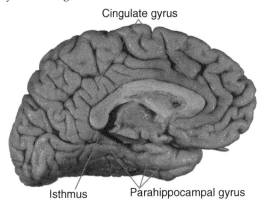

Limen insulae. Limen is Latin for "threshold" and in this case refers to the transition point from *anterior perforated substance* to *insula.* The circular sulcus, which surrounds almost the entire *insula,* ends on either side of the limen insulae, allowing access for the *middle cerebral artery.*

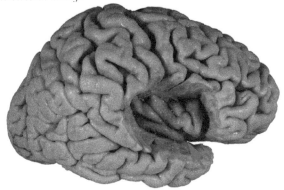

Lingual gyrus. The gyrus forming the inferior bank of the *calcarine sulcus*. The lingual gyrus overlaps the posterior part of the *occipitotemporal gyrus*, separated from it by the *collateral sulcus*.

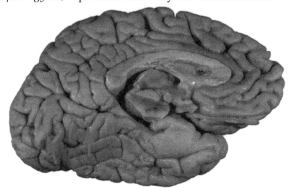

Lissauer's tract. A pale-staining area of white matter between the *substantia gelatinosa** (capping the *posterior horn* of the spinal gray matter) and the pial surface of the cord. Lissauer's tract stains more lightly than the rest of the spinal white matter because it contains finely myelinated and unmyelinated pain and temperature fibers (derived from the lateral division of each *dorsal root* filament) that then distribute into the underlying substantia gelatinosa over several segments.

Locus ceruleus. A column of pigmented, blue-black neurons (locus ceruleus is Latin for "blue place") near the floor of the *fourth ventricle*, extending through the rostral *pons*. Locus ceruleus neurons provide most of the far-flung noradrenergic innervation of the forebrain.

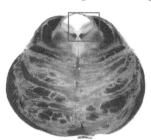 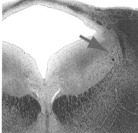

Longitudinal fissure. An extensive vertical cleft, oriented sagittally and occupied by the falx cerebri, separating the two cerebral hemispheres around the margin of the undivided *corpus callosum*.

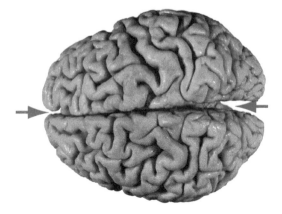

Mammillary body. A prominent component of the posterior *hypothalamus*. The mammillary body receives afferents from the *hippocampus* (chiefly the subiculum) via the *fornix* and sends efferents to the anterior nucleus of the *thalamus* via the *mammillothalamic tract*. This is part of a historic neural circuit proposed by James Papez in 1937 as an anatomical substrate for emotion. Although derided by some then and viewed as simplistic by others now, the

Papez circuit—a grand loop from *hippocampus* through *hypothalamus*, *thalamus*, and cortex back to *hippocampus* again—was unquestionably the impetus for the decades of research that led to the limbic system concept of today.

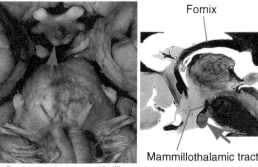

Fornix

Mammillothalamic tract

Provided by Dr. Norman Koelling, University of Arizona

Mammillothalamic tract. The projection from the *mammillary body** to the anterior nucleus of the *thalamus*; part of the Papez circuit.

Medial geniculate nucleus (MGN). See *thalamus**.

Medial forebrain bundle. A collection of thinly myelinated and unmyelinated fibers running longitudinally through the lateral *hypothalamus* and reaching the *basal forebrain* and the *brainstem tegmentum*. It interconnects the *hypothalamus* with both these areas and also conveys monoaminergic fibers on their way from the *brainstem* to widespread forebrain areas.

Medial lemniscus. Somatosensory afferents originating from the contralateral *posterior column nuclei* and *trigeminal main sensory nucleus* and ascending through the brainstem to the *thalamus* (VPL/VPM). The medial lemniscus is the principal ascending pathway for tactile and proprioceptive information.

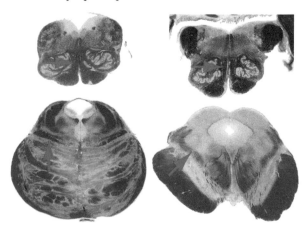

Medial longitudinal fasciculus (MLF). A longitudinal fiber bundle involved in coordinating eye and head movements. Each MLF

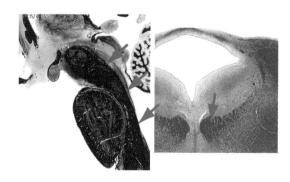

includes fibers from contralateral *abducens* interneurons to medial rectus motor neurons in the *oculomotor nucleus*. It is also the route of descent for fibers of the medial vestibulospinal tract.

Medial striate artery. A large penetrating branch of the *anterior cerebral artery*, also known as the recurrent artery of Heubner. It supplies the *striatum* and *internal capsule* in the region of *nucleus accumbens* and some posterior parts of *orbital* cortex.

Medial vestibular nucleus. See *vestibular nuclei.*

Median aperture. One of the three apertures through which the *fourth ventricle* communicates with subarachnoid space. The median aperture (also called the foramen of Magendie) opens into *cisterna magna.*

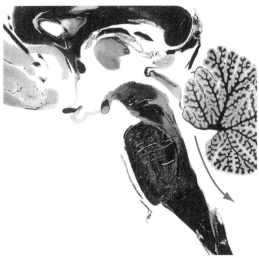

Median eminence. A swelling at the base of the *hypothalamus*, in the middle of the *tuber cinereum*, from which the *infundibulum* arises. The median eminence lacks a blood-brain barrier and is the site at which hypothalamic releasing hormones and inhibiting hormones gain access to the portal system that delivers them to the anterior *pituitary.*

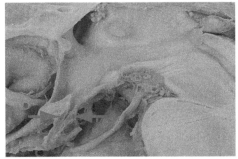

Medulla (medulla oblongata). The most caudal of the three subdivisions of the *brainstem*, continuous rostrally with the *pons*

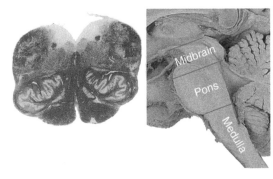

and caudally with the *spinal cord*. This small structure is important out of proportion to its size: it is crucial to vital functions (respiratory, cardiovascular, visceral activity) and other integrative activities. In addition, most sensory and motor tracts of the CNS run up and down through it.

Midbrain (mesencephalon). The most rostral of the three subdivisions of the *brainstem*. The midbrain remains tubular in plan but features a great variety of structures: the *superior* and *inferior colliculi* in its roof (tectum), *aqueduct* and *periaqueductal gray*, *oculomotor* and *trochlear nuclei* and *pretectal area*, upper part of the *reticular formation*, red nuclei, *substantia nigra*, and *cerebral peduncles*. Like the *medulla*, a small region of enormous importance.

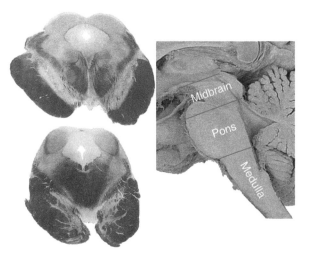

Middle cerebellar peduncle. The largest of the cerebellar peduncles, containing fibers that arise in the *basal pons** from contralateral *pontine nuclei* and end as mossy fibers in almost all areas of cerebellar cortex. Sometimes referred to as the brachium pontis (the "arm of the pons").

Middle cerebral artery. The more posterior of the two terminal branches of the *internal carotid artery**. The middle cerebral artery runs laterally beneath the *basal forebrain* to reach the *lateral sulcus*, where many branches arise. It supplies the *insula*, most of the lateral surface of the cerebral hemisphere, and the anterior tip of the *temporal lobe.*

Middle frontal gyrus. One of three longitudinally oriented gyri in the anterior part of the *frontal lobe**, situated between the *superior* and *inferior frontal gyri*. It includes part of premotor cortex, as well as the frontal eye field, which is involved in initiating voluntary eye movements to the contralateral side.

Middle temporal gyrus. One of three longitudinally oriented gyri on the lateral surface of the *temporal lobe** between the *superior* and *inferior temporal gyri*. It contains some visual association cortex, as well as multimodal or heteromodal association cortex.

MLF. See *medial longitudinal fasciculus**.

Nucleus accumbens. The most inferior part of the *striatum**, with predominantly limbic connections. Nucleus accumbens was traditionally known as nucleus accumbens septi but is now recognized as a major component of the *ventral striatum*. (The original, longer name reflects its position immediately lateral to the base of the *septum pellucidum*, as if leaning against it.)

Nucleus ambiguus. A collection of motor neurons for laryngeal and pharyngeal muscles, and preganglionic parasympathetic neurons for the heart. So called because these neurons are somewhat scattered in the *reticular formation* of the rostral *medulla* and do not form a compact, easily seen nucleus.

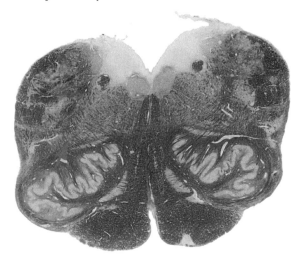

Nucleus cuneatus. The more lateral of the *posterior column nuclei**. Site of termination of *fasciculus cuneatus* and origin of the arm region of the *medial lemniscus*.

Nucleus gracilis. The more medial of the *posterior column nuclei**. Site of termination of *fasciculus gracilis* and origin of the leg region of the *medial lemniscus*.

Nucleus of the solitary tract. The principal visceral sensory nucleus of the *brainstem*; the site of termination of the visceral and gustatory primary afferents in the *solitary tract*, which it surrounds, doughnut-like, in cross section.

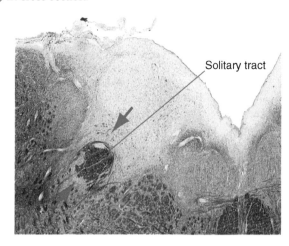

Solitary tract

Obex. Apex of the V-shaped caudal *fourth ventricle*, where the ventricle narrows into the *central canal* of the caudal *medulla* and the *spinal cord*.

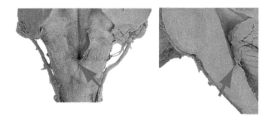

Occipital lobe. The most posterior lobe of each cerebral hemisphere. The occipital lobe includes the primary visual cortex in the banks of the *calcarine sulcus*, as well as adjoining areas of visual association cortex.

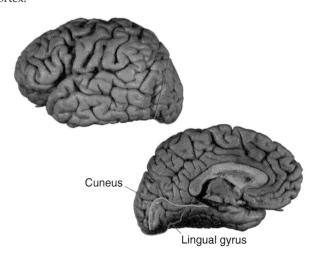

Cuneus

Lingual gyrus

Occipitotemporal gyrus (fusiform gyrus). A long gyrus, beginning just lateral to the *uncus* and running posteriorly along the inferior surface of the *temporal lobe* into the *occipital lobe*. Along its course in the *temporal lobe*, the occipitotemporal gyrus is bounded laterally by the *inferior temporal gyrus* and medially by the *parahippocampal gyrus*.

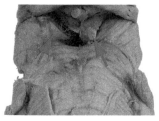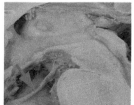

Oculomotor nerve. The 3rd cranial nerve, emerging into the *interpeduncular fossa* of the *midbrain*. The oculomotor nerve innervates most of the extrinsic ocular muscles (see also *oculomotor nucleus*): superior, medial, and inferior recti, inferior oblique, and levator palpebrae superioris. It also conveys preganglionic parasympathetic fibers to the ciliary ganglion, where postganglionic fibers arise to innervate the pupillary sphincter and ciliary muscle.

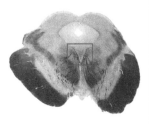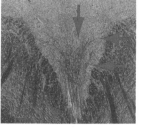

Oculomotor nucleus. Motor neurons for the ipsilateral medial and inferior recti and inferior oblique, the contralateral superior rectus, and the levator palpebrae of both sides. Preganglionic parasympathetic neurons in one of its columns, the *Edinger-Westphal nucleus**, control the ipsilateral pupillary sphincter and ciliary muscle.

Oculomotor nerves

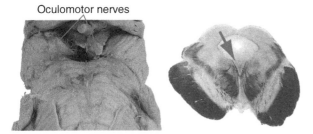

Olfactory bulb. The knoblike anterior end of the *olfactory tract** on the *orbital* surface of the *frontal lobe*. The olfactory bulb is the site of central termination of incoming olfactory fibers (cranial nerve I) from the olfactory epithelium in the nasal cavity. It is large and well laminated in animals that depend heavily on the sense of smell (e.g., rats, dogs), but relatively small and poorly differentiated in the human brain.

Olfactory sulcus. A sulcus on the *orbital* surface of the *frontal lobe*, immediately lateral to *gyrus rectus* and harboring the *olfactory bulb* and *tract**.

Olfactory tract. Projections from *olfactory bulb* neurons (mitral and tufted cells) to olfactory (*piriform*) *cortex* and the *amygdala*. The olfactory tract also conveys modulatory efferents traveling from deeper CNS centers back to the *olfactory bulb*.

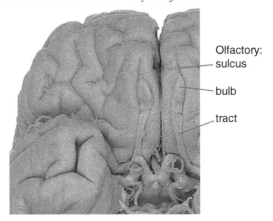

Olfactory:
— sulcus
— bulb
— tract

Olfactory tubercle. A restricted area of the *anterior perforated substance* where some *olfactory tract* fibers terminate. The olfactory tubercle forms a distinct elevation in some animals but is not very apparent in human brains.

Olive. Protuberance on the lateral aspect of the rostral *medulla*, just dorsolateral to the *pyramid*, caused by the underlying *inferior olivary nucleus*.

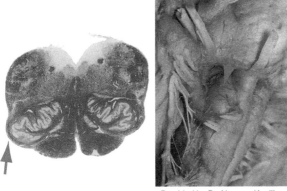

Provided by Dr. Norman Koelling,
University of Arizona

Opercula (singular, **operculum**). The parts of the *frontal*, *parietal*, and *temporal lobes* bordering the *lateral sulcus* and overlying the *insula*, hiding it from view.

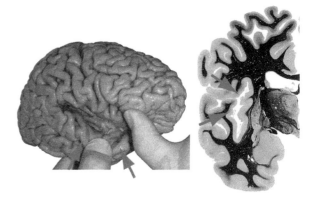

Opercular part (of the inferior frontal gyrus). The most caudal part of the *inferior frontal gyrus*, the most inferior of three longitudinally oriented gyri in the anterior part of the *frontal lobe**. In the dominant hemisphere, it forms the posterior half of Broca's area.

Optic chiasm. The site at which *optic nerve* fibers from ganglion cells in the nasal half of each retina decussate, so that each *optic tract* contains fibers arising in the temporal retina of the ipsilateral eye and the nasal retina of the opposite eye.

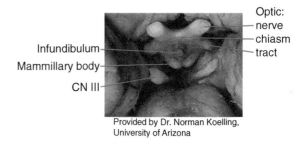

Optic:
— nerve
— chiasm
— tract

Infundibulum—
Mammillary body—
CN III—

Provided by Dr. Norman Koelling,
University of Arizona

Optic nerve. The 2nd cranial nerve, containing axons of the various types of retinal ganglion cells projecting to the lateral geniculate nucleus of the *thalamus*, the *superior colliculus*, *pretectal area*, suprachiasmatic nucleus of the *hypothalamus*, and a few other sites.

Optic radiation. A conspicuous, sharply defined, and heavily myelinated bundle of visual fibers originating in the lateral geniculate nucleus of the *thalamus*, departing through the retrolenticular and sublenticular parts of the *internal capsule*, curving in a broad fan around the atrium and the posterior and inferior horns of the *lateral ventricle*, and terminating in the primary visual cortex in the upper and lower banks of the *calcarine sulcus*.

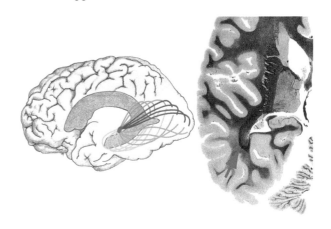

Optic tract. Axons of ganglion cells from corresponding (homonymous) halves of each retina on their way to the lateral geniculate nucleus of the *thalamus, superior colliculus, pretectal area,* and a few other sites.

Orbital gyri. The variably sulcated (in a pattern often resembling the letter H) group of gyri that make up most of the orbital surface of the *frontal lobe.* The orbital gyri usually are not named individually, in contrast to the *gyrus rectus* immediately medial to them. (*Gyrus rectus* is on the orbital surface but is usually not included among the orbital gyri.)

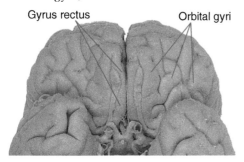

Gyrus rectus   Orbital gyri

Orbital part (of the inferior frontal gyrus). The most anterior part of the *inferior frontal gyrus,* the most inferior of three longitudinally oriented gyri in the anterior part of the *frontal lobe**, so named because it merges with the *orbital gyri.*

Parabrachial nuclei. A collection of nuclei adjacent to the *superior cerebellar peduncle* (brachium conjunctivum) as the latter traverses the rostral *pons.* Various parts of the parabrachial nuclei are involved in transferring visceral, pain, and temperature information to the *hypothalamus* and *amygdala.*

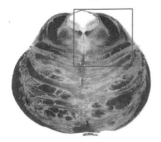
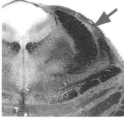

Paracentral lobule. The extensions of the *precentral* and *postcentral gyri* onto the medial surface of the hemisphere, forming a lobule that surrounds the end of the *central sulcus.*

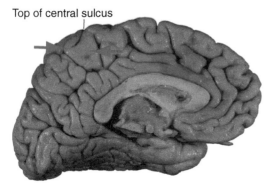

Top of central sulcus

Parafascicular nucleus (PF). See *thalamus**.

Parahippocampal gyrus. The gyrus immediately adjacent to (and continuous with) the *hippocampus,* forming a major part of the *limbic lobe**. Its anterior region contains the *entorhinal cortex,* a meeting ground for cortical projections from multiple areas and the source of most afferents to the *hippocampus.*

Paraterminal gyrus. A small patch of cortex adjacent to the *lamina terminalis,* continuous with the *subcallosal gyrus** and through it with the rest of the *limbic lobe.*

Parietal lobe. A cerebral lobe bounded by the *frontal, temporal,* and *occipital lobes* on the lateral surface of each hemisphere, and by the *frontal, limbic,* and *occipital lobes* on the medial surface. The parietal lobe contains primary somatosensory cortex in the *postcentral gyrus,* areas involved in language comprehension (in the *inferior parietal lobule,* usually on the left), and regions involved in complex aspects of spatial orientation and perception.

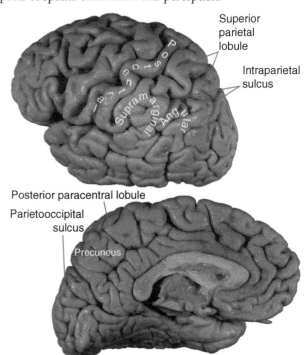

Superior parietal lobule

Intraparietal sulcus

Posterior paracentral lobule

Parietooccipital sulcus

Precuneus

Parietooccipital sulcus. A deep fissure separating the *parietal** and *occipital lobes* on the medial aspect of the cerebral hemisphere. Inferiorly, the parietooccipital sulcus joins the *calcarine sulcus**, which continues into the *temporal lobe* as a common stem for both these sulci.

Periamygdaloid cortex. A cortical area covering part of the *amygdala* and merging with it; part of primary olfactory cortex. (See *lateral olfactory tract**.)

Periaqueductal gray. An area of gray matter and poorly myelinated fibers surrounding the *aqueduct* in the *midbrain.* The periaqueductal

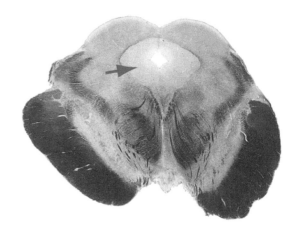

gray is the site of origin of a descending pain-control pathway that relays in nucleus *raphe* magnus (among other connections).

Periventricular gray. The continuation of the *periaqueductal gray* into the floor of the *fourth ventricle*.

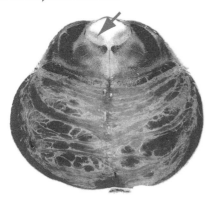

Pineal gland. A dorsal outgrowth of the *diencephalon*, protruding from the *third ventricle* immediately caudal to the paired *habenulae*. The pineal is an endocrine gland important in seasonal cycles of some animals. In humans it secretes the hormone melatonin, which is involved in the synchronization of circadian rhythms.

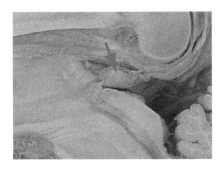

Piriform cortex. A cortical area adjacent to the *lateral olfactory tract** as it moves toward the *temporal lobe*; part of primary olfactory cortex.

Pituitary gland. The two-part gland through which the *hypothalamus* controls most other endocrine glands. The posterior lobe of the pituitary is an outgrowth of the *diencephalon* and remains connected to the *median eminence* through the *infundibulum*. Neurons of the hypothalamic supraoptic and paraventricular nuclei release oxytocin and vasopressin into the bloodstream in the posterior lobe. The anterior lobe, although attached to the posterior lobe and *infundibulum*, is derived embryologically from the roof of the oral cavity.

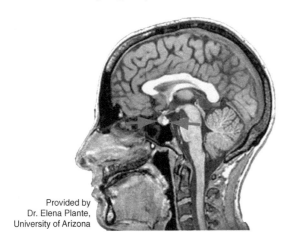

Provided by
Dr. Elena Plante,
University of Arizona

It secretes a variety of hormones that control other endocrine glands at rates dictated by releasing hormones and inhibiting hormones that reach it from the *median eminence* via the pituitary portal system.

Pons. The second of the three parts of the *brainstem*, continuous rostrally with the *midbrain* and caudally with the *medulla*. The pons is overlain by the *cerebellum* and includes an enlarged basal region (see *basal pons*).

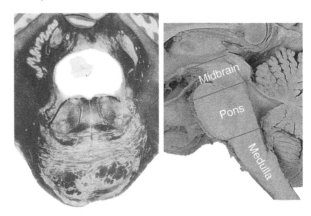

Pontine nuclei. A collective term for the many small nuclei in the *basal pons** that receive afferents from the cerebral cortex (via the *internal capsule* and *cerebral peduncle*) and project to the contralateral cerebellar cortex (via the *middle cerebellar peduncle*).

Pontocerebellar fibers. Projections from *pontine nuclei* that cross in the *basal pons**, traverse the *middle cerebellar peduncle*, and enter the contralateral cerebellar cortex, where they terminate as mossy fibers (as do all cerebellar afferents except those from the *inferior olivary nucleus*).

Postcentral gyrus. A vertically oriented convolution of the *parietal lobe** immediately posterior to the *central sulcus*. The postcentral gyrus is the site of the primary somatosensory cortex.

Posterior cerebral artery. A prominent artery that arises from the bifurcation of the *basilar artery* at the level of the *midbrain*. The posterior cerebral artery forms the caudal part of the *circle of Willis* and supplies the rostral *midbrain*, much of the *thalamus*, the medial *occipital lobe*, and inferior and medial surfaces of the *temporal lobe*.

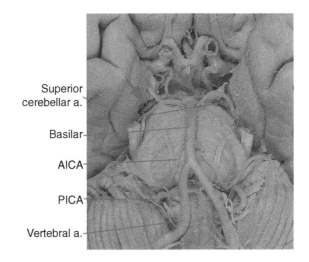

Superior
cerebellar a.

Basilar

AICA

PICA

Vertebral a.

Posterior column. The entire contents of one *posterior funiculus* except for its share of the propriospinal tract (a thin shell of white matter around the gray matter).

Posterior column nuclei. *Nuclei gracilis* and *cuneatus*, the principal collections of second-order neurons receiving touch and position information from the body. Site of termination of *fasciculi gracilis* and *cuneatus* and origin of the contralateral *medial lemniscus*.

lemniscus system, the major pathway to cerebral cortex for low-threshold cutaneous, joint, and muscle receptor information.

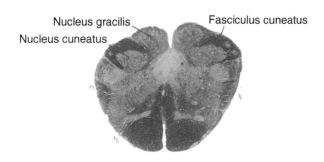

Nucleus gracilis — Fasciculus cuneatus
Nucleus cuneatus

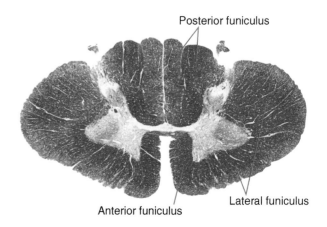

Posterior funiculus

Anterior funiculus   Lateral funiculus

Posterior commissure. Crossing fibers interconnecting the two sides of the rostral *midbrain* and *pretectal area*. These crossing fibers are involved in the consensual pupillary light reflex and in coordinating vertical eye movements.

Posterior horn. One of the three general divisions of the spinal gray matter, the others being the *anterior horn* and the *intermediate gray*; contains second-order sensory neurons of multiple types and is capped at all levels by the *substantia gelatinosa*.

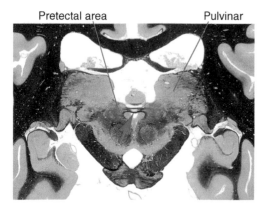

Pretectal area   Pulvinar

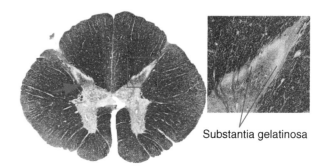

Substantia gelatinosa

Posterior communicating artery. A short vessel connecting the *posterior cerebral artery* to the *internal carotid*, thereby forming one link in the *circle of Willis*. These arteries are often asymmetrical, with one being considerably larger than the other. Normally pressures in the *internal carotid* and *posterior cerebral arteries* are balanced so that little or no blood flows around the circle, but if one vessel is occluded, the posterior communicating artery may allow anastomotic flow and thus prevent neurologic damage.

Posterior inferior cerebellar artery. A long, circumferential branch of the *vertebral artery*, arising before the two vertebrals fuse to form the *basilar artery*. It supplies much of the inferior surface of the *cerebellar hemisphere* and *vermis*, en route sending shorter branches to the *choroid plexus* of the *fourth ventricle* and to much of the lateral *medulla*; commonly referred to by the acronym PICA.

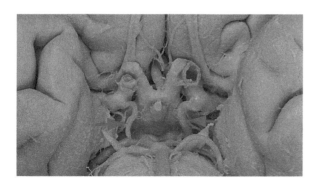

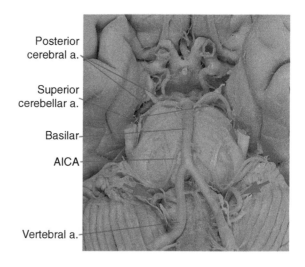

Posterior cerebral a.

Superior cerebellar a.

Basilar

AICA

Vertebral a.

Posterior funiculus. One of the three major divisions of the spinal white matter, the others being the *anterior* and *lateral funiculi*. Principally occupied by ascending collaterals of large myelinated primary afferents carrying impulses from various kinds of mechanoreceptors. This is the first stage of the *posterior column–medial*

Posterior root. See *dorsal root*.

Posterior spinocerebellar tract. Uncrossed fibers from *Clarke's nucleus*, carrying proprioceptive information from the arm to the ipsilateral half of the *cerebellar vermis* and medial *hemisphere* via the *inferior cerebellar peduncle*.

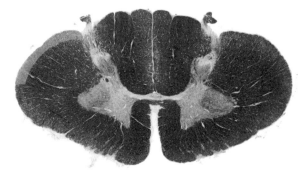

Precentral gyrus. A vertically oriented convolution of the *frontal lobe** immediately anterior to the *central sulcus*. The precentral gyrus is the site of primary motor cortex.

Precuneus. The part of the *parietal lobe** on the medial surface of the hemisphere, excluding the posterior *paracentral lobule* (the medial extension of the *postcentral gyrus*).

Preoccipital notch. The midpoint of a shallow, curved indentation along the inferior margin of the lateral aspect of each cerebral hemisphere. The preoccipital notch serves as a landmark for synthesizing boundaries for the *parietal*, *occipital*, and *temporal lobes* on the lateral and medial surfaces of hemisphere.

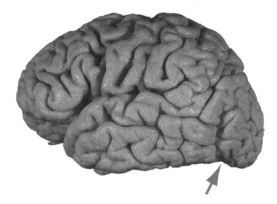

Preoptic area. The area in the walls of the *third ventricle* immediately anterior to the *optic chiasm*, continuing into the *lamina terminalis*; once considered a telencephalic region, but structurally and functionally continuous with the *hypothalamus** of the *diencephalon*.

Pretectal area. The region between the *superior colliculus* and posterior *thalamus*. The pretectal area receives afferents from the retina and visual association cortex. It projects efferents bilaterally to the *Edinger-Westphal nuclei*, crossing both in the *posterior commissure** and in the ventral *periaqueductal gray*. It is important in the pupillary light reflex.

Pulvinar. See *thalamus**.

Putamen. The part of the *striatum** involved most prominently in the motor functions of the *basal ganglia*. The putamen receives afferents from cerebral cortex (primarily motor and somatosensory areas) and from the *substantia nigra* (compact part) and the centromedian nucleus of the *thalamus*. It projects efferents to the *globus pallidus*, which in turn projects via the *thalamus* (VA, VL)

to premotor and supplementary motor areas. The putamen forms the outer component of the *lenticular nucleus* (the *globus pallidus* is the inner part).

Pyramid. *Corticospinal* fibers from the ipsilateral *precentral gyrus* and adjacent areas of cerebral cortex, forming a prominent fiber bundle (roughly triangular in cross section, which gave rise to the name) on the ventral surface of the *medulla*.

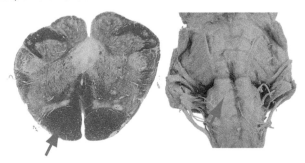

Pyramidal decussation. The site, located at the spinomedullary junction, at which most fibers in each *pyramid* cross the midline to form the contralateral *lateral corticospinal tract*.

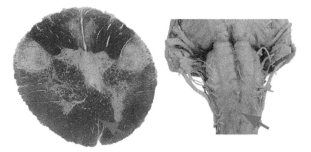

Raphe nuclei. A series of nuclei extending through the *brainstem* near the midline of the *tegmentum*, collectively providing the serotonergic innervation of the CNS.

Red nucleus. The site of termination of part of the *superior cerebellar peduncle*, and the site of origin of uncrossed fibers to the *inferior olivary nucleus* and of the crossed rubrospinal tract.

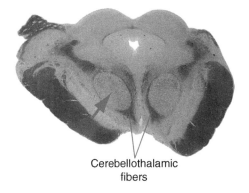

Cerebellothalamic
fibers

Reticular formation. The central region of the *brainstem*, forming most of the *tegmentum* of the *midbrain*, *pons*, and *medulla*, with a complex netlike fabric of nerve cell bodies and interwoven processes; its myriad multimodal afferents, profusely collateralizing efferents running upward and downward to every level of the CNS, and involvement in virtually every activity from visceral functions to consciousness, make it a core integrating structure of the brain.

Reticular nucleus. See *thalamus**.

Rhinal sulcus. A sulcus demarcating the lateral boundary of the *uncus* on the medial aspect of the *temporal lobe*; sometimes continuous with the *collateral sulcus* behind it.

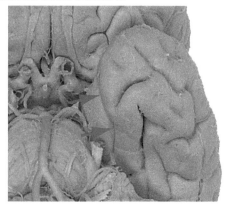

Septal nuclei. A component of the medial wall of each cerebral hemisphere just beneath the base of the largely glial *septum pellucidum*. The septal nuclei are continuous inferiorly with the *preoptic area* of the *hypothalamus* and are reciprocally connected with the *hippocampus, amygdala, hypothalamus,* and other limbic structures via the *fornix, stria terminalis,* and other tracts. They are also the source of cholinergic input to the *hippocampus*.

Septum pellucidum   Septal vein

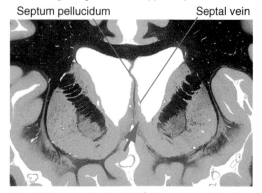

Septal vein. A deep cerebral vein that runs posteriorly across the *septum pellucidum* to join the *terminal* (thalamostriate) *vein* and form the *internal cerebral vein*.

Septum pellucidum. A thin, chiefly glial, almost transparent, paired membrane separating the two *lateral ventricles*, grading inferiorly into the *septal nuclei**. (In most brains the two septa pellucida are so closely apposed as to appear as a single structure, and for simplicity they are so labeled in most of the illustrations in this book.)

Solitary tract. Primary afferents conveying visceral and gustatory information from cranial nerves VII, IX, and X to the adjacent *nucleus of the solitary tract**, which surrounds it.

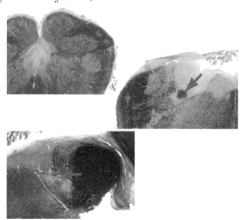

Spinal cord. The most caudal subdivision of the CNS, extending from the *pyramidal decussation* to the *conus medullaris* at about vertebral level L1-L2. The human spinal cord has 31 segments and 2 enlargements (cervical, C5-T1, and lumbar, L2-S3).

Spinothalamic tract. Crossed fibers from neurons in the *posterior horn* of the *spinal cord* conveying pain and temperature information to the *thalamus* (VPL and other nuclei).

Straight sinus. A venous channel in the line of attachment between the falx cerebri and tentorium cerebelli. The straight sinus collects blood from the deep cerebral veins, which reaches it primarily by way of the *great vein*. The straight and *superior sagittal sinuses** then meet at the confluence of the sinuses and empty into the transverse sinuses.

Stria medullaris (of the thalamus). The site of attachment of the roof of the *third ventricle* and a route through which efferents from the *septal nuclei* reach the *habenula*.

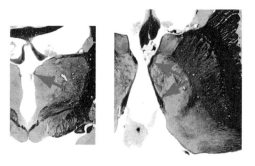

Stria terminalis. A slender, poorly myelinated tract following a long C-shaped course within the thalamostriate groove that separates the *caudate nucleus* from the *thalamus*. The stria terminalis plays a role analogous to that played by the *fornix* for the *hippocampus*: it conveys efferents from the *amygdala* to the *septal nuclei* and *hypothalamus*.

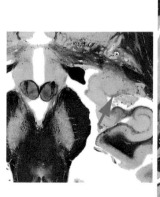
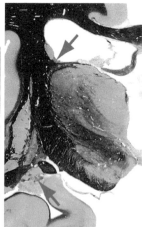

Striatum. An inclusive term for the caudate nucleus, putamen, and nucleus accumbens.

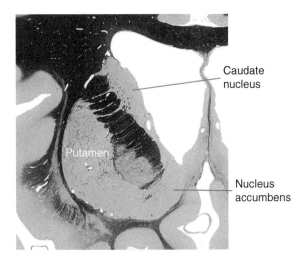

Caudate nucleus

Putamen

Nucleus accumbens

Stripe of Gennari. A sheet of myelinated fibers that run through one of the middle layers of primary visual cortex, giving it the distinctive appearance that gave rise to its alternate name, striate cortex. Named for the medical student who first described it in the 18th century.

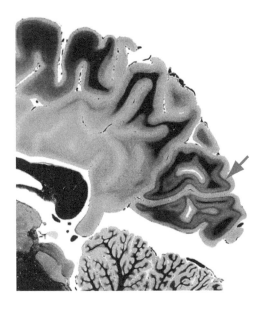

Strumus (commonly misspelled "strumous"). A primitive telencephalic extension that, unlike structures such as the neocortex that have expanded greatly in primates, has remained constant in size and position. It is located rostral to the *lamina terminalis*, medial to *gyrus rectus*, and ventromedial to the *substantia innominata*. Only the anterior and ventral nuclear groups are developed in humans, and these are subdivided cytoarchitectonically into four discrete nuclei: the anteroventral, the anterior ventral, and the subdivided anterior and ventral anterior nuclei.

The interconnections of the strumus are extensive and complex, but their importance cannot be underestimated. There are four major afferent pathways: a substantial input from a variably present limbic nucleus, the effluvium, traveling through the superior and inferior effluviostrumular tracts; and minor inputs from the trivium and nimbus in the *temporal lobe*. Because the strumus has no known efferent pathways, however, its functional importance has been difficult to justify anatomically. (The frequently mentioned strumulotrivionimboeffluviostrumular loop apparently does not exist.)

The clinical importance of the strumus is based on the disorder subacute combined strumuloma. This is an idiopathic disease of exquisitely rare occurrence and indeterminate symptomatology that forms the basis for the identification of the strumus as the center controlling involuntary higher cortical functions.

Subcallosal fasciculus. A compact group of lightly staining myelinated fibers in the white matter of each cerebral hemisphere (visible mainly in the *frontal lobe*). The subcallosal fasciculus forms a pale, arched band adjacent to the *corpus callosum* and *caudate nucleus* and contains afferents on their way from the cerebral cortex (mainly association areas) to the *caudate nucleus*. Nearby association fibers that interconnect the *frontal lobe* and the *occipital, parietal,* and *temporal lobes* are sometimes considered separately as the superior occipitofrontal fasciculus.

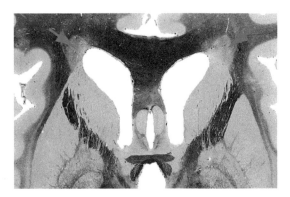

Subcallosal gyrus. The continuation of the *cingulate gyrus* under the rostrum of the *corpus callosum*, in turn continuing into the *paraterminal gyrus*.

Paraterminal gyrus

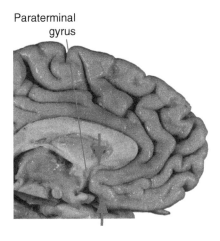

Subiculum. See *hippocampus*.

Subparietal sulcus. A variable sulcus on the medial surface of the hemisphere, separating the *precuneus* from the posterior part of the *cingulate gyrus*. The subparietal sulcus is roughly in line with the *cingulate sulcus*, and in about a third of hemispheres the two are continuous with each other (see Fig. 1.8A).

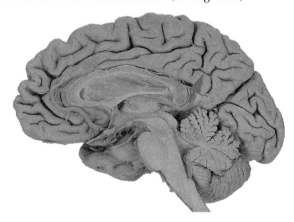

Substantia gelatinosa. A distinctive region of gray matter, adjacent to *Lissauer's tract*, that caps the *posterior horn* of the *spinal cord* at all levels. The substantia gelatinosa looks pale in myelin-stained material because its inputs are poorly myelinated or unmyelinated. It deals mostly with pain and temperature sensation.

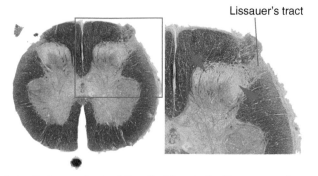

Lissauer's tract

Substantia innominata. Literally "the stuff with no name," a now seldom-used term roughly synonymous with *basal forebrain*, left over from an era when the components of the *basal forebrain* were less well understood.

Substantia nigra. A large, flattened nucleus in the *midbrain*, interposed between the *red nucleus* and *cerebral peduncle*. The substantia nigra has two parts: a compact part, containing closely packed, pigmented (with neuromelanin) dopaminergic neurons that project to the *striatum*, and a reticular part, containing more loosely arranged neurons, receiving inputs from the *striatum* and projecting to the *thalamus*.

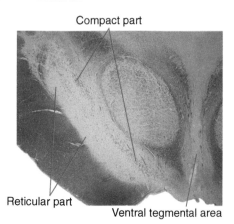

Compact part

Reticular part

Ventral tegmental area

Subthalamic fasciculus. Small bundles of fibers that cross the *internal capsule* like the teeth of a comb. Fibers of the subthalamic fasciculus interconnect the *globus pallidus* and *subthalamic nucleus**, which face each other on either side of the *internal capsule*.

Subthalamic nucleus. A lens-shaped, biconvex mass of gray matter just medial and superior to the junction of the *internal capsule* and *cerebral peduncle*. The subthalamic nucleus is a major link in an indirect route through the *basal ganglia*: *striatum* → *globus pallidus (external segment)* → subthalamic nucleus → *globus pallidus (internal segment)* → *thalamus*. The *globus pallidus*–subthalamic nucleus connections travel in the *subthalamic fasciculus*.

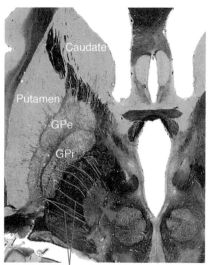

Caudate

Putamen

GPe

GPi

Subthalamic fasciculus

Sulcus limitans. A longitudinal groove in the embryonic neural tube that separates sensory nuclei from motor nuclei. In the adult brain it persists as a groove in the floor of the *fourth ventricle* that separates motor nuclei of cranial nerves (medial to it) from sensory nuclei of cranial nerves.

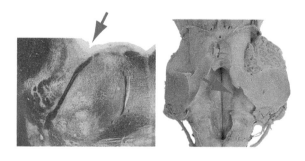

Superior brachium. See *brachium of the superior colliculus**.

Superior cerebellar artery. A branch of the *basilar artery** that arises just caudal to the bifurcation of the *basilar artery* into the *posterior cerebral arteries*. Long circumferential branches supply the superior surface of the *cerebellum*, and shorter branches supply much of the rostral *pons* and caudal *midbrain*.

Superior cerebellar peduncle. The major efferent route from the *cerebellum*, containing projections from deep cerebellar nuclei on their way to the *red nucleus* and the *thalamus* (mainly VL). Sometimes referred to as the brachium conjunctivum (a "conjoined arm," named for its course through a decussation with its contralateral counterpart).

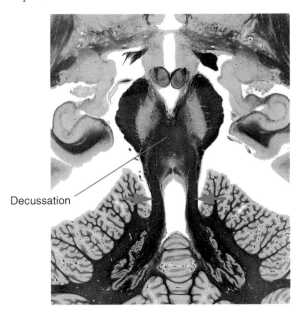

Decussation

Superior cistern. The enlarged, CSF-filled subarachnoid cistern above the *midbrain*, also termed the quadrigeminal cistern and the cistern of the great cerebral vein. The superior cistern is an important radiological landmark, continuous anteriorly and posteriorly with the *transverse fissure* and laterally with thin, curved spaces that partially encircle the midbrain before joining its underlying interpeduncular cistern (see *interpeduncular fossa*). (The combination of the superior cistern and these sheetlike extensions is known as the *ambient cistern*.)

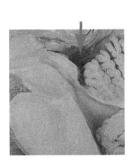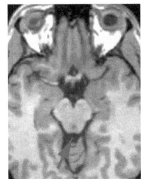

Provided by Dr. Elena Plante,
University of Arizona

Superior colliculus. A large, rounded mass of gray matter in the roof of the rostral *midbrain*. The superior colliculus receives afferents from the retina and visual cortex (via the *brachium of the superior colliculus**), sends efferents to the pulvinar of the *thalamus* and other structures, and plays a role in visual attention and control of eye movements.

Superior frontal gyrus. The most superior of three longitudinally oriented gyri in the anterior part of the *frontal lobe**, continuing on to the medial surface of the hemisphere. The superior frontal gyrus includes supplementary motor cortex and part of premotor cortex.

Superior olivary nucleus. A complex of nuclei near the rostral end of the *facial nucleus* in the caudal *pons*. The superior olivary nucleus is the first site of convergence of fibers representing the two ears and is the source of many fibers of the *lateral lemniscus*. It is also the origin of olivocochlear fibers that travel centrifugally in the *vestibulocochlear nerve* and terminate in the organ of Corti, modulating hair cell activity.

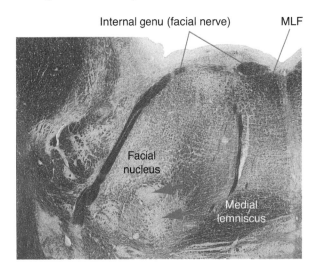

Internal genu (facial nerve)   MLF

Facial
nucleus

Medial
lemniscus

Superior parietal lobule. The upper part of the lateral surface of the *parietal lobe**, above the *intraparietal sulcus*. The superior parietal lobule contains somatosensory association cortex.

Superior sagittal sinus. A venous channel in the superior line of attachment of the falx cerebri, providing the major outflow pathway for superficial cerebral veins.

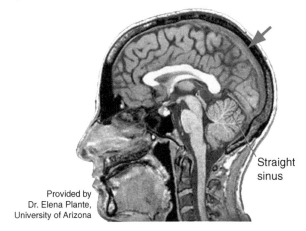

Straight
sinus

Provided by
Dr. Elena Plante,
University of Arizona

Superior temporal gyrus. The uppermost gyrus of the *temporal lobe**, bordering on the *lateral sulcus*. The superior temporal gyrus includes primary auditory cortex (actually located in the wall of the lateral sulcus, in *transverse temporal gyri* crossing the top of the superior temporal gyrus), auditory association cortex, and (usually on the left) Wernicke's area. This is one example of a region of visibly different size and configuration in the two cerebral hemispheres, typically being more extensive in the left hemisphere.

Superior vestibular nucleus. See *vestibular nuclei*.

Supramarginal gyrus. The part of the *inferior parietal lobule** surrounding the upturned end of the *lateral sulcus*. Although variable in size and shape, the supramarginal gyrus (usually on the left) is important in language function.

Tegmentum. A general anatomical term for the area anterior to the ventricular spaces of the *medulla*, *pons*, and *midbrain*. Tegmentum (Latin for "covering") is a useful umbrella term for all structures covering the basal components of the *brainstem* (*pyramids*, *basal pons*, *cerebral peduncles*) and includes the *reticular formation*, nuclei of cranial nerves, most ascending and descending tracts, the *red nuclei*, and *substantia nigra*.

Temporal lobe. The most inferior lobe of each cerebral hemisphere, inferior to the *lateral sulcus* and anterior to the *occipital lobe*. The temporal lobe includes primary auditory and auditory association cortex, part of posterior language cortex, visual and higher-order association cortex, primary and association olfactory cortex, the *amygdala*, and the *hippocampus*. (The *parahippocampal gyrus*, a major part of the *limbic lobe*, is also commonly referred to as part of the medial temporal lobe.)

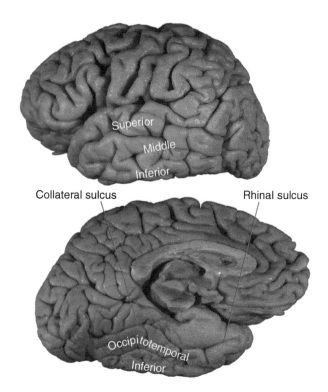

Terminal vein. A deep cerebral vein that travels with the *stria terminalis* in the groove between the *thalamus* and adjacent *caudate nucleus* and drains much of these two structures. (Because of the location of this groove, the terminal vein is also referred to as the thalamostriate vein.)

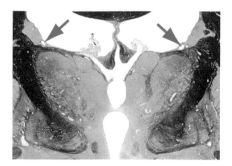

Thalamic fasciculus. Projections from the *cerebellum* (via the *superior cerebellar peduncle*) and *basal ganglia* (via the *ansa lenticularis* and lenticular fasciculus), gathered together beneath the ventral anterior and ventral lateral nuclei (VA/VL) of the *thalamus*.

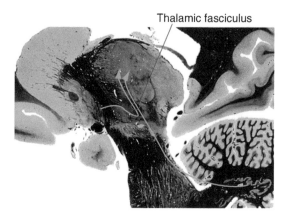

Thalamic fasciculus

Thalamostriate vein. See *terminal vein**.

Thalamus. A collection of nuclei that collectively are the source of most extrinsic afferents to the cerebral cortex. Some thalamic nuclei (relay nuclei) receive distinct input bundles and project to discrete functional areas of the cerebral cortex. Others (association nuclei) are primarily interconnected with association cortex. Still others have diffuse cortical projections, and one (the reticular nucleus) has no projections to the cortex at all.

Anterior nucleus. The thalamic relay nucleus for part of the *limbic lobe*. Afferents from the *mammillary body* and other limbic structures, efferents to the *cingulate gyrus*.

Centromedian nucleus (CM). The largest of the intralaminar nuclei (so called because they are embedded in the *internal medullary lamina*); afferents from the *globus pallidus*, efferents to the *striatum* (with branches projecting diffusely to widespread cortical areas).

Dorsomedial nucleus (DM). Interconnections with prefrontal association cortex and parts of the *limbic lobe*.

Lateral dorsal nucleus (LD). Efferents to the posterior part of the *cingulate gyrus*; in many ways an extension of the anterior nucleus.

Lateral geniculate nucleus (LGN). The thalamic relay nucleus for vision. Afferents from the retina via the *optic tract*, efferents to primary visual cortex above and below the *calcarine sulcus*.

Lateral posterior nucleus (LP). Interconnections, similar to those of the pulvinar, with posterior association cortex.

Medial geniculate nucleus (MGN). The thalamic relay nucleus for hearing. Afferents from the *inferior colliculus* via the *brachium of the inferior colliculus*, efferents to auditory cortex in the *transverse temporal gyri*.

Parafascicular nucleus (PF). An intralaminar nucleus with connections similar to those of the centromedian nucleus.

Pulvinar. The largest thalamic nucleus, interconnected with parietal-occipital-temporal association cortex.

Reticular nucleus. An unusual thalamic nucleus with no projections to the cortex. Afferents from the thalamus and cerebral cortex, GABAergic efferents back to the thalamus.

Ventral anterior nucleus (VA). A thalamic relay nucleus for the motor system. Afferents from the *globus pallidus* and *cerebellum*, efferents to motor areas of cortex.

Ventral lateral nucleus (VL). A thalamic relay nucleus for the motor system. Afferents from the *cerebellum* and *globus pallidus*, efferents to motor areas of cortex.

Ventral posterolateral nucleus (VPL). The thalamic relay nucleus for somatic sensation from the body. Afferents from the *medial lemniscus* and *spinothalamic tract*, efferents to somatosensory cortex in the *postcentral gyrus*.

Ventral posteromedial nucleus (VPM). The thalamic relay nucleus for somatic sensation from the head and for taste. Afferents from the trigeminal regions of the *medial lemniscus* and *spinothalamic tract* and from the *nucleus of the solitary tract*; efferents to somatosensory cortex in the *postcentral gyrus* and to gustatory cortex in and near the *insula*.

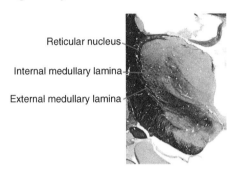

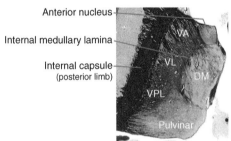

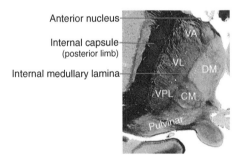

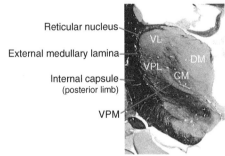

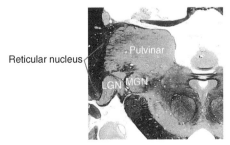

Third ventricle. The single, median, vertically oriented cavity of the *diencephalon*, separating the *thalamus* and *hypothalamus* of the two hemispheres. The third ventricle is confluent anteriorly with both *lateral ventricles* through the *interventricular foramina* and posteriorly with the *aqueduct* and has four small outpocketings:

  Infundibular recess. Leads into the hollow *infundibulum*.
  Optic recess. Small recess just above and anterior to the *optic chiasm*.
  Pineal recess. Leads into the stalk of the *pineal gland*.
  Suprapineal recess. An outpocketing of the roof of the third ventricle just anterior to the *pineal gland*.

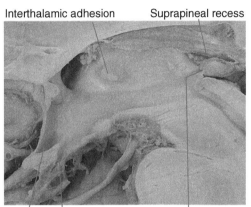

Transverse fissure. An extension of subarachnoid space, situated above the roof of the *third ventricle* and containing the *internal cerebral veins*. We use the term in a more extended sense in this book: to refer to the long slit intervening between the cerebral hemispheres and structures below them—the cleft normally occupied by the tentorium cerebelli, continuing into the *superior cistern*, and from there into the subarachnoid space above the roof of the *third ventricle*.

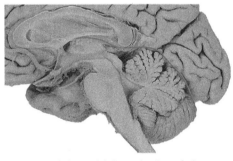

Transverse temporal (Heschl's) gyri. Gyri (often two) that run transversely across the lower bank of the *lateral sulcus*. The location of primary auditory cortex.

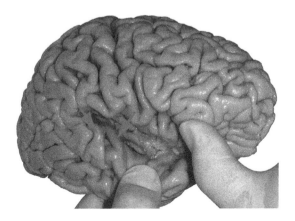

Trapezoid body. Auditory fibers from the *cochlear nuclei* to the contralateral *superior olivary nucleus* or *lateral lemniscus* that cross the midline in a trapezoid-shaped area of the pontine *tegmentum*.

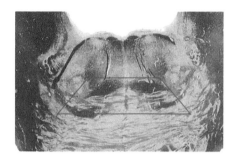

Triangular part (of the inferior frontal gyrus). The middle of the three parts of the *inferior frontal gyrus*, the most inferior of three longitudinally oriented gyri in the anterior part of the *frontal lobe**. In the dominant hemisphere, it forms the anterior half of Broca's area.

Trigeminal nerve. The 5th cranial nerve, emerging anterolaterally from the *basal pons*. The trigeminal nerve conveys somatosensory (and some chemosensory) fibers from the ipsilateral half of the head, as well as efferents to ipsilateral muscles of mastication.
   Motor root. Small, anterior root containing efferent fibers that distribute through the mandibular division of the nerve.
   Sensory root. Massive, posterior root containing afferent fibers that arrive through all three divisions of the nerve.

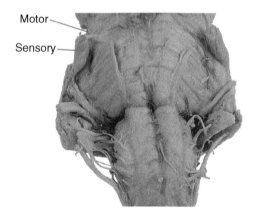

Motor
Sensory

Trigeminal nuclei.
   Main sensory. Termination site of large-diameter afferents (the equivalent of a *posterior column nucleus* for the trigeminal system). Most of its efferents project to the contralateral VPM via the *medial lemniscus*; some, however, project to the ipsilateral VPM via the dorsal trigeminal tract.
   Mesencephalic. The cell bodies of primary afferents from muscle spindles in muscles of mastication and from other oral mechanoreceptors.
   Motor. Motor neurons for ipsilateral muscles of mastication.
   Spinal. The termination site of the spinal *trigeminal tract*. The most caudal part of the nucleus (in the caudal *medulla*) looks like the spinal *posterior horn*, has a component similar to the *substantia gelatinosa*, and processes pain and temperature information. Its efferents project to VPM (and other thalamic nuclei) through the *spinothalamic tract*.

Motor   Main sensory   Spinal nucleus & tract

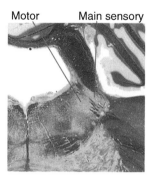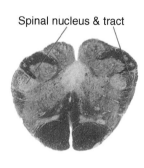

Trigeminal tracts.
   Mesencephalic. Processes of cell bodies in the adjacent mesencephalic *trigeminal nucleus* that send one branch to innervate mechanoreceptors in and around the mouth, and others to central termination sites such as the *trigeminal main sensory nucleus*.

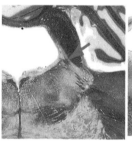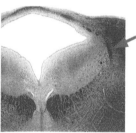

   Spinal. Central processes of primary afferents from the ipsilateral side of the face, conveying information about pain and temperature (and some tactile information) to the *spinal trigeminal nucleus**.

Trochlear nerve. The 4th cranial nerve, emerging as an already-crossed small bundle from the posterior aspect of the *midbrain*, just caudal to the *inferior colliculus*. The trochlear nerve innervates the superior oblique, which helps to intort the eyeball and turn it downward and laterally.

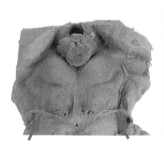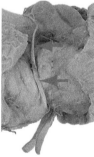

Trochlear nucleus. Motor neurons for the contralateral superior oblique muscle, located in the caudal *midbrain* just caudal to the *oculomotor nucleus*. Trochlear axons exit the paired nuclei, turn caudally in the overlying *periaqueductal gray*, arch posteriorly to decussate (like old-time ice tongs used to handle large blocks of ice), and leave the *brainstem* at the *pons-midbrain* junction.

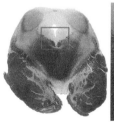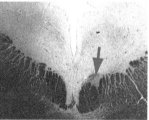

Tuber cinereum. A low mound of gray matter on the inferior surface of the *hypothalamus*, bounded by the *optic chiasm*, *optic tracts*, and anterior edge of the *mammillary bodies*. The tuber cinereum contains the *median eminence* and the beginning of the *infundibulum* and is a region of great importance in hypothalamic hormonal regulation of the anterior *pituitary*.

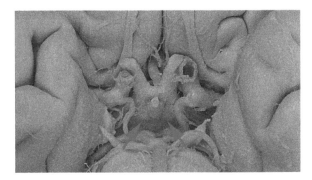

Uncus. A medial protuberance from the anterior end of the *parahippocampal gyrus* caused by the underlying *amygdala* and anterior end of the *hippocampus*. The proximity of its surface to the adjacent *cerebral peduncle* can cause clinical problems during cerebral edema or as a result of space-occupying masses.

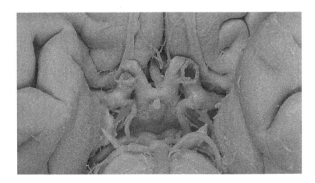

Vagal trigone. A small elevation in the floor of the caudal *fourth ventricle* forming a narrow triangle just lateral to the *hypoglossal trigone*. Each vagal trigone is a fusiform swelling produced by the underlying *dorsal motor nucleus of the vagus*.

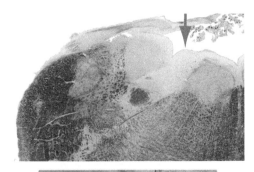

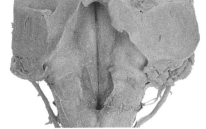

Vagus nerve. The 10th cranial nerve, emerging as a series of filaments from a groove dorsal to the *olive*. The vagus has diverse components: efferents to muscles of the pharynx and larynx arise from *nucleus ambiguus* in the *medulla* and mediate swallowing and phonation; efferents to parasympathetic ganglia for thoracic and abdominal viscera arise from the *dorsal motor nucleus of the vagus* and *nucleus ambiguus* in the *medulla*; afferent fibers mediate general visceral sensation, taste from the epiglottis, and cutaneous sensation in and near the outer ear.

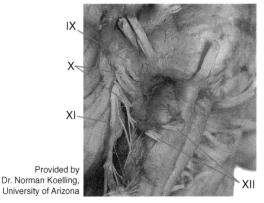

IX
X
XI
XII

Provided by
Dr. Norman Koelling,
University of Arizona

Vein of Galen. See *great vein**.

Venous angle. The point at which the newly formed *internal cerebral vein* turns sharply caudally as it leaves the *interventricular foramen*. This is an important radiological landmark indicating the location of the genu of the *internal capsule* and the anterior end of the *thalamus*.

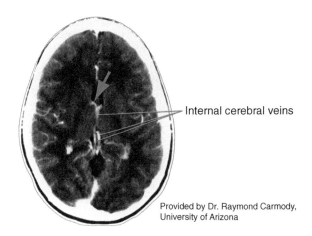

Internal cerebral veins

Provided by Dr. Raymond Carmody,
University of Arizona

Ventral amygdalofugal pathway. A massive but loosely organized fiber bundle running transversely in the *basal forebrain*. It interconnects the *amygdala* with the *hypothalamus*, *septal nuclei*, *thalamus*, and even the *brainstem*, and is thus an important pathway of the limbic system. The name is somewhat misleading, because the pathway contains fibers traveling both from and to the amygdala.

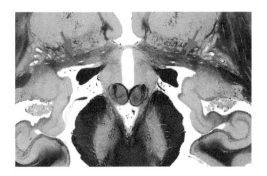

Ventral anterior nucleus (VA). See *thalamus**.

Ventral lateral nucleus (VL). See *thalamus**.

Ventral pallidum. A limbic extension of the *globus pallidus*, located beneath the *anterior commissure*, with inputs from the *ventral striatum*. The ventral pallidum is part of a basal ganglia circuit similar to that involved in motor functions, but in this case has limbic inputs (*amygdala, hippocampus* → *ventral striatum* → ventral pallidum) and outputs (via the dorsomedial nucleus of the *thalamus*) to prefrontal and *orbital* cortex.

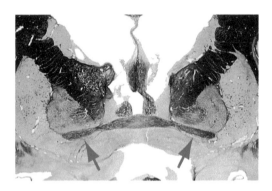

Ventral posterolateral nucleus (VPL). See *thalamus**.

Ventral posteromedial nucleus (VPM). See *thalamus**.

Ventral root. The anterior (motor) root of a spinal nerve, coalescing from a variable number of unevenly spaced rootlets that depart the spinal cord along its anterolateral sulcus.

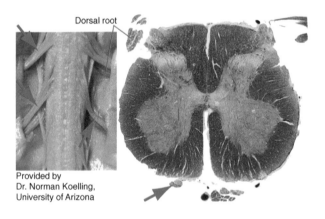

Dorsal root

Provided by
Dr. Norman Koelling,
University of Arizona

Ventral striatum. The primarily limbic subdivision of the *striatum*, comprising *nucleus accumbens* and adjacent parts of the *caudate nucleus* and *putamen*.

Ventral tegmental area. An unpaired region of the *midbrain* medial to the compact part of the *substantia nigra**, containing dopaminergic neurons that project to various limbic and neocortical areas.

Vermis. Midline, sinuous (vermis is Latin for "worm") zone of the *cerebellum** between the two *cerebellar hemispheres*. The vermis includes a representation of the trunk conveyed by the spinocerebellar tracts; its outputs, primarily through the *fastigial nucleus*, reach the *vestibular nuclei* and *reticular formation*.

Vertebral artery. One of the two major arteries that supply each side of the CNS (see also *internal carotid artery*). The vertebral artery originates as the first branch of the subclavian, runs cranially through foramina in cervical vertebrae, enters the base of the skull through the foramen magnum, and ascends along the *medulla*. At the pontomedullary junction it unites with its contralateral counterpart to form the *basilar artery*. The vertebral artery and its *posterior inferior cerebellar* branch (PICA) supply blood to the *medulla* and inferior part of the *cerebellum*, and it supplies the cervical spinal cord via the posterior and *anterior spinal arteries*.

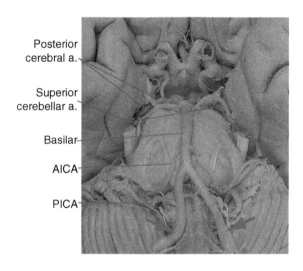

Posterior
cerebral a.

Superior
cerebellar a.

Basilar

AICA

PICA

Vestibular nuclei. Four elaborately subdivided secondary sensory nuclei of the vestibular division of the 8th cranial nerve in the floor of the *fourth ventricle*, extending through much of the *medulla* and into the caudal *pons*. They reach their greatest extent near the pontomedullary junction, medial to the *inferior cerebellar peduncle*. Collectively the vestibular nuclei project to the nuclei of extraocular muscles (mostly via the *medial longitudinal fasciculus*), the *cerebellum*, the *reticular formation*, and the *spinal cord*:
   Inferior. Peppered with small bundles of vestibular primary afferents that run through it.
   Lateral. Origin of the lateral vestibulospinal tract to ipsilateral extensor motor neurons.
   Medial. Origin of the medial vestibulospinal tract, projecting bilaterally to cervical motor neurons.
   Superior. Ascending and descending connections with nuclei of extraocular muscles (other vestibular nuclei also share in this).

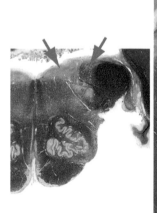
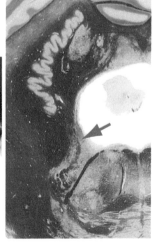

Vestibulocochlear nerve. The 8th cranial nerve, emerging antero-laterally from the *brainstem* in the cerebellopontine angle. It has vestibular and cochlear divisions innervating hair cells in vestibular organs (semicircular ducts and maculae of the utricle and saccule) and the auditory spiral organ of Corti in the cochlear duct, respectively.

Zona incerta. A small sheet of gray matter interposed between the *subthalamic nucleus* and *thalamus*, enveloped by efferent fibers of the *globus pallidus*. The zona incerta has widespread connections, including direct inputs to cerebral cortex, but its function is largely unknown.

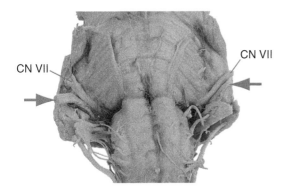

CN VII   CN VII

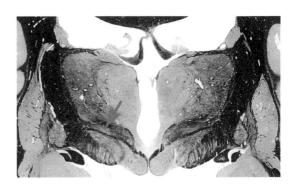

Page numbers followed by "*f*" indicate figures.